Acute
Obstetrics

A Practical Guide

THIRD EDITION

Acute Obstetrics

A Practical Guide

Martha C. S. Heppard, MD, FACOG
Consultants in Obstetrics and Gynecology, PC
Clinical Instructor
University of Colorado
Denver, Colorado

Thomas J. Garite, MD, FACOG
Professor and Chairman
Department of Obstetrics and Gynecology
University of California at Irvine Medical Center
Orange, California

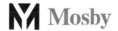

A Harcourt Health Sciences Company

St. Louis   London   Philadelphia   Sydney   Toronto

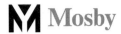

A Harcourt Health Sciences Company

Acquisitions Editor: Dolores Meloni
Production Manager: Donna L. Morrissey

THIRD EDITION

Mosby, Inc.
A Harcourt Health Sciences Company
11830 Westline Industrial Drive
St. Louis, Missouri 63146

Printed in the United States of America

Library of Congress Cataloging in Publication Data

Heppard, Martha C. S.
    Acute obstetrics : a practical guide / Martha C. S. Heppard, Thomas J.
Garite. — 3rd ed.
        p. cm.
    Includes index.
    ISBN 0-323-01202-7
    1. Pregnancy—Complications—Handbooks, manuals, etc. I. Garite,
Thomas J. II. Title.
RG571 .H42   2002
618.3—dc21
                                                        2001030420

Last digit is the print number: 9   8   7   6   5   4   3   2   1

To my twin sons
Matthew and Patrick
who made it possible for me to experience a high-risk pregnancy
and who gave me three months of bedrest
to write the first edition of this book; and to my third son
Daniel
who proved that 90% of pregnancies are indeed low risk.

This third edition is dedicated to my husband
Kurt
who for the past 18 years has provided
love, inspiration, and support. Thank you.

— *Martha*

PREFACE

This book provides practicing physicians and their obstetric staff with a quick and accurate reference concerning the management of high-risk obstetric patients. The management schemes described here are based on the most recent literature and standard practices to which I was exposed initially during my residency at the University of California Irvine (UCI) Medical Center and have continued to encounter throughout my career. Although patient management varies among hospitals, this book provides fundamental information upon which treatment may be initiated.

The book fills a void in reference material supporting the management of high-risk obstetric patients. At the beginning of my internship I found myself relying on old notes and various handouts to develop patient management schemes. Researching through texts and current literature proved to be too time consuming in an acute care setting. This book provides patient care guidelines for residents, nursing students, staff, and physicians who labor under similar time constraints.

I first distributed an abbreviated version of this book as an informal guide in 1988 and found that it was well received by my fellow residents and other physicians associated with UCI Medical Center. The first edition was formally published in 1992. Medical students and residents have continually commented on the book's value as a tool for providing quality patient care. In addition to being a quick and practical reference, the book can be useful for practicing physicians in reviewing for obstetric and gynecology board examinations.

I would like to thank Dr. Thomas J. Garite, Dr. Phillip J. DiSaia, the Department of Obstetrics and Gynecology staff, and my fellow residents for their help and encouragement, which made it possible to transform my informal guide into this book. My colleagues and friends throughout the world but especially here in Colorado have been equally supportive and gracious in offering advice for this book. Jeanne Nieto, Kate Lof, RN, Dr. Nicole Nilson, Katie Travis, and Beverly Cline have been invaluable in preparing the manuscript for the third edition. I also want to thank the staff at Mosby and Harcourt for their patience and support.

Martha C. S. Heppard

CONTENTS

PART I
EVALUATION OF THE PATIENT

1 Prenatal Evaluation, 3
   Background, 3
   Contributors to Perinatal Mortality, 3
   Prenatal Evaluation, 4
   Initial Problem List, 6
   Identifying Risk Factors, 6
   Follow-up Prenatal Care, 7

2 Intrapartum Evaluation: Admission Note, 11

PART II
MEDICAL COMPLICATIONS OF PREGNANCY

3 Acute Abdominal Pain, 17
   Acute Appendicitis, 17
   Cholelithiasis and Cholecystitis, 20
   Acute Pancreatitis, 23
   Peptic Ulcer Disease (PUD), 25
   Pyelonephritis, 28

4 Asthma, 29
   Background, 29
   Evaluation, 30
   Therapeutic Management, 33

5 Diabetes, 37
   Background, 37
   Evaluation, 39
   Diagnostic Evaluation, 40
   Therapeutic Management, 40
   Antepartum Surveillance, 43
   While the Patient Is Antepartum, 44
   Diabetic Patients in Labor at Term or in Whom Induction of Labor Is Being
      Undertaken, 44
   Diabetic Patient Scheduled for Elective Cesarean Delivery, 44
   Immediate Postpartum Management, 46
   Special Discharge Orders, 47

6 Hepatitis, 49
   General Information for All Types of Viral Hepatitis, 49
   Hepatitis A Virus (HAV), 49
   Hepatitis B Virus (HBV), 52
   Hepatitis C Virus (HCV; Formerly Non-A, Non-B Hepatitis [NANBH]), 59
   Hepatitis D Virus (Delta Agent), 60
   Hepatitis E Virus (Formerly Called Epidemic NANBH), 61
   Hepatitis G Virus (Also Known as GB Virus C [HGV-GBV-C]), 61

7 Chronic Hypertension, 63
   Background, 63
   Evaluation, 63
   Therapeutic Management, 67

8 Chronic Immunologic Thrombocytopenia, 73
   Background, 73
   Evaluation, 74
   Therapeutic Management, 74

9 Seizure Disorders, 79
   Background, 79
   Evaluation, 79
   Therapeutic Management, 80

10 Urinary Tract Infections, 85
   Background, 85
   Evaluation of Patients with Pyelonephritis, 85
   Therapeutic Management of Patients with Pyelonephritis, 86

PART III
OBSTETRIC COMPLICATIONS

11 Hyperemesis Gravidarum, 91
   Background, 91
   Evaluation, 92
   Therapeutic Management, 92

12 Incompetent Cervix, 95
   Background, 95
   Antenatal Evaluation, 95
   Second-Trimester Evaluation on Presentation to Emergency Room, 96
   Therapeutic Management, 97

13 Isoimmunization in Pregnancy, 101
   Background, 101
   Evaluation, 105
   Therapeutic Management, 107
   Prevention of D Isoimmunization, 112

14 Group B Streptococcal Infections, 115
   Background, 115
   Evaluation, 117
   Therapeutic Management, 117
   Prevention, 118

15 Chorioamnionitis, 123
   Background, 123
   Evaluation, 123
   Therapeutic Management, 125

16 Premature Rupture of the Fetal Membranes, 127
   Background, 127
   Perinatal and Maternal Morbidity, 127
   Patient Evaluation, 128
   Therapeutic Management, 130

17 **Preterm Labor, 135**
    Background, 135
    Evaluation, 135
    Therapeutic Management, 137
    Prevention, 151

18 **Pregnancy-Induced Hypertension and Preeclampsia, 155**
    Background, 155
    Evaluation, 157
    Therapeutic Management, 158

19 **Antepartum Hemorrhage, 167**
    Background, 167
    Hemorrhage Assessment, 167
    Abruptio Placentae, 168
    Placenta Previa, 179
    Vasa Previa, 184
    Summary, 185

20 **Venous Thromboembolism in Pregnancy, 187**
    Background, 187
    Evaluation, 189
    Therapeutic Management, 192
    After Recovery and Treatment for VTE, 194

21 **Pregnancy Loss: Spontaneous Abortion and Stillbirths, 195**
    Preclinical Losses, 195
    First-Trimester Losses, 195
    Early Second-Trimester Losses, 199
    Stillbirth/Fetal Death, 200

PART IV
APPENDICES

Maternal Physiology, 207
A   Temperature Conversion Chart, 207
B   Common Laboratory Values in Pregnancy, 209
C   Analgesia and Anesthesia in Labor and Delivery, 215

Fetal Physiology, 225
D   Chromosomal Abnormalities, 225
E   Diagnostic Radiology and the Fetus, 229
F   Fetal Circulation, 235
G   Blood Gases: Normal and Abnormal, 237
H   Ultrasound Evaluation: Fetal Growth, 241
I   Ultrasound Evaluation: Amniotic Fluid Volume, 247
J   Ultrasound Evaluation: Placental Grading, 253
K   Intrapartum Fetal Heart Rate Monitoring, 257
L   Antepartum Fetal Surveillance, 265
M   Fetal Lung Maturity: Glucocorticoids for Accelerated Fetal
    Lung Maturation, 277
N   Fetal Lung Maturity: Assessment Before Repeat
    Cesarean Delivery, 287

Medical Administration, 289

O   Medications in Pregnancy: FDA Guidelines, 289
P   Immunizations During Pregnancy, 291
Q   Sexually Transmitted Disease Treatment Guidelines, 301
R   Drugs of Abuse: Urine Drug Screens, 319
S   Drug Use During Pregnancy: Maternal and Embryonic Effects, 325
T   Drug use During Pregnancy: Perinatal Characteristics, 329
U   Definition of Terms: Street Names of Drugs of Abuse, 331
V   Definition of Terms: Vital Statistics, 335
W   Definition of Terms: Symbols, 337
X   Definition of Terms: Abbreviations, 339
Y   Useful Telephone Numbers, 363

Index, 365

PART I

Evaluation of the Patient

PRENATAL EVALUATION

I. BACKGROUND

Prenatal care is one of the few routine examples of regularly provided preventive health care commonly accepted in Western medicine. From a cost-benefit standpoint, prenatal care is most effective at lowering perinatal mortality and morbidity. It accomplishes this goal by identifying pregnant women and their fetuses at increased or high risk for specific adverse outcomes and applying appropriate diagnostic and therapeutic measures. The purposes and goals of prenatal care include the following:

A. Prevention of perinatal morbidity and mortality

B. Application of other preventive health measures not specifically related to pregnancy but instituted because the patients are now in the health care system (e.g., Pap smears, tuberculosis skin testing)

C. Provision of appropriate psychosocial counseling

D. Patient education and preparation

E. Contraceptive planning

II. CONTRIBUTORS TO PERINATAL MORTALITY

Because reduction of perinatal mortality and morbidity is the most realistic goal, the physician must first be aware of the main contributors to such adverse outcomes and then be able to assess the risk for these specific contributors.

A. ANTEPARTUM FETAL DEATH

1. Etiology
   a. Uteroplacental insufficiency
   b. Fetal anomalies
   c. Cord accidents
   d. Abruptio placentae
   e. Hydrops fetalis
   f. Fetal infections

2. Prevention
   a. Risk assessment
   b. Ultrasound and genetic testing
   c. Antepartum fetal testing

B. INTRAPARTUM FETAL DEATH. This is now rare, largely because of routine electronic or frequent auscultative fetal heart rate monitoring in labor.

C. NEONATAL DEATH

1. Etiology
   a. Prematurity (accounts for the vast majority)
   b. Asphyxia
   c. Anomalies
   d. Infections

2. **Prevention**
   a. Risk identification[1-4]
   b. Education and detection of early premature labor
   c. Initiate 0.4 mg of folic acid per day orally starting 6 weeks before anticipated conception[5,6]

III. PRENATAL EVALUATION

A. **HISTORY.** Of all antenatal high-risk factors, 80% are identified on the **first visit.**

1. **History of present illness**
   a. Ascertain the state of the woman's present health and well-being.
   b. Identify any pregnancy complications that occurred before the first visit.
   c. **Accurate dating** may be accomplished by evaluating the following:
      (1) Patient's menstrual history
      (2) Patient's uterine size on the first prenatal examination
      (3) Patient's fetal ultrasound
      (4) Gestation at which fetal heart tones were first detected by Doppler echocardiography and fetoscopic examination
      (5) Patient's quickening date

2. **Obstetric history**
   a. Place special emphasis on the following:
      (1) Complications of previous pregnancies
      (2) Size of previous babies
      (3) Course of previous labors and deliveries
   b. Other medical and surgical history

3. **Family history**
   a. Emphasize the following:
      (1) History of genetic diseases or anomalies
      (2) Obstetric problems
      (3) Diabetes
      (4) Hypertension
   b. Other significant family history

4. **Social history**
   a. How is the pregnancy welcomed, wanted, and perceived?
   b. How is the pregnancy impacting the family emotionally and economically?
   c. What are the plans for future pregnancies and contraception?
   d. Use of illicit drugs,[7] alcohol, caffeine,[8,9] and nicotine[10]
   e. Occupation[11] and impact of pregnancy
   f. Support of family and friends
   g. Other

5. **Review of systems.** Generally is limited to likely current problems (e.g., morning nausea) and is directed at any actual positive medical history

B. PHYSICAL EXAMINATION
1. Routine complete physical examination
2. Uterine size and location of pregnancy
3. Establish fetal viability (fetal heart tones [FHTs])
4. Pelvic measurements to determine likelihood of a successful vaginal birth
5. **Initial laboratory assessment** (Table 1-1)

TABLE 1-1

INITIAL LABORATORY ASSESSMENT

1. Complete blood cell count
2. Urinalysis
3. Screening test or routine culture for urinary tract infection
4. Venereal Disease Research Laboratory or rapid plasma reagin testing
5. Blood type, Rh, antibody screen
6. Hepatitis B surface antigen
7. Rubella titer
8. Pap smear
9. Population-dependent routine tests
   a. Purified protein derivative
   b. Vaginal swabs to evaluate for bacterial vaginosis and *Trichomonas**
   c. *Chlamydia* culture of cervix (obtain on all women 16-26 years of age in addition to others at high risk)
   d. Cervical culture for gonorrhea, enteropharyngeal pathogens, other organisms as indicated
10. One-hour post-Glucola test for patients at risk for diabetes (Only patients at risk will have screening at the initial visit in addition to the routine screening of all patients at 28 wk' gestation.)
   a. Family history of diabetes
   b. Maternal age >25 years
   c. Glucosuria
   d. Marked obesity
   e. Accelerated fetal growth
   f. Polyhydramnios
   g. History of any of the following:
      (1) Macrosomic baby
      (2) Baby with a congenital anomaly
      (3) Preeclampsia
      (4) Previous gestational diabetes
      (5) Previous stillborn
      (6) Polyhydramnios

*Affirm VPIII DNA probe testing is the preferred method of evaluation, if available, because of its significantly higher sensitivity and specificity than wet mount and at least equal sensitivity and specificity but more rapid turnaround time than culture for *Candida* species, *Trichomonas vaginalis*, and bacterial vaginosis.

IV. INITIAL PROBLEM LIST

After the initial history, physical, and laboratory assessment, the patient's initial problem list can be constructed. Problems should include the following:

A. INTRAUTERINE PREGNANCY. Excellent, good, fair, or poor dates at (_) weeks' gestation

B. DIAGNOSIS-BASED PROBLEMS

1. Hypertension
2. Diabetes
3. Other

C. IDENTIFIED RISK FACTORS

V. IDENTIFYING RISK FACTORS

Because 80% of all antenatal high-risk patients are identified on the first visit, this is the best time to identify patients at risk for the three major factors that contribute to perinatal mortality.

A. RISK FACTORS FOR PERINATAL DEATH CAUSED BY HYPOXIA OR ASPHYXIA

1. Diabetes
2. Hypertension (chronic and pregnancy induced)
3. Post dates
4. Collagen vascular disease
5. Previous stillbirth
6. Chronic renal disease
7. Chronic hypoxia
   a. Pulmonary origin
   b. Cardiac origin
8. Severe anemia
9. Thyrotoxicosis
10. Intrauterine growth retardation

B. RISK FACTORS FOR PERINATAL DEATH CAUSED BY PREMATURITY

1. Multiple gestation
2. Previous premature birth
3. Two or more midtrimester abortions
4. Teenager (<17 years of age)
5. In utero diethylstilbestrol exposure
6. Uterine malformation
7. Cervical cerclage or cervical incompetence
8. Uterine fibroids
9. Polyhydramnios
10. Thyrotoxicosis
11. Acute and chronic infections
    a. Genital tract infection (upper and lower)
    b. Pyelonephritis
    c. Hepatitis

12. Acute medical illnesses
13. Abdominal surgery with current pregnancy
14. Premature contractions (5 per hour)
15. Previous cervical cone biopsy
16. Cervical dilation >2 cm
17. Vaginal bleeding

C. **RISK FACTORS FOR ANOMALIES AND GENETIC DISEASES**[12]
1. Race
   a. Southeast Asian: α-thalassemia
   b. Ashkenazi Jews: Tay-Sachs disease
   c. Mediterranean: β-thalassemia
   d. Black
      (1) Sickle cell disease
      (2) Glucose-6-phosphate dehydrogenase deficiency
2. Advanced maternal age: trisomies
3. Advanced paternal age: new autosomal dominant mutations
4. Family history of genetic disease or multifactorial birth defect
5. Previous pregnancy with birth defect or genetic disease
6. Teratogen exposure (TORCH: toxoplasmosis, other [viruses], rubella, cytomegalovirus, herpes [simplex viruses] infections)
7. Diabetes
8. Elevated or low maternal serum α-fetoprotein, abnormal triple screen
9. Polyhydramnios or oligohydramnios
10. Intrauterine growth retardation

VI. FOLLOW-UP PRENATAL CARE

A. **MONITORING FOR PROBLEMS.** The majority of problems that appear after the first prenatal visit but before hospital admission will be picked up by monitoring the following:
1. Routine blood pressure
2. Routine fundal height
3. Simple history for new patient problems (i.e., "Any problems?")
4. Ultrasound (Because ultrasound has become nearly routine, many unexpected problems will be identified on a sonogram.)

B. **ROUTINE FOLLOW-UP VISITS FOR LOW-RISK PATIENTS**
1. **First visit.** Initial history, physical, laboratory assessment, and problem list development as described previously
2. **Subsequent visits**
   a. Frequency
      (1) Every month until 26 to 28 weeks' gestation
         (a) If no FHTs are detected with use of Doppler echocardiography on the first visit, the patient should return more frequently until FHTs are documented.
         (b) At 18 to 20 weeks' gestation, FHTs should be detectable with fetoscopic examination. If not, the patient should return every 1 or 2 weeks until they are heard.

      (2) Every 2 to 3 weeks until 36 weeks' gestation

      (3) After 36 weeks' gestation, every week until term

  b. At each visit, review the patient's problem list and obtain the following:

      (1) Weight

      (2) Blood pressure

      (3) Urine (for sugar and albumin levels)

      (4) Fundal height

      (5) FHTs

      (6) Fetal presentation after about 32 weeks' gestation

      (7) New complaints

  c. Follow-up laboratory assessment

      (1) Maternal serum α-fetoprotein or triple screen at 15 to 18 weeks' gestation[13]

      (2) One-hour post-Glucola (diabetes screen) at 28 weeks' gestation

      (3) For all Rh-negative patients at 28 weeks' gestation:

         (a) Repeat the antibody titer.

         (b) Administer RhoGAM if the antibody titer test results are negative.

      (4) Repeat a complete blood cell count (CBC) at 28 weeks' gestation in all patients.

      (5) Obtain a vaginal or rectal culture for group B beta strep (GBS) between 35 and 37 weeks if your GBS prevention policy is screening based.

  d. Topics for discussion—at some time during the entire prenatal course, discuss each of the following with the patient:

      (1) Weight gain[14]

      (2) Diet

      (3) Exercise[15,16]

      (4) Sexual activity

      (5) Common complaints of pregnancy

      (6) Explanation of any risk factors

      (7) Toxin and teratogen avoidance

         (a) Smoking

         (b) Alcohol

         (c) Prescribed and unprescribed drugs used during pregnancy

      (8) Travel during pregnancy

      (9) Signs and symptoms of toxemia

      (10) Signs and symptoms of premature labor

      (11) Prenatal classes

         (a) Prenatal/Lamaze method

         (b) Baby care

         (c) Cesarean birth

         (d) Breast feeding

      (12) Fetal movement counting

(13) Labor and delivery instructions
    (a) When to come in
    (b) Where to go
(14) Anesthesia
(15) Contraception and sterilization
(16) Breast and bottle feeding
(17) Choice of pediatrician
(18) Circumcision

REFERENCES

1. ACOG Committee Opinion: Bacterial vaginosis screening for prevention of preterm delivery, 198:1-2, Feb 1998.
2. Goldenberg RL et al: The Preterm Prediction Study: the value of new versus standard risk factors in predicting early and all spontaneous preterm births, *Am J Public Health* 88:233-238, 1998.
3. McGregor JA, French JI, Witkin S: Infection and prematurity: evidence-based approaches, *Curr Opin Obstet Gynecol* 8:428-432, 1996.
4. Saling E: Prevention of prematurity: a review of our activities during the last 25 years, *J Perinat Med* 25:406-417, 1997.
5. Czeizel AE, Dudas I: Prevention of the first occurrence of neural-tube defects by periconceptional vitamin supplementation, *N Engl J Med* 327(26):1832-1835, 1992.
6. Werler MM, Shapiro S, Mitchell AA: Periconceptional folic acid exposure and risk of occurrent neural tube defects, *JAMA* 269(10):1257-1261, 1993.
7. Mattison DR: Minimizing toxic hazards to fetal health, *Contemp Ob/Gyn* 37:81-100, 1992.
8. James JE, Paull I: Caffeine and human reproduction, *Rev Environ Health* 5(2):151-167, 1985.
9. Mills JL et al: Moderate caffeine use and the risk of spontaneous abortion and intrauterine growth retardation, *JAMA* 269(5):593-597, 1993.
10. Kelly J: Smoking in pregnancy: effects on mother and fetus, *Am J Obstet Gynecol* 91:111-117, 1984.
11. Simpson JL: Are physical activity and employment related to preterm birth and low birth weight? *Am J Obstet Gynecol* 168(4):1231-1238, 1993.
12. D'Alton ME, DeCherney AH: Prenatal diagnosis, *N Engl J Med* 328(2):114-120, 1993.
13. Phillips OP et al: Maternal serum screening for fetal Down syndrome in women less than 35 years of age using alpha-fetoprotein, hCG, and unconjugated estriol: a prospective 2-year study. Part 1, *Obstet Gynecol* 80(3):353-358, 1992.
14. Johnson JWC, Longmate JA, Frentzen B: Excessive maternal weight and pregnancy outcome, *Am J Obstet Gynecol* 167(2):353-372, 1992.
15. Artal R et al: Pulmonary responses to exercise in pregnancy, *Am J Obstet Gynecol* 154(2):378-383, 1986.
16. Boschetto-Schick B, Rose NC: Exercise in pregnancy, *Obstet Gynecol Surv* 47(1):10-13, 1991.

SUGGESTED READING

Adams MM et al: The Prams working group: pregnancy planning and pre-conception counseling, *Obstet Gynecol* 82(6):955-959, 1993.

PRENATAL EVALUATION

1

INTRAPARTUM EVALUATION: ADMISSION NOTE

When a pregnant patient is admitted to the hospital because of antepartum complications, it is vital that the condition of the mother and the fetus be thoroughly documented. The admission note serves as the cornerstone for future treatment and care. Because of its importance, this note may be complex and may detail many problems. The following example demonstrates a complete evaluation in a format that is clear and easy to read.

A. DATE AND TIME _____

B. HISTORY OF PRESENT ILLNESS

1. Mrs/Miss (name) is a (age, nationality, gravida, para, aborta) with (number) living children.
2. Her last menstrual period (LMP) was on (date).
3. Her estimated date of confinement is (date), placing her estimated gestational age at (weeks).
4. She presented to the obstetric emergency room with complaints of _____.
5. If she was transported from another hospital, give the name of the hospital from which she was transported and the reason for transport.
6. Provide a brief paragraph of the history of her present illness. Use the problem list to fill in details of labor status (i.e., preterm labor [PTL]).
7. Her problems include the following:
   a. **Intrauterine pregnancy (IUP)**
      LMP (date). Estimated gestational age (weeks).
      Her menses were (regular/irregular).
      She is (sure/unsure) of her LMP.
      Oral contraceptive pills were (taken/not taken) within the 3 months preceding conception.
      Her first urine pregnancy test was on (date).
      Her first examination was on (date) at (weeks' gestation). Her uterine size (was/was not) appropriate for her gestational age.
      She has had (number) follow-up examinations. Size = dates? (yes/no).
      Her triple screen (date/weeks' gestation) was (normal/abnormal, list exact values and their interpretation).
      A 1-hour post-Glucola was performed on (date) at (weeks' gestation) and revealed a value of (detail results and results of 3-hour glucose testing if it was performed).
      A sonogram performed on (date/weeks' gestation) revealed (list all parameters measured and their equivalency in weeks).
      Her fundal height (FH) is (cm), and her fetal heart tones (FHTs) in beats per minute (bpm) are (rate).

Her estimated gestational age is (weeks), by (excellent, good, fair, or poor) dates.

b. **Primary reason for admission.** Example: PTL.

c. **Briefly detail her history (uterine contractions, dysuria, fever).** If she was transported from another hospital, describe her medical course before admission to your hospital (e.g., tocolysis with magnesium sulfate [MgSO$_4$] for [hours]).

Explain the current status of her labor, her pertinent physical examination (cervix, fundal firmness), and laboratory findings (complete blood cell count [CBC] with differential, urinalysis, cervical and amniotic fluid cultures, Gram's stain).

C. **MEDICAL HISTORY.** Detail the patient's illnesses, operations, allergies, and medication use. Provide her obstetric history (date, place, method of termination if an abortion occurred or was performed, gestational age, weight, route of delivery if pregnancy progressed to viability, prenatal problems, complications).

D. **FAMILY HISTORY.** Inquire especially into the patient's family history of hypertension, diabetes mellitus, twins, congenital anomalies, and genetic diseases.

E. **SOCIAL HISTORY.** Determine the patient's use of tobacco, alcohol, and prescribed and nonprescribed drugs. Does the patient have a stable marriage? Is there evidence of social problems? Has she planned for postpartum contraception or sterilization?

F. **REVIEW OF SYSTEMS.** Limit to pertinent positive findings only.

G. **PHYSICAL EXAMINATION**

1. Vital signs (include weight)
2. Head, eyes, ears, nose, and throat (HEENT) and funduscopic examination (especially important for patients with diabetes mellitus and hypertension)
3. Throat, lungs, breast, and heart
4. Abdominal examination:
   a. FH
   b. Contraction frequency, duration, and strength
   c. Fetal position on Leopold's maneuver
   d. Estimated fetal weight (EFW)
5. Pelvic examination (to be done on all patients **except for those with third-trimester bleeding, patients in whom placenta previa has not yet been ruled out, and those with premature rupture of membranes [PROM]**)
6. Sterile speculum examination on patients with premature rupture of membranes and who have third-trimester bleeding
7. Extremities (edema, tenderness)
8. Neurologic examination (deep tendon reflexes)

H. **LABORATORY EVALUATION AND DIAGNOSTIC DATA**

1. Include prenatal laboratory examinations in addition to those tests ordered during this admission.
2. Determine uterine and fetal heart rate monitoring patterns.

I. **ASSESSMENT.** Example: patient with PTL
1. IUP at weeks' gestation
2. PTL
3. Other problems
J. **PLAN.** Example: patient with PTL
1. Bed rest
2. Tocolysis with $MgSO_4$. Then attempt to wean to oral terbutaline (or obtain consent for a study protocol). (Always check updated study lists at your institution to see if the patient is eligible.)
3. Initiate antibiotic while awaiting cervical culture results.
4. Consider steroid administration.
5. Laboratory tests: CBC with differential; serum electrolytes (if indicated); urinalysis with culture and sensitivity; cervical, vaginal, and perineal swab for Gram's stain and group B β-streptococcus culture; and cervical culture for *Neisseria gonorrhoeae.*

_____
Signature

PART II

Medical Complications of Pregnancy

ACUTE ABDOMINAL PAIN

The diagnosis of acute abdominal pain in pregnancy is challenging to the obstetrician, internist, and general surgeon. Maternal physiologic and anatomic changes during pregnancy affect the patient's symptoms, signs, and laboratory parameters during an acute illness. Many common causes of acute abdominal pain may be associated with increased maternal and fetal morbidity and mortality if not treated early in the disease process. The following discussion focuses on the more common causes unrelated to the gestation.

3

ACUTE APPENDICITIS

I. BACKGROUND
A. **DEFINITION.** Inflammation of the vermiform appendix.
B. **INCIDENCE.** Approximately 1 in 2000 pregnancies (unchanged from the general population). The frequency of appendicitis is constant through all trimesters.
C. **PERINATAL MORBIDITY AND MORTALITY.** The fetal loss rate is 15%. Abortion and preterm labor are increased, especially in the presence of peritonitis, particularly with a ruptured appendix.[1]
D. **MATERNAL MORBIDITY AND MORTALITY.** Maternal mortality is 2% in the first trimester and rises to 7.3% in the third trimester. Mortality in nonpregnant patients is less than 0.1% for uncomplicated acute appendicitis and 5% when perforation has occurred.[2]

II. EVALUATION
A. **HISTORY.** A history of anorexia, nausea, vomiting, and right-side abdominal pain is usually present.
B. **PHYSICAL EXAMINATION.** Perform a thorough physical examination. With appendicitis, the patient may have a fever and will most often, but not always, demonstrate abdominal tenderness (Table 3-1), guarding, and rebound. Figure 3-1 illustrates the usual position of the appendix throughout pregnancy.
C. **DIAGNOSTIC DATA.** Obtain a complete blood cell count (CBC) with differential (a left shift of the white blood cell count [WBC] is usually present) and a urinalysis (pyuria may be present with appendicitis).
D. **DIAGNOSIS.** Diagnosis of acute appendicitis is often difficult to make in pregnancy.
1. The presenting symptoms of acute appendicitis mimic the common symptoms of early pregnancy (anorexia, nausea, vomiting).

TABLE 3-1

COMPARISON OF FINDINGS IN PREGNANT AND NONPREGNANT PATIENTS
WITH APPENDICITIS

	Pregnant	Nonpregnant
Diagnostic accuracy	72%	75%
Symptoms	Nausea, vomiting, increased frequency of urination, abdominal pain, anorexia	
Physical findings	Abdominal pain (100%)	Abdominal pain (100%)
	First trimester: right lower quadrant (100%)	Right lower quadrant (65%)
	Second trimester: right lower quadrant (80%)	Pelvis (30%)
	Third trimester: right upper quadrant (20%)	Flank (5%)
	Rebound tenderness (75%)	Present
	Guarding (60%)	Present
	Fever >38°C (100.2°F) (18%)	High 38°C (100.4°F)
Laboratory findings		
White blood cell count (WBC)	Normal pregnancy: 12,500-16,000/mm³ with 80% bands	Normal WBC: 3000-10,000/mm³
		Most patients demonstrate a shift to the left. Not all demonstrate leukocytosis. Fewer than 4% have a normal WBC and no shift to the left.
Urinalysis	Pyuria is present if the ureter or renal pelvis is in contact with the inflamed appendix	Pyuria: rare

From DeVore GR: *Clin Perinatol* 7:349-369, 1980.

2. As the gestation advances, the appendix moves upward and laterally in the abdomen (Fig. 3-1).
3. The leukocytosis commonly seen with acute appendicitis is normally present during pregnancy.
4. During pregnancy the abdominal signs of appendicitis are often atypical of those noted in a nonpregnant patient.

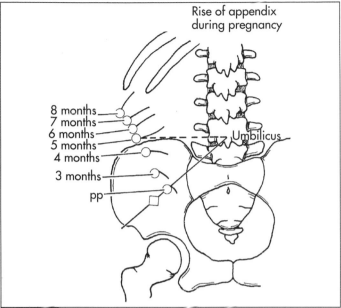

Rise of appendix
during pregnancy

8 months
7 months
6 months
5 months
4 months
3 months
pp

Umbilicus

FIGURE 3-1

Schematic representation of the location of the appendix during pregnancy in relationship to McBurney's point. *PP,* Prepregnant position. *(Redrawn from Baer JL, Reis RA, Arens RA: JAMA 98:1359, 1932.)*

3

ACUTE ABDOMINAL PAIN

E. DIFFERENTIAL DIAGNOSIS

1. Pyelonephritis is the diagnosis most commonly confused with acute appendicitis, especially as pregnancy progresses. Bacteriuria is present with pyelonephritis but absent in appendicitis.
2. Other disorders that may present with similar findings include a ruptured ovarian cyst or corpus luteum, ovarian torsion, preterm labor (PTL), abruptio placentae, degenerating myoma, cholecystitis, pneumonia, and, rarely, appendiceal endometriosis.
3. When undiagnosed, appendicitis stimulates PTL, and after delivery the contracted uterus may disrupt a previously walled-off infection, spilling purulent material into the abdomen and creating a surgical abdomen postpartum.

III. THERAPEUTIC MANAGEMENT (TABLE 3-2)

A. **Surgical intervention** is mandatory. A vertical midline incision between the symphysis pubis and umbilicus, or a right paramedian incision, provides adequate exposure for removal of the appendix or treatment of

TABLE 3-2			
RECOMMENDATION OF SURGICAL APPROACH IN PREGNANT PATIENTS WITH APPENDICITIS			
Surgical Technique	Uncomplicated	Gangrenous	Perforated
Bury stump if possible	X		
Double ligate stump	X	X	X
Close all layers with nonabsorbable suture	X	X	X
Do not place suture in subcutaneous fat	X	X	X
Irrigate wound with antibiotics	X	X	X
Close skin with locking mattress suture	X		
Leave skin and subcutaneous tissue open		X	X
Place intraabdominal drain			X

From DeVore GR: *Clin Perinatol* 7:349-369, 1980.

other gynecologic disorders that mimic appendicitis. The preoperative diagnosis of appendicitis is correct less than half the time.

B. Cesarean delivery should be avoided in the presence of appendicitis unless absolutely necessary.

C. Antibiotics are unnecessary in uncomplicated appendicitis. When gangrene or perforation occurs, antibiotics directed against bowel flora are indicated.

D. Postoperatively the patient should be observed on labor and delivery for at least the first 24 hours. If contractions occur, tocolysis should be considered, depending on the gestational age and the patient's status. If the patient has septic complications, she may be unable to tolerate the cardiovascular and hemodynamic side effects of some tocolytic agents.

CHOLELITHIASIS AND CHOLECYSTITIS

I. BACKGROUND
A. DEFINITIONS
1. **Cholelithiasis:** gallstones
2. **Cholecystitis:** inflammation of the gallbladder
B. ETIOLOGY. Cholesterol crystals retained in the gallbladder may form stones (gallstones), subsequently obstruct the cystic duct, and result in inflammation of the bladder wall. When repeated episodes of acute inflammation occur, the gallbladder may become chronically infected and develop edematous, rigid walls.

C. INCIDENCE
1. **Asymptomatic gallstones** are identified in 2% to 4% of women under-going a routine obstetric ultrasonic examination.
2. **Acute cholecystitis** occurs in 1 of 1000 pregnancies.
3. Pregnancy is thought to increase the prevalence of gallstones by the following mechanisms[3]:
   a. Progesterone-mediated decrease in gallbladder emptying
   b. Increasing cholesterol saturation in the bile (resulting from the 50% increase in esterified and free cholesterol in the bloodstream)
   c. Decreasing bile salt pool, which may result in a relative cholesterol excess, thus leading to gallstone formation
4. In the general population, 2% of patients with previously silent gall-stones develop symptoms. This figure is thought to be unchanged in pregnancy.

II. EVALUATION
A. HISTORY. The symptoms of cholecystitis are the same in pregnant and nonpregnant patients. The patient will usually complain of anorexia, nausea, vomiting, and pain of abrupt onset (usually lancing, occasionally deep and cramping), originating in the midportion of the epigastrium and radiating to the upper right area of the abdomen or back. The pain may be colicky or steady for up to 1 hour.

B. PHYSICAL EXAMINATION. Although one third of nonpregnant patients with cholecystitis have a palpable gallbladder, this is found in less than 5% of pregnant patients. Localized tenderness may suggest pancreatitis or abscess formation around the gallbladder, whereas rebound tenderness may suggest perforation.

C. DIAGNOSTIC DATA
1. Obtain a CBC with differential, amylase, and an alkaline phosphatase level. If the alkaline phosphatase level is not elevated above that found in a normal pregnancy, consider obtaining specific alkaline phosphatase isoenzymes, nucleotidase, and blood and urine samples for an amylase/creatinine clearance ratio (Fig. 3-2), which is normal in this disease but elevated in pancreatitis.
2. **Ultrasound** evaluation of the gallbladder demonstrates stones in 96% of patients in whom acute cholecystitis has been diagnosed clinically.
3. **Cholescintigraphy** (technetium 99m creates a minimal radiation exposure for the fetus) has excellent sensitivity and specificity in the diagnosis of cholecystitis. This is the diagnostic procedure of choice in a non-pregnant patient and may be used during pregnancy when the benefits are thought to outweigh the risks.

D. CLINICAL CHALLENGES OF DIAGNOSING CHOLECYSTITIS IN PREGNANCY. The diagnosis of cholecystitis may be difficult to make in pregnancy because of the following:
1. Anorexia, nausea, and vomiting are commonly seen in the first trimester of pregnancy.

$$Cam/Ccr \% = \frac{\text{Amylase clearance}}{\text{Creatinine clearance}} \times 100$$

$$Cam/Ccr \% = \frac{\dfrac{(\text{Amylase}) \text{ urine} \times (\text{Volume}) \text{ urine}}{(\text{Amylase}) \text{ serum}} \times \text{Time}^*}{\dfrac{(\text{Creatinine}) \text{ urine} \times (\text{Volume}) \text{ urine}}{(\text{Creatinine}) \text{ serum}} \times \text{Time}^*} \times 100$$

$$Cam/Ccr \% = \frac{\text{Amylase urine}}{\text{Amylase serum}} \times \frac{(\text{Creatinine}) \text{ serum}}{(\text{Creatinine}) \text{ urine}} \times 100$$

FIGURE 3-2

Formula for calculating the amylase/creatinine clearance ratio (*volume and time cancel). *Cam*, Amylase clearance; *Ccr*, creatinine clearance. *(From DeVore GR: Clin Perinatol 7:349-369, 1980.)*

2. A moderate leukocytosis, which is usually found with this disorder, is often present during pregnancy.
3. Alkaline phosphatase is produced by the placenta and elevated in uncomplicated pregnancies.
E. **DIFFERENTIAL DIAGNOSIS.** Hepatitis (severe acute viral vs. alcoholic), duodenal ulcer perforation, acute pancreatitis, pyelonephritis, appendicitis, pneumonia, and myocardial infarction.

III. THERAPEUTIC MANAGEMENT

A. **MEDICAL MANAGEMENT.** Successful in the majority of patients; thus an initial attempt at conservative management should be made. This therapy consists of the following:
1. Intermittent nasogastric suction
2. Intravenous colloids
3. Narcotics for pain control
4. Antibiotics if there is evidence of sepsis or if the patient does not respond to conservative therapy within 4 days
B. **SURGICAL MANAGEMENT.** Necessary when, at initial presentation, the patient has a surgically "acute" abdomen and when medical management fails. The second trimester is the optimal period in which to perform surgery because the uterus is below the operative field and thus at decreased risk for abortion or PTL. When surgery is indicated, the rate of maternal and fetal morbidity and mortality increases with delay. Laparoscopic cholecystectomy has been performed safely during pregnancy.[4,5]
C. **ASYMPTOMATIC GALLSTONES.** Require only clinical observation during pregnancy; the risks of surgical management outweigh any potential benefit.

ACUTE PANCREATITIS

I. BACKGROUND

A. DEFINITION. Inflammation of the pancreas.

B. INCIDENCE. Acute pancreatitis occurs in 0.01% to 0.1% of pregnancies (the incidence in nonpregnant patients is 0.5%). Although this disorder is seen in all trimesters, it is more frequent in the third trimester and postpartum.[6]

C. PATHOPHYSIOLOGY. Pancreatitis arises from pancreatic autodigestion by enzymes that are inappropriately activated by alcohol abuse, gallstones, infection, ischemia, trauma, vasculitis, hyperlipidemia, and hypercalcemia. Alcohol abuse and gallstones are thought to be associated with 80% of cases of acute pancreatitis in nonpregnant patients. In the majority of cases of pancreatitis in pregnancy, the disease is thought to be related to **gallstones.** It is usually self-limiting and resolves within 1 week when medically managed.

D. PERINATAL MORBIDITY AND MORTALITY. Abortion and PTL may be triggered by disease complications such as hypovolemia, hypoxia, and acidosis.

E. MATERNAL MORBIDITY AND MORTALITY. Maternal mortality in mild and moderate pancreatitis is unchanged from that noted in uncomplicated pregnancies. When severe pancreatitis develops, the mortality is greater when managed medically than when managed surgically.

II. EVALUATION

A. HISTORY. Elicit information regarding the risk factors detailed in the previous section. The patient may complain of severe midepigastric pain radiating through to her back, as well as nausea, vomiting, and fever.

B. PHYSICAL EXAMINATION. A thorough physical examination may reveal fever and may confirm the presence of midepigastric pain or tenderness radiating posteriorly.

C. DIAGNOSTIC DATA

1. Obtain a CBC with differential, serum amylase, lipase, glucose, electrolyte panel (include creatinine, calcium, magnesium, phosphorus); urine (spot sample) amylase; and creatine.

2. Amylase and lipase levels are elevated with appendicitis (and other gastrointestinal and reproductive tract disorders), but this change may be masked by the normal elevation of amylase (up to fourfold its normal value) in midpregnancy. Serial amylase and lipase values may be helpful in diagnosing pancreatitis. The magnitude of the values does not correlate with disease severity. When these values remain elevated longer than 1 to 2 weeks, a pancreatic pseudocyst or ascites may be developing.

3

ACUTE ABDOMINAL PAIN

3. **An amylase/creatinine clearance ratio** may assist in this diagnosis. It is elevated with this disease and remains elevated after the acute rise of serum amylase, which occurs within the first 2 days of acute pancreatitis. The ratio is 1% to 4% in a healthy nonpregnant patient and 2% to 3.5% in uncomplicated pregnancies. The ratio of serum amylase to creatinine is decreased compared with that in the nonpregnant state as a result of the increased creatinine clearance during pregnancy (Fig. 3-2).

4. **Hypocalcemia** is commonly present and can be corrected with intravenous (IV) calcium gluconate.

5. **Hyperglycemia** may be present. Administration of regular Humulin insulin, depending on the severity of the patient's condition, should be considered.

6. An **ultrasonic examination or computed tomographic** scan may assist in diagnosis when the patient's presentation or recovery is atypical.

D. **DIFFERENTIAL DIAGNOSIS.** Acute cholecystitis, perforated ulcer, renal colic, dissecting aortic aneurysm, pneumonia, and vasculitis complicating a connective tissue disorder, intestinal obstruction, and diabetic ketoacidosis.

III. THERAPEUTIC MANAGEMENT

A. **MILD AND MODERATE PANCREATITIS**

1. **Nasogastric suction** (to avoid stimulation of the pancreas) and IV hydration are mandatory until the patient has improved symptomatically and biochemically (usually 3 to 5 days). When the patient's condition has improved, she may receive a clear liquid diet and then gradually advance during the next 2 days to regular food.

2. **Meperidine** (Demerol), 75 to 100 mg intramuscularly (IM) every 4 hours, may be administered for pain relief.

3. **Antibiotics** are indicated only if infection develops (e.g., ascending cholangitis or pancreatic abscess).

4. **Avid monitoring of vital signs, fluid intake and output, and electrolytes** is necessary because some degree of third spacing and dehydration occurs in each patient. The need for large fluid replacement coincident with hypotension and respiratory insufficiency indicates that the disease is worsening and that surgical intervention is necessary.

5. **Complications**. Pancreatic pseudocysts occur in 2% to 10% of patients. These may be complicated by pancreatic ascites, abscess development, hemorrhage and rupture, or pleural effusion.

B. **SEVERE PANCREATITIS.** Mild and moderate disease may worsen despite conservative medical management. Surgical intervention is necessary in the event of the following[7]:

1. **Cardiovascular collapse or respiratory insufficiency.** In these cases, either a wide sump drain may be placed or peritoneal lavage via a laparotomy incision may be performed to remove the toxic exudate from the pancreas.

2. Common bile duct obstruction with **cholangitis**
3. **Pancreatic abscess**
4. Life-threatening **hemorrhagic pancreatitis**

PEPTIC ULCER DISEASE (PUD)

I. BACKGROUND

A. DEFINITION. A peptic ulcer is a defect in the mucosa of the esophagus, stomach, or duodenum caused by gastric acid.

B. INCIDENCE. PUD occurs in 5% of the population and is rare in pregnancy. PUD occurs so infrequently in pregnancy that any newly diagnosed case during pregnancy mandates evaluation for its cause (cancer and Zollinger-Ellison syndrome must be considered).

C. ETIOLOGY. An increase in stomach secretion of hydrochloric acid and pepsin may initiate or maintain an ulcer. *Helicobacter pylori* is recognized as an etiologic agent in PUD. Disease improvement may be seen in pregnancy because of the elevated level of progesterone, which results in decreased gastric acid production and increased gastric mucous secretion. In addition, the placenta produces plasma histaminase, which inactivates, or blocks, the effect of histamine (an activator of hydrochloric acid secretion).

D. PERINATAL AND MATERNAL MORBIDITY AND MORTALITY. Mild PUD and moderate PUD have a morbidity and mortality equivalent to those in uncomplicated pregnancies. When surgery is indicated, medical management results in a 44% mortality (maternal and fetal) and surgical management in a 13% maternal and 26% fetal mortality. The mortality from PUD in the general population is 2 to 5 per 100,000 people per year.

II. EVALUATION

A. HISTORY. The patient may complain of moderate to severe midepigastric pain (boring, burning, or cramping) lasting 15 to 60 minutes. The pain is often relieved by ingesting food or antacids and exacerbated by alcohol, aspirin, or coffee. If the lesion is in the pyloric region (or if several ulcers are present elsewhere), vomiting may occur. Complaints of hematemesis or melena signify erosion of blood vessels at the ulcer base.

B. PHYSICAL EXAMINATION. A complete examination is often significant only for minimal tenderness in the midepigastric region.

C. DIAGNOSTIC DATA

1. Serum electrolytes, liver enzymes, and CBC with differential are usually at normal levels. If iron deficiency anemia is present, it may be a result of poor dietary intake of iron or gastrointestinal bleeding (if hematemesis or melena is present).

2. Detection of *H. pylori* may be done with the ^{13}C-urea breath test.

ACUTE ABDOMINAL PAIN

3

H. pylori secretes urease, which hydrolyzes ^{13}C-urea and produces NH_3 and ^{13}CO. $^{13}CO_2$ is then detected by mass spectroscopy in expired air.[8] However, the gold standard for its detection is endoscopic biopsy specimen histology and culture.[9,10]

D. DIFFERENTIAL DIAGNOSIS. Acute pancreatitis, chronic cholecystitis, and acute appendicitis.

III. THERAPEUTIC MANAGEMENT

A. MILD DISEASE

1. Patients with uncomplicated PUD are instructed to refrain from gastric acid stimulants, such as alcohol and decaffeinated coffee. In addition, they are encouraged to avoid late night snacks to prevent gastric acid stimulation during sleep. Research indicates that other than the previously mentioned items, no specific diet has been found to assist in the resolution of PUD.

2. *H. pylori* is easily suppressed with bismuth Pepto-Bismol (525 mg four times per day) plus metronidazole (250 mg three times per day, pregnancy category B) for 4 weeks.[9]

3. **Antacids**
   a. Magnesium hydroxide, calcium carbonate, and aluminum hydroxide may all be safely used during pregnancy (Table 3-3). Sodium bicarbonate may cause fluid retention and cardiac disease.
   b. Recommended dosage of magnesium hydroxide, calcium carbonate, or aluminum hydroxide is 80 mmol 1 hour after meals and every 1 to 2 hours thereafter, with 160 mmol at bedtime.

4. **Histamine analogs** should be used.
   a. **Famotidine** (Pepcid, category B), 40 mg per day orally at bedtime or 20 mg twice daily. After the ulcer improves, the dosage may be decreased to 20 mg once daily.

TABLE 3-3

ANTACIDS AND THEIR CHARACTERISTICS

Ingredient	Characteristics
Sodium bicarbonate	Rapid and potent neutralizer; yields large absorbable sodium; may produce milk-alkali syndrome
Magnesium hydroxide	Slow but prolonged action; poorly absorbed; osmotic laxative; serum magnesium must be monitored in renal insufficiency
Calcium carbonate	Potent neutralizer; causes constipation; may produce hypercalcemia, milk-alkali syndrome, or late acid rebound
Aluminum hydroxide	Slow; not very potent; causes constipation; absorbs phosphate and some drugs

From DeVore GR: *Clin Perinatol* 7:349-369, 1980.

b. **Ranitidine hydrochloride** (Zantac, category B), 300 mg per day at bedtime or 150 mg orally twice per day.

c. **Cimetidine hydrochloride** (Tagamet, category B), 800 mg per day orally at bedtime, 300 mg four times per day (with meals and at bedtime), or 400 mg twice per day.

d. **Nizatidine** (Axid, category C) is not recommended in pregnancy because of the effectiveness of the histamine receptor antagonists listed previously.

5. **Anticholinergics** are used infrequently. They may provide relief to patients who are unresponsive to antacids and to patients who have epigastric pain during the night. The most frequently used anticholinergic is propantheline bromide (Pro-Banthine). It is administered as a 15-mg tablet orally 30 minutes before each meal and two tablets (30 mg total dose) at bedtime.

6. Sedation with **phenobarbital** may be required during an acute episode of discomfort.

B. **Peptic ulcer complications** are rare in pregnancy.

1. When **bleeding** occurs from the ulcer base, do the following:
   a. **Initiate treatment** with the following:
      (1) Nasogastric suction
      (2) Cold isotonic saline lavage
      (3) Blood replacement
   b. Consult a **gastroenterologist** and consider using the following diagnostic and therapeutic procedures:
      (1) **Diagnostic endoscopy** to localize the bleeding vessel (90% accuracy), with possible electrocoagulation (90% successful) of the bleeding site
      (2) **Selective angiography** with **embolization** of the affected vessel
         (a) This exposes the fetus to radiation.
         (b) Maternal complications include liver and stomach necrosis.
         (c) When the patient is severely ill and has lost 30% or more of her blood volume within 12 hours, **vagotomy, pyloroplasty,** or **partial gastrectomy** may be indicated.

2. Patients with **luminal obstruction** require continuous nasogastric suction for a minimum of 3 days. If the patient does not respond within this time, a surgical drainage procedure (e.g., pyloroplasty with vagotomy) may be required.

3. Ulcer **perforation** during pregnancy mandates immediate surgical treatment. If perforation is managed conservatively, maternal mortality approaches 100%.

4. When surgical treatment is necessary during the third trimester, fetal maturity should be documented and concurrent cesarean delivery should be considered to allow improved visualization of the upper area of the abdomen and to avoid fetal distress resulting from hypotension that may occur during the procedure.

PYELONEPHRITIS
See Urinary Tract Infections, Chapter 10.

REFERENCES

1. Mazze RI: Appendectomy during pregnancy: a Swedish registry study of 778 cases, *Obstet Gynecol* 77(6):835-840, 1991.
2. DeVore GR: Acute abdominal pain in the pregnant patient due to pancreatitis, acute appendicitis, cholecystitis, or peptic ulcer disease, *Clin Perinatol* 7:349-369, 1980.
3. Landers D et al: Acute cholecystitis in pregnancy, *Obstet Gynecol* 69:131-133, 1987.
4. Soper NJ, Hunter JG, Petrie O: Laparoscopic cholecystectomy during pregnancy, *Surg Endosc* 6:115-117, 1992.
5. Schorr RT: Laparoscopic cholecystectomy and pregnancy, *J Aparendosc Surg* 3(3):291-293, 1993.
6. Lowe TW, Cunningham FG: Surgical diseases complicating pregnancy. In Cunningham FG, MacDonald PC, Gant NF, editors: *Williams obstetrics*, ed 18, suppl 3, Raritan, NJ, 1990, Ortho Pharmaceutical.
7. Kammerer WS: Nonobstetric surgery in pregnancy, *Med Clin North Am* 71:551-559, 1987.
8. Cave DR: Therapeutic approaches to recurrent peptic ulcer disease, *Hosp Pract* 27:33-49, 1992.
9. Peterson WL: Helicobacter pylori and peptic ulcer disease, *N Engl J Med* 324(15):1043-1048, 1991.
10. Martinez E, Marcos A: Helicobacter pylori and peptic ulcer disease, *N Engl J Med* 325:727-738, 1991.

ASTHMA

A. DEFINITION. Asthma is a disorder in which paroxysmal dyspnea occurs in the presence of spasmodic bronchial contractions. Wheezing is common.

1. Mild: infrequent exacerbations, good exercise tolerance

2. Moderate: more frequent exacerbations, symptomatic (coughing and wheezing) a few times per week

3. Severe: daily wheezing, with sudden exacerbations necessitating more than three emergency room visits per year[1]

B. ETIOLOGY. Asthma may have an allergic or idiosyncratic cause, with overlap between these categories.

1. Allergic

    a. One third of all persons with asthma and a higher proportion of pregnant women with asthma have an allergic trigger to their asthma.

    b. Elevated serum immunoglobulin E (IgE) levels. Comprehensive antibody testing measuring relative IgE antibody levels to food and environmental allergens, as well as IgG antibody levels to foods, may now be performed at certain laboratories.

    c. Positive skin reactions and positive responses to provocative tests (airborne allergens, exercise, emotional stress) identify IgE-mediated immediate allergic and possible asthmatic triggers.

    d. A family history of asthma is common

2. Idiosyncratic

    a. Two thirds of **all** persons with asthma and a smaller proportion of pregnant women with asthma have been classified as having an idiosyncratic etiology to their asthma. Now, with enzyme-linked immunoabsorbent assay (ELISA) assessment of relative IgG antibody levels, some asthmatics classified as having an idiosyncratic etiology might soon be reclassified. IgG antibodies may induce reactions whose onset is delayed by hours or days (thus making a causal relationship between allergen and asthmatic symptom difficult to establish).

    b. Normal serum IgE levels

    c. Negative provocative and skin test results

C. INCIDENCE

1. Asthma is present in 1% to 4% of pregnancies.[2]

2. Status asthmaticus occurs in 0.05% to 0.2% of pregnancies.

D. PERINATAL MORBIDITY AND MORTALITY

1. Perinatal mortality is unchanged from that noted in uncomplicated pregnancies.[3]

2. The only fetal complication is an increased incidence of intrauterine growth retardation,[4] which is attributed to hypoxemia in the mother, with resultant hypoxemia in the fetus. Intrauterine growth retardation occurs exclusively in those patients with severe disease and in those whose disease has not been properly treated. Low birth weight has also been noted.[4,5]

3. An infant born to an asthmatic mother has a 5% to 7% risk of developing asthma during the first year of life and a 58% risk of developing it during his or her lifetime.

E. MATERNAL MORBIDITY AND MORTALITY. An increased rate of preterm delivery and preterm premature rupture of membranes occurs in all women with asthma, in addition to an increase in cesarean deliveries for fetal distress.[4] Women with steroid-dependent asthma have an increased risk for gestational (1.5% vs. 12.9%) and insulin-requiring (0% vs. 9.7%) diabetes.[4] An association between asthma and pregnancy-induced hypertension has also been noted.[6]

II. EVALUATION

A. HISTORY. Assess the severity of the attack. Has the patient been hospitalized previously for asthma? Needed corticosteroids? Been intubated? How does this attack compare with previous attacks? Were there any precipitating factors? Has the patient been compliant with medications?

B. PHYSICAL EXAMINATION

1. Evaluate whether the patient is using accessory muscles in her breathing effort. Agitation or somnolence indicates decompensation.

2. Vital signs consistent with a severe episode include a pulse greater than 120 bpm, respirations more than 30/min, and a pulsus paradoxus more than 18 mm Hg.

3. Perform a complete physical examination, and pay special attention to the airway. The intensity of wheezing does not correlate with the severity of the asthma. Rule out upper and lower respiratory infections.

C. DIFFERENTIAL DIAGNOSIS. Asthma usually is not difficult to diagnose, especially with a good history and physical examination. The differential diagnosis includes the following:

1. Left ventricular failure

2. Pulmonary embolism

3. Upper airway obstruction (tumor or edema)

4. Chronic bronchitis

5. Pneumonia

6. Dehydration

D. DIAGNOSTIC DATA

1. Arterial blood gases (ABGs) are useful in evaluating the severity and chronicity of an attack. Mild hypoxemia and mild respiratory alkalosis are present early in an asthmatic attack. Metabolic alkalosis occurs gradually, and with a severe, prolonged attack, muscle exhaustion produces respiratory acidosis (Tables 4-1 and 4-2).

2. IMPORTANT: If the patient's Pco_2 is elevated, she is in respiratory failure and may need endotracheal intubation and mechanical ventilation.

3. Pulmonary function tests are useful to assess the severity of the attack

TABLE 4-1

ACID-BASE BALANCE AND BLOOD GASES

	Nonpregnant	Pregnant
P_{O_2} (mm Hg)	98-100	101-104
P_{CO_2} (mm Hg)	35-40	25-30
Arterial pH	7.38-7.44	7.40-7.45
Bicarbonate (mmol/L)	24-30	18-21
Base deficit (mEq/L)	0.07	3-4

From Gleicher N, editor: *Principles of medical therapy in pregnancy,* New York, 1985, Plenum.

4

ASTHMA

TABLE 4-2

METABOLIC AND RESPIRATORY ACIDOSIS AND ALKALOSIS

The primary acid-base disturbances result from conditions that initially affect the HCO_3^- (metabolic acidosis and alkalosis) or from states that initially alter the P_{CO_2} (respiratory acidosis and alkalosis). Each of these primary disturbances causes the blood pH (H^+ concentration) to shift away from normal by changing the ratio of P_{CO_2} (HCO_3^-) and evokes compensatory responses that return pH **toward,** but not completely to, normal.

1. **Metabolic acidosis** results from a reduction in HCO_3^- that reflects the accumulation of nonvolatile acids. The compensatory response is increased ventilation, leading to a fall in P_{CO_2}.
2. **Metabolic alkalosis** occurs from a primary increase in the HCO_3^-. The compensatory response is hypoventilation, causing a rise in P_{CO_2}.
3. **Respiratory acidosis** is the result of insufficient pulmonary removal of CO_2 (increased P_{CO_2}), leading to an increase of H_2CO_3. The compensatory response is an increase in renal recovery and generation of HCO_3^-, leading to a rise in serum HCO_3^- concentration.
4. **Respiratory alkalosis** occurs as a result of hyperventilation (decreased P_{CO_2}). The compensatory response is increased renal HCO_3^- loss and reduced regeneration, leading to a fall of serum HCO_3^- concentration.

	Primary Change	pH	Compensatory Response
Metabolic acidosis	$\downarrow HCO_3^-$	$\downarrow$ pH	$\downarrow P_{CO_2}$
Metabolic alkalosis	$\uparrow HCO_3^-$	$\uparrow$ pH	$\uparrow P_{CO_2}$
Respiratory acidosis	$\uparrow P_{CO_2}$	$\downarrow$ pH	$\uparrow HCO_3^-$
Respiratory alkalosis	$\downarrow P_{CO_2}$	$\uparrow$ pH	$\downarrow HCO_3^-$

Metabolic acidosis results from accumulation of fixed (nonvolatile) acid (as a result of ingestion and endogenous production) or from loss of alkali.

From Orland MJ, Saltman RJ: *Manual of medical therapeutics,* Boston, 1986, Little, Brown.

and the degree of improvement with treatment. Spirometry may be performed at the bedside to measure the volume of forced air expired in the first second of expiration (FEV_1).[2] This value, expressed as a percentage of forced vital capacity (FVC), exceeds 75% in healthy people. When this ratio declines below 30%, severe disease is present and hospitalization is indicated (Table 4-3 and 4-4 and Fig. 4-1).

TABLE 4-3		
LUNG VOLUMES AND CAPACITIES		
Test	Definition	Change in Pregnancy
Respiratory rate	—	No significant change
Tidal volume	The volume of air inspired and expired at each breath	Progressive rise throughout pregnancy of 0.1-0.2 L. In late pregnancy the tidal volume is probably 40% greater than before conception and mixes with a (functional) residual volume nearly 20% smaller, a change making for greatly increased efficiency of gas mixing
Expiratory reserve volume	The maximal volume of air that can be additionally expired after a normal expiration	Lowered by approximately 15% (0.55 L in late pregnancy compared with 0.65 L postpartum). The increased depth of respiration takes place at the expense of the expiratory reserve.
Residual volume	The volume of air remaining in the lungs after a maximal expiration	Falls considerably (0.77 L in late pregnancy compared with 0.96 L postpartum, a fall of approximately 20%)
Vital capacity	The maximal volume of air that can be forcibly inspired after a maximal expiration	Unchanged except for possibly a small terminal diminution
Inspiratory capacity	The maximal volume of air that can be inspired from the resting expiratory level	Increased by approximately 5%
Functional residual capacity	The volume of air in the lungs at the resting expiratory level	Lowered by approximately 18% (see remarks under tidal volume)
Minute ventilation	The volume of air inspired or expired in 1 min	Increased by approximately 40% as a result of the increased tidal volume and unchanged respiratory rate (10.34 L in late pregnancy compared with 7.27 L postpartum).

From Main DM, Main EK: *Obstetrics and gynecology: a pocket reference,* St Louis, 1984, Mosby.

TABLE 4-4

TESTS OF RESPIRATORY FUNCTION

Test	Definition	Change in Pregnancy
Maximal voluntary ventilation (maximal breathing capacity)	The maximal minute ventilation attainable by voluntary hyperventilation	Unchanged
Timed vital capacity	The proportion of the vital capacity that can be expired in the first second	Unchanged
Diffusing capacity	The rate at which a gas passes from the alveoli into the blood at a partial pressure difference of 1 mm Hg	Unchanged (measured with carbon monoxide)
Airway resistance	Resistance to flow in the airways	Reduced. Both mean and maximal flow rates are unaltered, but the pressure required to achieve these is less

Modified from Hytten FE, Lind T: Diagnostic indices in pregnancy. In Main DM, Main EK: *Obstetrics and gynecology: a pocket reference,* St Louis, 1984, Mosby.

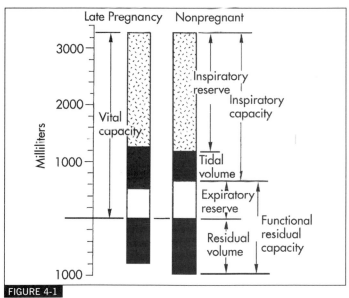

FIGURE 4-1

Lung volume and capacities in pregnancy. (*From Hytten FE, Leitch I: The physiology of human pregnancy, ed 2, Oxford, England, 1971, Blackwell Scientific.*)

4. **A chest x-ray** is useful to rule out conditions that may be exacerbating the asthma. Asthmatic lungs often demonstrate hyperinflation.
5. Obtain a **sputum** sample and examine it for eosinophils, white blood cells, bacteria, and Charcot-Leyden crystals.
6. Obtain serum for a complete blood cell count (CBC) with differential and an electrolyte panel.

III. THERAPEUTIC MANAGEMENT

A. **ACUTE MANAGEMENT.** In general, this is the same whether the patient is or is not pregnant.
1. Provide **oxygen** at 2 to 3 L/min by nasal cannula. Maintain the Po_2 above 60 mm Hg.
2. **Hydrate** the patient with 5% dextrose in water at 100 to 200 ml/h.
3. If this is an acute attack, administer the following:
   a. **Aerosolized bronchodilator**
      (1) **Metaproterenol** (Alupent, category B),[7] 0.3 ml in 2.5 ml normal saline by nebulized inhaler. If neither subcutaneous terbutaline nor epineprine is used, this may be repeated every 2 hours for three total doses and then every 4 to 6 hours, **or**
      (2) **Isoetharine** (Bronkosol, category B), 0.5 ml in 2.5 ml normal saline by nebulized inhaler every 2 to 4 hours, **or**
      (3) **Metaproterenol** (Alupent) and **isoetharine** (Bronkosol) may be alternated every 2 hours for three total doses.
   b. **Parenteral sympathomimetics**
      (1) **Terbutaline** (category B). This drug should not be used to initiate treatment because of its delayed onset of action (30 to 60 minutes). It has a longer serum half-life than epinephrine and therefore may be used for long-term treatment. It may be administered subcutaneously in a 0.25-ml dose. The dose may be repeated once in 20 minutes. Hold for a pulse of >115 bpm.
      (2) **Epinephrine** may be used in place of terbutaline, although it is not recommended because of the possibility of uterine vasoconstriction. It is also administered subcutaneously, but the dose is 0.3 to 0.5 ml of a 1:1000 dilution. The dose may be repeated every 30 minutes (hold for a pulse of >115 bpm) up to three times to achieve a symptomatic response. Relative contraindications (as with terbutaline) are severe hypertension and cardiac disease.
      (3) **Aminophylline** (80% theophylline, category B) may be given in addition to terbutaline (as severity warrants) in a loading dose of 5 to 6 mg/kg (IV) for a period of 20 to 30 minutes and then followed by a continuous infusion of 0.9 mg/kg/h. If the patient has taken oral theophylline intermittently, decrease the loading dose by half (measure the theophylline level, and adjust it accordingly). The therapeutic theophylline plasma concentration is

10 to 20 mg/ml. Serious complications may arise if the theophylline level exceeds 30 μg/ml. Side effects of aminophylline include anorexia, nausea, vomiting, nervousness, and headache. The theophylline half-life is shortened in cigarette smokers.

4. **Glucocorticoids. Do not hesitate to administer these to a pregnant patient if an indication for their use is present.**
   a. **Methylprednisolone** (Solu-Medrol, category B) may be administered in a loading dose of 2 mg/kg by intravenous push (IVP). The average loading dose is 120 mg, and the maximum is 200 mg.
   b. Follow the loading dose with a maintenance dose of Solu-Medrol. Frequently used regimens include the following:
      • 0.75 mg/kg (average dose 40 mg) IVP every 4 hours
      • 60 mg IVP every 6 hours
   c. After 2 to 3 days, Solu-Medrol may be discontinued and 30 mg of **oral prednisone** (category B) may be initiated twice a day, with gradual tapering by 5 mg every other day, beginning with the evening dose.
   d. **Hydrocortisone** (Solu-Cortef, category B) may be used instead of Solu-Medrol. The relative intravenous strength is 4:1 (Solu-Medrol/Solu-Cortef).

5. **Antibiotics** are not routinely used unless a bacterial infection is strongly suspected.

6. If the patient responds to emergency treatment with metaproterenol and parenteral sympathomimetics, she may be discharged home with an **Alupent** inhaler (two puffs every 4 to 6 hours) and continuation of theophylline if previously prescribed. The patient should return to the physician's office within 1 week (sooner if symptomatic) to have her **theophylline** level and pulmonary function reevaluated.

7. If the patient requires aminophylline, glucocorticoids, or antibiotics, consider admitting her for further treatment and observation.

B. **CHRONIC/LONG-TERM MANAGEMENT.** In pregnant patients, chronic/long-term management is similar to that of nonpregnant patients. The goal is to optimize pulmonary function and prevent acute attacks.

1. **Educate** the patient and her family so that they understand the disease, avoid precipitating factors (e.g., exercise, cold, dust, animal dander, tartrazine, aspirin, nonsteroidal antiinflammatory agents), and seek care at the beginning of an attack.

2. **Bronchodilators** are useful in controlling mild asthmatic attacks.
   a. Aerosolized agents, such as **Alupent** and **Bronkosol,** are usually the first line of therapy and are taken two to four times a day, as indicated, for rapid resolution of mild exacerbations.
   b. **Terbutaline,** 2.5 to 5 mg taken three times per day orally, and **theophylline,** 200 to 400 mg taken twice a day orally, may be used when inhalants no longer control the attacks.

4

ASTHMA

    c. Hepatic clearance of theophylline during the third trimester of pregnancy is decreased by 20% to 30% in comparison with the nonpregnant state. Thus theophylline levels must be monitored periodically.

3. Corticosteroids may be used in those patients with frequent, severe attacks despite bronchodilator treatment.

    a. Do not hesitate to use steroids in pregnant patients if they are indicated. The risks associated with maternal hypoxia are greater than those with steroid use.

    b. Consider using beclomethasone, two puffs (100 μg) four times per day.

4. If clinically indicated, **cromolyn sodium** may be used prophylactically for patients with asthma induced by exercise and cold. The usual dosage is 20 mg (one capsule) via aerosol inhaler (e.g., Intal inhaler) four times per day. Experience with cromolyn sodium in pregnancy is limited.[8]

C. DELIVERY

1. The vaginal route is preferable.

2. An epidural anesthetic is the one of choice.

3. If the patient is taking steroids for a long time, increase levels to stress doses (25 mg Solu-Medrol **IVP** or 100 mg Solu-Cortef **IVP**). Gradually taper the steroids postpartum as described in section IIIC1d(4) above.

REFERENCES

1. Greenberger PA: Asthma in pregnancy, *Clin Chest Med* 13(4):597-605, 1992.
2. Clark SL: Asthma in pregnancy, *Obstet Gynecol* 82(6):1036-1040, 1993.
3. Coutts II, White RJ: Asthma in pregnancy, *J Asthma* 26(6):433-436, 1991.
4. National Asthma Education Program: *Report of the working group on asthma & pregnancy: management of asthma during pregnancy,* NIH Pub No. 93-3279:1-3, Washington, DC, 1993, National Institutes of Health.
5. Perlow JH et al: Severity of asthma and perinatal outcome. Part I, *Am J Obstet Gynecol* 167(4):963-967, 1992.
6. Lehrer S et al: Association between pregnancy-induced hypertension and asthma during pregnancy, *Am J Obstet Gynecol* 168(5):1463-1466, 1993.
7. Matsuo A, Kast A, Tsunenari Y: Teratology study with orciprenaline sulfate in rabbits, *Arzneimittelforschung* 32(8):808-810, 1982.
8. Clark B et al: Nedocromil sodium preclinical safety evaluation studies: a preliminary report, *Eur Respir J* 69(suppl):248-251, 1986.

DIABETES

I. BACKGROUND

A. **DEFINITION.** Diabetes mellitus (DM) is a metabolic disorder of carbohydrate intolerance that is usually caused by insufficient insulin secretion or a lack of normal response to insulin at the cellular level. Hormonal changes and consequent alterations in carbohydrate, fat, and protein metabolism during pregnancy may exacerbate existing diabetes or uncover latent diabetes.

B. **INCIDENCE.** Insulin-dependent (type 1) diabetes occurs at a rate of 0.1% to 0.5% in the general population. The incidence of gestational diabetes (carbohydrate intolerance first recognized in pregnancy; classes A_1 and A_2 as defined in Table 5-1) is 3% of pregnancies. These account for 90% of patients with diabetes that complicates pregnancy.

C. **ETIOLOGY.** Patients who are older than 25 years of age; are markedly obese and have glucosuria, accelerated fetal growth, or a history of macrosomia, anomalous fetus, or stillbirth; or have a family history of diabetes, preeclampsia, previous gestational diabetes, previous stillbirth, or polyhydramnios are at high risk of developing diabetes during pregnancy. One or more of these risk factors are present in almost half of the patients who develop gestational diabetes.[1]

1. Screen high-risk patients for diabetes at their initial prenatal care visit.

2. At 24 to 28 weeks' gestation,[2] screen all other patients, including those high-risk patients whose first screen results were within normal range (universal screening for diabetes is controversial, and some centers elect to screen only high-risk patients).

3. Screen with a 1 hour post-Glucola test in which 50 g of glucose is ingested orally and a venous blood specimen is drawn 1 hour later.
   a. The screen is within normal limits if the plasma glucose level is ≤140 mg/dl (sensitivity 80% and specificity 90%). Adjustment of this threshold has been recommended according to race.[3]
   b. If the plasma glucose level is >140 mg/dl, obtain a 3-hour glucose tolerance test (GTT). Approximately 15% of these patients will have an abnormal GTT.

4. A normal GTT is defined as follows:
   a. Fasting blood sugar (FBS) ≤105 mg/dl
   b. 1-hour plasma glucose ≤190 mg/dl
   c. 2-hour plasma glucose ≤165 mg/dl
   d. 3-hour plasma glucose ≤145 mg/dl

5. Gestational DM is present if two of the three GTT plasma glucose values (excluding the FBS) exceed the normal range.

D. **WHITE'S CLASSIFICATION OF DIABETES IN PREGNANCY.**[4] This is the most commonly used system (Table 5-1).

TABLE 5-1

WHITE'S CLASSIFICATION OF DIABETES IN PREGNANCY

		Pregestational Diabetes		
Class	Age of Onset (y)	Duration (y)	Vascular Disease	Therapy
A	Any	Any	0	A_1, diet only A_2, insulin
B	≥20	<10	0	Insulin
C	10-19 or	10-19	0	Insulin
D	<10	≥20	Benign retinopathy	Insulin
F	Any	Any	Nephropathy	Insulin
R	Any	Any	Proliferative retinopathy	Insulin
H	Any	Any	Heart disease	Insulin

	Gestational Diabetes		
Class	Fasting Glucose Level		Postprandial Glucose Level
A_1	<105 mg/dl	and	<120 mg/dl
A_2	≥105 mg/dl	and/or	≥120 mg/dl

From American College of Obstetricians and Gynecologists: Tech Bull No. 92, Washington, DC, May 1986, The College.

E. PERINATAL MORBIDITY AND MORTALITY

1. Perinatal mortality is 2% to 5%. Intrauterine fetal death occurs at an increased rate in women with insulin-dependent diabetes.
2. The increased rate of malformations seen in women with insulin-dependent diabetes is believed to correlate with poor control of diabetes.[5-8]
   a. Most malformations noted in infants of diabetic mothers occur during the first 7 weeks of pregnancy (Table 5-2).
   b. Diabetic women who require insulin have a 6% to 8% chance of delivering an infant with a major malformation (two to four times the rate in the general population). Class A_1 diabetic women do not have an increased rate of fetal anomalies.
3. Fetal macrosomia in insulin-dependent diabetic patients increases the risk of birth trauma.
4. Additional neonatal complications include hypoglycemia, hyperbilirubinemia, hypocalcemia, polycythemia, and transient respiratory distress.
5. Decreased neonatal and perinatal morbidity, particularly macrosomia and hypoglycemia, are seen when glucose is adequately controlled. In addition, improved metabolic control may increase fetal pulmonary maturity to nondiabetic levels near term.[9]

F. MATERNAL MORBIDITY

1. Of class A_1 insulin-dependent diabetic patients, 10% will progress to class A_2 during the current pregnancy.
2. All insulin-dependent diabetic patients are at risk of developing vascular

---

TABLE 5-2

CONGENITAL MALFORMATIONS IN INFANTS OF DIABETIC MOTHERS

Cardiovascular system
   Transposition of the great vessels
   Ventricular septal defect
   Atrial septal defect
   Hypoplastic left ventricle
   Situs inversus
   Anomalies of the aorta
Central nervous system
   Anencephaly
   Encephalocele
   Meningomyelocele
   Microcephaly
Skeletal system
   Caudal regression syndrome
   Spina bifida
Genitourinary system
   Absent kidneys (Potter's syndrome)
   Polycystic kidneys
   Double ureter
Gastrointestinal system
   Tracheoesophageal fistula
   Bowel atresia
   Imperforate anus

From Gabbe SG, Niebyl JR, Simpson JL, editors: *Obstetrics: normal and problem pregnancies*, ed 2, New York, 1991, Churchill Livingstone.

5

DIABETES

   disease with specific involvement of the eyes (retinopathy, macular edema), kidneys, heart, and extremities.
3. The rate of preeclampsia rises in diabetic patients.
4. Infection and dehydration may precipitate diabetic ketoacidosis (DKA).
5. Hypothyroidism is a frequent finding during pregnancy in diabetic patients.
6. Diabetes will develop 2 to 11 years postpartum in 17% of women who experience gestational diabetes.[10]
7. Diabetic patients are more likely to require cesarean delivery for dystocia, fetal distress, and macrosomia.

II. EVALUATION

A. **HISTORY.** Elicit information regarding the patient's previous pregnancies (e.g., history of macrosomia, stillbirth, insulin use), history of polyuria and vaginitis (*Candida* infections are seen more frequently in diabetic patients), and results of screening tests and GTTs.
B. **PHYSICAL EXAMINATION.** Particular attention needs to be directed to the patient's vital signs (her blood pressure should be carefully

evaluated because pregnancy-induced hypertension is more common in diabetic patients), funduscopic examination, fundal height (size and dates), and neurologic examination (especially the vibration sense in extremities, which is the most sensitive test for detecting neuropathy).

III. DIAGNOSTIC EVALUATION

A. LABORATORY STUDIES INDICATED FOR ALL DIABETIC PATIENTS

1. Plasma blood sugar (BS). Any random BS level higher than 200 mg/dl is diagnostic for diabetes.
2. Baseline complete blood cell count (CBC) with differential
3. Electrolyte panel
4. Clean-catch urinalysis with culture and sensitivity (avoid catheterization in diabetic patients in the absence of pyelonephritis)
5. Consider obtaining a 24-hour urine collection for protein and creatinine clearance if the patient has either an elevated creatinine or a class F DM.
6. See Appendix L.

B. ADDITIONAL EVALUATIONS INDICATED FOR CLASSES A_2, B, C, D, E, AND F

1. Electrocardiogram (ECG) for patients with vascular or renal disease
2. Thyroid panel
3. Genetic counseling
4. Hemoglobin A_{1c}
5. Ophthalmologic examination

IV. THERAPEUTIC MANAGEMENT

Therapeutic management depends on diagnostic data. The following discussion does not apply to patients in DKA, who require more aggressive management. If the patient is in DKA, the physician should refer to a standard medical textbook or consult an internist or a perinatologist.

A. AMERICAN DIABETIC ASSOCIATION (ADA) DIET

1. Adherence to the ADA diet is important for therapeutic success of all patients with diabetes.
2. The ADA recommends that 30 calories per kilogram of actual body weight (2200 to 2400 calories) be consumed as 45% carbohydrate, 20% protein, and 35% fat. In the first trimester, however, calorie intake may be lower.
3. Calorie intake should be balanced throughout the day: 25% at breakfast, 30% at lunch, 30% at dinner, and 15% as a bedtime snack.
4. Instruct the patient to eat all her meals.

B. INSULIN ADMINISTRATION

1. If the patient's disease is **newly diagnosed as class A_1 or A_2** diabetes and if her FBS is between 105 and 125 mg/dl, recommend an ADA diet for 1 week; then reexamine her FBS. If her FBS is 105 mg/dl, start her on a regimen of insulin therapy.*

---

*Some authorities advocate routine insulin therapy for class A_1 diabetes.

2. Oral hypoglycemic medications are not used during pregnancy because they may cause fetal hyperinsulinemia.
3. Calculate the patient's **24-hour insulin dosage** according to trimester. Modifications may be made if this is the first time the patient has been on insulin (decrease dosage) and if the patient is markedly obese (increase dosage).
    a. First trimester: 0.6 U of insulin per kilogram of body weight. Second trimester: 0.7 U of insulin per kilogram of body weight. Third trimester: 0.8 U of insulin per kilogram of body weight.
    b. The 24-hour insulin requirement is **divided into morning and evening injections,**[10] with all insulin administered subcutaneously 20 to 30 minutes before meals. When ordering insulin, specify **human** insulin (i.e., Humulin [Lilly]). Human insulin (made by monoclonal techniques) is less allergenic than that obtained from other sources such as pork.
        (1) **Morning:** administer two thirds of the total daily dose as follows:
            (a) Two-thirds neutral protamine Humulin (NPH) insulin (peaks in 6 to 8 hours)
            (b) One-third regular Humulin insulin (peaks in 2 to 4 hours)
        (2) **Evening:** administer one third of the total daily dose as follows:
            (a) One-half NPH insulin
            (b) One-half regular insulin
            (c) Frequently, a **three-dose regimen** is employed: NPH insulin ± regular insulin at breakfast, regular insulin with dinner, and NPH insulin at bedtime. An **alternative for new borderline class A$_2$ diabetic patients** is to treat the patients with a single dose of NPH insulin in the morning. In an attempt to normalize BS levels throughout the day, 20 U of NPH insulin is a good starting dose. If the patient is obese, a larger dose may be required. If the FBS remains >105 mg/dl, give additional NPH insulin at bedtime.
C. **OUTPATIENT CARE.** If the patient's **FBS is <250 mg/dl** and she is spilling no or minimal ketones, her disease can be managed on an outpatient basis, with insulin and outpatient education.
D. **POSSIBLE INPATIENT CARE.** If the patient's **FBS is >250 mg/dl or she is spilling a moderate or large amount of ketones** (or if both conditions exist), consider admission, including inpatient education and continuous insulin infusion.
1. If the patient has a moderate or large amount of ketones, check her **venous bicarbonate** level.
    a. If the patient's condition is indicative of acidosis, examine her **serum acetone** level and **arterial blood gas.**
    b. The **diagnosis of DKA** includes the following:
        (1) Plasma glucose >300 mg/dl

      (2) Plasma bicarbonate <15 mg/dl

      (3) Serum acetone positive at a 1:2 dilution

      (4) Arterial pH <7.30

    c. During pregnancy, DKA may develop with hyperglycemia as mild as 200 to 300 mg/dl.

    d. If the patient has DKA, obtain a medical or perinatal consultation.

2. Patients with DKA are often extremely **dehydrated.** Fluid administration needs to be individualized; however, 1 L of normal saline (NS) over the first hour followed by 4 to 10 L of fluid over the first 24 hours may be administered. Potassium chloride is added to the NS as the **serum potassium** begins to decrease. This is expected because as cells become acidotic, they allow K^+ and H^+ to move from intracellular to extracellular space. Potassium is then excreted by the kidneys into the urine and lost. As the condition is treated, the cells begin to hold onto all the potassium they can, and thus extracellular spaces such as the vascular system experience hypokalemia. As the serum **glucose** declines to <200 mg/dl, change the intravenous injection to 5% dextrose in normal saline (D_5NS) solution so the insulin can help clear the ketones.

3. Continuous insulin infusion: Place 50 U of regular Humulin insulin into 500 ml of NS. Administer a bolus of 10 to 20 U, and then start the infusion at a rate appropriate for the patient (3 to 8 U/h). Continue the infusion for approximately 1 day, adjusting the dosage and drip rate as needed.

4. Capillary glucose testing should be performed every 2 hours. The treating physician should be notified of all values.

5. Check the patient's urine at each void for sugar and acetone.

6. When changing to subcutaneous insulin therapy, calculate the patient's total 24-hour insulin requirement by adding the hourly amounts of intravenous insulin infused on the previous day. Use this as a starting point to calculate appropriately divided subcutaneous doses.

E. REQUIREMENTS FOR ALL PATIENTS RECEIVING INSULIN SUBCUTANEOUSLY

1. Capillary glucose testing every day before or after breakfast, lunch, dinner, and bedtime snack. Therapeutic objectives are for maternal plasma glucose values to be in the range of those seen in nondiabetic pregnant patients (Table 5-3).

2. Urine examined for **sugar** and **acetone** at each void.

F. INSULIN ADJUSTMENT GUIDELINES

1. If the serum glucose level is elevated, increase the insulin dose as detailed below (alterations in calorie distribution are also sometimes useful alternatives):

If elevated before:	Then increase:
Breakfast	Evening NPH insulin
Lunch	Morning regular insulin
Dinner	Morning NPH insulin
Bedtime snack	Evening regular insulin

TABLE 5-3

NORMAL PLASMA GLUCOSE VALUES DURING PREGNANCY

Meal Status	Range (mg/dl)	Maximum (mg/dl)
Fasting	60-90	105
Before lunch, dinner, and bedtime snack	60-105	120
2 h postprandial	120	135

NOTE: The patient receives an evening snack with the ADA diet. Monitor the number of meals and snacks that the patient is actually eating and whether friends and family are bringing extra food to the patient.

2. Increase insulin by 20% to a maximum of 4 U at a time.

3. If the FBS is persistently high despite increased insulin, obtain a capillary glucose test at 2 AM to rule out the possibility of rebound hyperglycemia.

V. ANTEPARTUM SURVEILLANCE*

A. CLASS A₁. Uncomplicated, without any other indications for antepartum testing

1. Perform weekly FBS.

2. Provide dietary counseling.

3. Perform ultrasound to rule out macrosomia at 37 to 38 weeks' gestation.[11]

4. Begin fetal surveillance (biophysical profile [BPP], contraction stress tests [CST], or modified BPP) at 40 weeks' gestation.

B. CLASSES A₂ AND B

1. Perform weekly FBS in the office and home capillary glucose testing after each meal and at bedtime.

2. Provide dietary counseling.

3. Perform ultrasound for gestational dating on admission and again in the second trimester at approximately 20 weeks' gestation to rule out fetal anomalies. Three-dimensional if available may be useful in the first and second trimester to better evaluate any fetal body areas not clearly seen or that demonstrate concern during two-dimensional ultrasonography. Consider a fetal echocardiogram at 20 to 22 weeks' gestation in institutions where this is available (strongly recommended for patients with elevated initial HbA_{1c}).[12]

4. Begin fetal surveillance at 32 to 34 weeks' gestation. Earlier antepartum testing (25 to 28 weeks' gestation) is indicated in patients with proteinuria, intrauterine growth retardation, or hypertension.[13]

---

*Antepartum surveillance of diabetic patients may be performed by various methods including (1) weekly contraction stress tests (CSTs) with an interval nonstress test (NST) and (2) twice per week biophysical profile (BPP) or modified BPP. Amniotic fluid volume may not be a reliable predictor of fetal status in diabetic patients because of the patients' propensity toward polyhydramnios.

C. CLASSES D, E, AND F

1. Begin antepartum testing as detailed for classes A_2 and B, but begin at 26 to 28 weeks' gestation.[14]
2. Deliver at 38 weeks' gestation or sooner in the presence of **intrauterine growth restriction, pregnancy-induced hypertension,** or abnormal test results.

VI. WHILE THE PATIENT IS ANTEPARTUM

Discuss sterilization. Special consents may be required in the antepartum period, depending on state laws.

VII. ON DISCHARGE HOME (ANTEPARTUM)

A. Be sure your patient has all her necessary prescriptions, supplies, and equipment and that she fully understands her dietary, insulin, and home testing instructions.
B. She must be seen weekly in the office. (Have blood drawn for an FBS on her arrival each week.)
C. Patients should be scheduled for antepartum testing as discussed in section V (p. 43).

VIII. DIABETIC PATIENTS IN LABOR AT TERM OR IN WHOM INDUCTION OF LABOR IS BEING UNDERTAKEN (TABLE 5-4)

A. Patients in whom labor is to be induced (e.g., preeclampsia) should have **documented fetal lung maturity**[9] unless induction is for maternal indications. In addition to routine labor care, **capillary glucose testing is performed every 2 hours** if values are normal and stable; otherwise, hourly. Maintain glucose values between 80 and 110 mg/dl.
B. Labor-induction patients are to consume **nothing by mouth (NPO) after midnight** the night before the induction is scheduled. Instruct her to continue capillary glucose testing but to **omit** her **bedtime and morning insulin.** Instruct her to arrive at the hospital's labor and delivery department early in the morning.
C. Some patients will require an **insulin infusion**[2,15] (i.e., patients who require prolonged inductions and those whose diabetes is not controlled on intermittent SC insulin dosing). The infusion may be run through her main line, which is recommended to be lactated Ringer's (LR) solution running at a minimum of 125 ml/h. Check her urine for ketones at each void. If ketones are present, place her on D_5LR (5% dextrose in lactated Ringer's solution) and increase the infusion rate until resolution of ketonuria. Continue to **evaluate her blood glucose every 2 hours** while the insulin drip is running (Table 5-5).

IX. DIABETIC PATIENT SCHEDULED FOR ELECTIVE CESAREAN DELIVERY

Within a reasonable time before admission:
A. Document fetal lung maturity.

B. Verify that the patient has no evidence of an upper respiratory infection.

C. Obtain routine laboratory tests (CBC, FBS, urinalysis, blood type, anti-body screen).

D. Check the patient's chart for a signed consent for surgery (and for sterilization if desired).

TABLE 5-4

BISHOP SCORE FOR INDUCIBILITY OF LABOR*

Factor	Score 0	Score 1	Score 2	Score 3
Cervical dilation (cm)	Closed	1-2	3-4	5+
Cervical effacement (%)	0-30	40-50	60-70	80+
Fetal station	−3	−2	−1.0	−1 + 2
Cervical consistency	Firm	Medium	Soft	
Cervical position	Posterior	Midposition	Anterior	

RANGE OF SCORES = 0-13

PREREQUISITES

Multiparity, gestation of at least 36 wk, vertex presentation, and a normal past and present obstetric history.

PREDICTIONS

Patients with scores of 9 or more will have safe, successful inductions with an average length of labor of less than 4 h*.

MODIFICATIONS OF THIS SCORE

To make it applicable to more patients and improve predictability†:

Add 1 point for:	Subtract 1 point for:
Preeclampsia	Postdatism
Totally elective	Nulliparity
Each prior vaginal delivery	Premature or prolonged rupture of membranes

PREDICTIVE VALUE

Score:	0-4	45% to 50% failure rate
	5-9	10% failure rate
	10-13	0% failure rate

From Main DM, Main EK: *Obstetrics and gynecology: a pocket reference*, St Louis, 1984, Mosby.
*Bishop EH: *Obstet Gynecol* 24:266, 1964.
†Hughey MJ, McElin TW, Bird CC: *Obstet Gynecol* 48.625, 1976.

TABLE 5-5

AN EXAMPLE OF HOW A CONTINUOUS INSULIN INFUSION MAY BE ADMINISTERED

Blood Glucose (mg/dl)	Insulin (U/h)	Fluids (125 U/h)
<100	0.5	D_5LR
100-140	1.0	D_5LR
141-180	1.5	NS
181-220	2.0	NS
>220	2.5	NS

D_5LR, 5% Dextrose in lactated Ringer's solution; *NS*, normal saline.

E. Instruct her to be NPO after midnight the evening before surgery and tell her she may shower in the morning if she wishes.

F. Instruct her to omit her morning insulin.

G. Obtain a capillary glucose test on admission, before surgery as needed, and immediately after surgery. If her blood glucose is <80 mg/dl, infuse D_5LR. If >120 mg/dl, administer insulin.

H. On admission, initiate an IV access and infuse LR at 125 ml/h.

I. Place a Foley catheter to gravity just before surgery. (This may be placed once she is anesthetized.)

J. Manage the postoperative period as for a normal postoperative cesarean delivery, except for blood glucose and insulin dosage as detailed in the next section.

X. IMMEDIATE POSTPARTUM MANAGEMENT

A. Examine the patient's capillary glucose immediately after delivery, again in 1 to 2 hours, and then before all meals and at bedtime (or every 4 to 6 hours in patients who are NPO). (Frequency may vary, depending on the last dose of insulin.) Check her urine for ketones at every void. If she becomes ketotic, replace LR with D_5LR.

B. The tight glycemic control needed antepartum to improve fetal outcome is loosened in the immediate postpartum period. Values of 150 to 200 mg/dl are acceptable.

C. Most diabetic patients, especially those in class A_2, will not require insulin for the first 24 hours after delivery. Insulin given at this time may trigger hypoglycemia.

D. Have her nurse call you or the physician covering her if her blood glucose is <60 or >200 mg/dl. Test all urine samples for glucose and acetone, and have her nurse notify her physician of all urine glucose levels >2+ or ketone levels >1+. A good empiric starting point for postpartum management of her diabetes is as follows:

1. If the patient's urine glucose is ≥2+, check her capillary glucose.

   a. If the capillary plasma value is <200 mg/dl, do not administer insulin (some prefer not to give insulin if BS is ≤250 mg/dl).

   b. If the capillary plasma value is >200 mg/dl, administer insulin according to the following sliding scale:

201-250	2 U regular
251-300	4 U regular
301-350	6 U regular
>350	Notify house officer

2. If ketonuria is present, increase her insulin dosage.

E. In those patients who **do require** postpartum insulin while on an ADA diet, the morning dose should be approximately 20 U NPH, or half the **prepregnancy insulin** requirements.

F. Her **ADA diet** is calculated as follows:

1. During pregnancy: 30 kcal/kg actual body weight

2. After pregnancy: 30 kcal/kg ideal body weight (up to 2600 calories)

3. Calculate the patient's ideal body weight according to the following formula:

   a. 45.5 + [2.3 (Height in inches − 60)] = kg

   b. For example: 45.5 + [2.3 (67 − 60)] = 61.6 kg (135.516)

4. If your patient is breast-feeding, an extra 500 kcal may be added to the calculated value.

XI. SPECIAL DISCHARGE ORDERS

A. CLASS A_1. Schedule an FBS or a 3-hour GTT to be performed just before the patient's 6-week follow-up visit. If test results are abnormal, refer her to an internist (or diabetologist). Advise and plan weight reduction.

B. CLASS A_2. If diabetes has resolved after delivery, schedule an FBS or 3-hour GTT for the patient in 6 weeks and arrange an appointment with an internist. If her diabetic condition persists after delivery, schedule the internal medicine appointment within 1 week for evaluation and follow-up.

C. Refer patients who were on a regimen of insulin therapy before pregnancy to their diabetologist within 1 to 2 weeks after delivery. Do not order a GTT.

D. Send all patients who are not on a regimen of insulin therapy home with urine glucose strips. Instruct them to check their morning urine for sugar every 1 or 2 days and, if glycosuria develops, to notify the physician immediately. Have these patients promptly evaluated for diabetes.

REFERENCES

1. American College of Obstetricians and Gynecologists: *Diabetes and pregnancy.* Tech Bull No. 200, Washington, DC, Dec 1994, The College.
2. Ryan EA: Pregnancy in diabetes, *Med Clin North Am* 82(4):823-845, 1998.
3. Nahum GG, Huffaker JB: Racial differences in oral glucose screening test results: establishing race-specific criteria for abnormality in pregnancy, *Obstet Gynecol* 81(4):517-522, 1993.
4. White P: Diabetes mellitus in pregnancy, *Clin Perinatol* 1:331-347, 1974.
5. Mills J, Baker L, Goldman AS: Malformations in infants of diabetic mothers occur before the seventh gestational week: implications for treatment, *Diabetes* 28:292-293, 1979.
6. Jovanovic-Peterson L, Peterson CM: Pregnancy in the diabetic woman, *Endocrinol Metab Clin North Am* 21(2):433-456, 1992.
7. Yukin JS: The Deidesheimer meeting: significance of classical and new risk factors in non-insulin-dependent diabetes mellitus, *J Diabetes Complications* 11:100-103, 1997.
8. Weintrob N, Karp M, Hod M: Short- and long-range complications in offspring of diabetic mothers, *J Diabetes Complications* 10:294-301, 1996.
9. Piper JM, Langer O: Does maternal diabetes delay fetal pulmonary maturity? *Am J Obstet Gynecol* 168:783-786, 1993.
10. Damm P et al: Predictive factors for the development of diabetes in women with previous gestational diabetes mellitus, *Am J Obstet Gynecol* 167(3):607-616, 1992.

5

DIABETES

11. Tamura RK, Dooley SL: The role of ultrasonography in the management of diabetic pregnancy, *Clin Obstet Gynecol* 34(3):526-534, 1991.
12. Shields LE et al: The prognostic value of hemoglobin A1c in predicting fetal heart disease in diabetic pregnancies, *Obstet Gynecol* 81(6):955-958, 1993.
13. Landon MB, Gabbe SG: Fetal surveillance in the pregnancy complicated by diabetes mellitus, *Clin Perinatol* 20(3):549-560, 1993.
14. Landon MB et al: Fetal surveillance in pregnancies complicated by insulin-dependent diabetes mellitus, *Am J Obstet Gynecol* 167:617-621, 1992.
15. Yeast JD, Porreco RP, Ginsberg HN: The use of continuous insulin infusion for the peripartum management of pregnant diabetic women, *Am J Obstet Gynecol* 131:861, 1978.

HEPATITIS

GENERAL INFORMATION FOR ALL TYPES OF VIRAL HEPATITIS

I. BACKGROUND

A. DEFINITION. The term *hepatitis* refers to inflammation of the liver. This may be caused by either an infectious agent or a toxicity (chemical or secondary to an infectious disease).

B. VIRAL HEPATITIS. Viral hepatitis is the most common cause of jaundice in pregnancy. The remainder of this chapter focuses on the specific hepatitis viruses (A, B, C, D, E). Four other viruses may also cause hepatitis: herpes simplex I and II, cytomegalovirus (CMV), and Epstein-Barr virus (EBV). Consider screening for these agents or toxins if appropriate.

II. PREVENTION OF DISEASE IN HEALTH CARE PROVIDERS

A. Wear gloves and protective covering when the potential for coming into contact with the patient's blood, excreta, and body secretions is present.

B. All patients and their specimens are to be regarded as infected and the disease considered contagious

HEPATITIS A VIRUS (HAV)

I. BACKGROUND (TABLE 6-1)

A. ETIOLOGY. HAV is caused by a 27-nm RNA virus.

B. INCIDENCE. Approximately 34,200 new cases occur each year in the U.S. general population.

C. TRANSMISSION. Usually fecal-oral (Table 6-2).

D. INCUBATION PERIOD. Ranges from 15 to 50 days, with a mean of 30 days. The virus is shed into the feces about 2 weeks before symptoms appear, persists for 1 to 2 weeks after the onset of clinical illness, and is absent after the patient develops jaundice. No carrier state exists. Long-term immunity follows recovery.[1]

E. PERINATAL MORBIDITY AND MORTALITY. HAV is associated with prematurity and an increased spontaneous abortion rate.

F. MATERNAL MORBIDITY AND MORTALITY from HAV are primarily due to the rare occurrence of fulminant hepatitis. No evidence exists to implicate HAV in progressing to chronic liver disease.

II. EVALUATION

A. HISTORY. Patients often have a 2- to 5-day prodrome of mild fever, generalized malaise, myalgias, fatigue, weakness, anorexia, nausea,

TABLE 6-1			
TYPES OF VIRAL HEPATITIS			
Infectious Agent	Hepatitis A	Hepatitis B	Hepatitis C
Causative agent	RNA virus (27 nm)	DNA virus (42 nm)	RNA virus (30-60 nm)
Transmission	Fecal-oral	Parenteral or body fluids	Parenteral or body fluids
Incubation period	15-50 d	45-160 d	18-100 d
Time of maximal infectivity	Prodrome	Prodrome (HB carrier: anytime)	Prodrome
Diagnosis	HA antibody (IgM, IgG)	HBsAg HBcAb HBsAb HBeAg (HB carrier:HBsAg)	HCAb
Carrier state	None	5%-10% become carriers	50%
Chronic forms	None	Chronic active hepatitis	Chronic active hepatitis

vomiting, and abdominal pain. After the prodrome, the icteric phase (icteric sclera, jaundice, light-colored stools, dark urine) occurs. This may be accompanied by increased anorexia, extreme fatigue, and mild pruritus. Symptoms last 10 to 15 days, followed by a gradual recovery. Rarely, fulminant hepatitis may occur (1 in 1000 cases).

B. DIAGNOSTIC DATA (FIG. 6-1)

1. The presence of immunoglobulin M (IgM) antibody to hepatitis A is diagnostic of a current HAV infection and is usually present at the onset of jaundice.

2. In a typical case, aspartate aminotransferase (AST/SGOT) may rise to 1000 and alanine aminotransferase (ALT/SGPT) may rise to 2000.

3. In some cases a cholestatic picture occurs, with an elevated alkaline phosphatase and bilirubin accompanied by marked pruritus and light stools.

4. Infrequently, the patient may become hypoalbuminemic and hypoglycemic and may develop a coagulopathy.

5. **Immunoglobulin G** (IgG) antibody to HAV persists after the infection has resolved. IgM antibody may last 4 to 6 months.

III. THERAPEUTIC MANAGEMENT

A. Pregnancy does not alter management. Treatment supports the goal of **adequate nutrition.** In severe cases, parenteral nutrition may be required. The patient should **avoid hepatotoxic drugs** and drugs requiring liver metabolism.

B. IgG should be given to all contacts without serologic documentation of

TABLE 6-2
VERTICAL TRANSMISSION OF HEPATITIS

Infectious Agent	Hepatitis A	Hepatitis B		Hepatitis C
		Active	Carrier	
Transmission risk to infant	Low	First and second trimesters: <10% Third trimester: 65%	HBeAg present: 75%-95% HBeAg absent: <5% HBcAg present: <5%	Unknown
Newborn disease	Rare—would manifest at 14-30 d of life	Manifests at 30-120 d; disease is mild, rarely severe	Manifests at 30-120 d; disease may be fatal	
Infant complications	None	Carrier state common	Carrier state is common; 10-20 y later cirrhosis or hepatoma may develop	

6

HEPATITIS

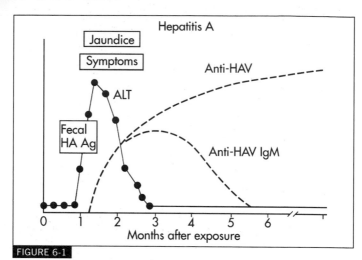

FIGURE 6-1

Clinical, serologic, and biochemical course of typical type A hepatitis. *HA Ag,* Hepatitis A antigen; *ALT,* alanine aminotransferase; *Anti-HAV,* antibody to hepatitis A virus.

infection (to facilitate rapid administration and to decrease the overall cost of care).

1. IgG may be administered prophylactically (0.02 ml/kg of body weight) if given within 2 weeks of exposure.
2. IgG is a sterilized pooled serum solution unable to transmit infection (including human immunodeficiency virus).
3. IgG is 80% to 90% effective in preventing or modifying the course of illness.

C. For high-risk contacts of patients with hepatitis A, consider administration of one of the two new inactivated hepatitis A vaccines: Havrix (Smith Kline Beecham) and Vaqta (Merck) (these are safe for use in pregnancy).[2]

HEPATITIS B VIRUS (HBV)

I. BACKGROUND

A. ETIOLOGY. HBV is caused by a 42-nm DNA virus.

B. INCIDENCE. Approximately 22,800 reported new cases develop each year in the U.S. general population. It is believed that this infection is underreported, with a possible actual occurrence of as many as 300,000 cases per year.

C. TRANSMISSION. Is by contact with blood or semen. This includes percutaneous transmission in intravenous drug abusers, health care workers with accidental percutaneous exposure, maternal-neonatal vertical transmission, and sexual promiscuity of affected individuals.

D. INCUBATION PERIOD. Ranges from 45 to 160 days, with a mean of 60 to 120 days.

E. PERINATAL MORBIDITY AND MORTALITY. It is thought by most experts on viral hepatitis that significant in utero infection of the fetus by HBV does not occur. This is because administration of hepatitis B immunoglobulin (HBIg) at birth dramatically reduces perinatal infection. The serologic findings of chronic infection in the newborn probably reflect contamination from the mother's blood.

F. MATERNAL MORBIDITY AND MORTALITY

1. Maternal mortality is the same as that experienced in the nonpregnant patient.

2. A **carrier state** may develop. A carrier is defined as a person who is hepatitis B surface antigen (HBsAg) positive on two occasions at least 6 months apart. In the United States the carrier rate is 0.1% to 0.5% (as high as 50% of adults in endemic areas). The resolution rate of chronic carriers is 1% per year.

3. Of HBV carriers, 25% develop chronic active hepatitis. Pregnancy does not increase the propensity of a patient to develop fulminant hepatitis.

4. Fulminant hepatitis associated with deep coma has an 80% mortality.

G. SCREENING. The Centers for Disease Control and Prevention (CDC)[2,3] and the American College of Obstetricians and Gynecologists (ACOG)[4] recommend that all pregnant women be screened for HbsAg. The following **high-risk groups** account for only 50% of carrier women:

1. Women of Asian, Pacific Islands, or Alaskan Eskimo descent, whether an immigrant or born in the United States

2. Women born in Haiti or sub-Saharan Africa

3. Women with histories of the following:
   a. Work in a health care or public safety field*
   b. Acute or chronic liver disease
   c. Work or treatment in a hemodialysis unit*
   d. Work or residence in an institution for mentally retarded people
   e. Rejection as a blood donor
   f. Repeated blood transfusions, as in sickle cell disease or thalassemia
   g. Frequent occupational exposure to blood in medical or dental settings (dental hygienist, nurse, physician)*
   h. Household contact with an HBV carrier or a hemodialysis patient*
   i. Multiple episodes of venereal diseases (prostitutes)
   j. Percutaneous use of illicit drugs

4. Women at risk for acquired immunodeficiency syndrome (AIDS)

*Denotes patients at highest risk.

6

HEPATITIS

II. EVALUATION

A. CLINICAL. The typical features of hepatitis detailed under HAV (part II) occur in the majority of patients; however, the prodrome in HBV usually lasts 2 to 4 weeks. A prodrome of arthralgia, arthritis, rash, angioedema, and, rarely, hematuria and proteinuria may occur in 5% to 10% of patients. Infrequently, fulminant hepatitis may develop with encephalopathy or coma (1 in 100 patients with HBV vs. 1 in 1000 patients with HAV).

B. DIAGNOSTIC DATA (FIG. 6-2)

1. Many serologic antigen markers exist for **HBV** (Table 6-3), but the three most important are **HBsAg,** hepatitis B core antigen (HBcAg), and hepatitis B early antigen (**HBeAg;** also known as soluble antigen).

2. **HBsAg** appears in the blood approximately 6 weeks after hepatitis exposure (2 weeks before clinical symptoms are present) and persists for about 3 months (1 to 2 weeks after symptoms resolve).

3. About the time that HBsAg disappears, **HBsAb** can be detected.

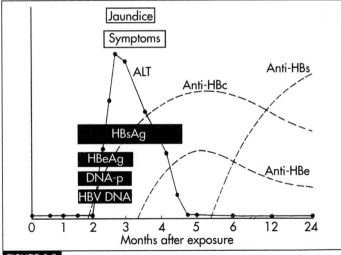

FIGURE 6-2

Clinical and serologic course of a typical case of acute type B hepatitis. *HBsAg,* Hepatitis B surface antigen; *HBeAg,* hepatitis B e antigen; *DNA-p,* DNA polymerase; *HBV DNA,* hepatitis B virus *DNA; ALT,* alanine aminotransferase; *Anti-HBc,* antibody to hepatitis B core antigen; *Anti-HBe,* antibody to hepatitis B e antigen; *Anti-HBs,* antibody to hepatitis B surface antigen. *(From Hoofnagle JH. In Mandell G, Douglas R, Bennett J, editors: Principles and practice of infectious diseases, ed 3, New York, 1990, Churchill Livingstone.)*

TABLE 6-3

HEPATITIS NOMENCLATURE

Viral Type	Terminology	Comments
Hepatitis A		
HAV	Hepatitis A virus	Eticlogic agent of "infectious" hepatitis, a picornavirus: single serotype
Anti-HAV	Antibody to HAV	Detectable onset of symptoms, lifetime persistence
IgM anti-HAV	IgM class antibody to HAV	Indicates recent infection with hepatitis A: positive up to 4-6 mo after infection
Hepatitis B		
HBV	Hepatitis B virus	Etiologic agent of "serum" or "long-incubation" hepatitis; also known as Dane particle
HBsAg	Hepatitis B surface antigen	Surface antigen(s) of HBV detectable in large quantity in serum: several subtypes identified
HBeAg	Hepatitis B e antigen	Soluble antigen: correlates with HBV replication, high-titer HBV in serum, and infectivity of serum
HBcAg	Hepatitis B core antigen	No commercial test available; present only in the liver, not serum
Anti-HBs (HBsAb)	Antibody to HBsAg	Indicates past infection with and immunity to HBV, passive antibody from HBIg, or immune response from HBV vaccine
Anti-HBe (HBeAb)	Antibody to HBeAg	Presence in serum of HBsAg carrier suggests low titer of HBV
Anti-HBc (HBcAb)	Antibody to HBcAg	Indicates past infection with HBV at some undefined time
IgM anti-HBc	IgM class antibody to HBcAg	Indicates recent infection with HBV; positive for 4-6 mo after infection

Continued

6

HEPATITIS

TABLE 6-3

HEPATITIS NOMENCLATURE—cont'd

Viral Type	Terminology	Comments
Delta hepatitis		
δ-Virus	Delta virus	Etiologic agent of delta hepatitis; may only cause infection in presence of HBV
δ-Ag	Delta antigen	Indicates past or present infection with delta virus (the delta antigen assay is not available commercially)
Anti-δ	Antibody to delta antigen	
Hepatitis C		
HCV	Hepatitis C virus	Causes at least 85% of non-A non-B (NANB) hepatitis; the remaining cases of NANB hepatitis are a diagnosis of exclusion: epidemiology parallels that of hepatitis
Anti-HC	Antibody to HCV	The antibody is detected 3-4 mo after an acute infection
Hepatitis E	Epidemic non-A, non-B hepatitis	Causes large epidemics in Asia, North Africa; fecal-oral or waterborne
Immune globulins		
Ig	Immune globulin (previously ISG [immune serum globulin] or gamma globulin)	Contains antibodies to HAV, low-titer antibodies to HBV
HBIg	Hepatitis B immune globulin	Contains a high titer of antibodies to HBV

From Immunization Practices Advisory Committee: *MMWR Morb Mortal Wkly Rep* 34:313-335, 1985.

4. **HBeAg** correlates with HBV replication and is a sign of high infectivity. It is only transiently present and occurs early in the infection.
5. **HBcAb** is present during the "window" phase, when HBsAg has cleared and the HBsAb has not appeared.

III. MANAGEMENT

A. As with HAV, management is supportive.
B. In the event of hepatic encephalopathy:
1. Dietary protein should be restricted.
2. **Lactulose syrup** should be administered in a 50-ml dose (65 g/dl) every 2 hours until diarrhea occurs. (It takes 24 to 48 hours to see the response to lactulose.) The dose may then be adjusted so that the patient has two to four loose stools per day.
3. Alternatively or in addition to the lactulose, **neomycin,** 0.5 g every 6 hours, should be administered orally.
4. Consider transferring the patient to a liver transplant center for observation.

IV. EFFECT ON PREGNANCY

A. The fetus may become infected more frequently from the viremia if the virus develops during pregnancy than in a mother who is chronically HBsAg positive.
B. More than 90% of maternal-fetal transmissions occur at delivery. Cesarean delivery does not reduce this risk.
C. Neonatal prophylaxis is mandatory for all infants born to HBsAg-positive mothers.

V. PREVENTION OF DISEASE IN THE NEONATE

A. The neonate of any mother who is HBsAg positive should be immunized, both passively with HBIg and actively with a hepatitis B vaccine at birth.[5] The status of the mother with respect to the HBeAg is not relevant to the decision to immunize the neonate, although if HBeAg is present, it is predictive of a higher transmission rate from the mother to the infant.
B. **PROCEDURE FOR NEONATAL IMMUNIZATION**
1. Wash the anterior aspect of the thighs of the neonate so that maternal blood is not inoculated with the needlestick.
2. Administer **HBIg** (0.5 ml) IM in the anterior aspect of one thigh and **hepatitis B vaccine** (0.5 ml) IM in the opposite thigh within 48 hours after birth (Table 6-4). (This is the ideal method; however, HBIg may be given up to 7 days after birth, and hepatitis B vaccine may be administered at any time.)
3. Repeat the hepatitis B vaccine at 1 and 6 months.
4. Test the infant for HBsAg and anti-HBsAg at 12 to 15 months of age.

TABLE 6-4

PROPHYLAXIS FOR INFANTS BORN TO MOTHERS WITH HEPATITIS

Type	Trimester		
	First	Second	Third
Hepatitis A (HA) acute infection	None	None	ISG, 0.5 ml at birth optional
Hepatitis B (HB) acute infection	None	None	HBIg, 0.5 ml at birth; HB vaccine at birth or within 1 mo; repeat 1 and 6 mo later
Carrier state, chronic hepatitis cirrhosis	HBIg, 0.5 ml at birth; HB vaccine at birth or within 1 mo; repeat 1 and 6 mo later	HBIg, 0.5 ml at birth or within 1 mo; repeat 1 and 6 mo later	HBIg, 0.5 ml at birth; HB vaccine at birth or within 1 mo; repeat 1 and 6 mo later
Hepatitis C acute infection	None	None	ISG, 0.5 ml at birth optional
High-risk mother but no prenatal care	—	—	HBIg, 0.5 ml at birth; await HBsAg test results for further prophylaxis

From Barron WM, Lindheimer MD: *Medical disorders during pregnancy*, ed 2, St Louis, 1995, Mosby.
ISG, Immune serum globulin; *HBIg,* HB immune serum globulin; *HBsAg,* HB surface antigen.

HEPATITIS C VIRUS (HCV; FORMERLY NON-A, NON-B HEPATITIS [NANBH])

I. BACKGROUND

A. INCIDENCE. Approximately 2400 new cases develop each year in the U.S. general population. This represents 5% of all cases of hepatitis. As with HBV, this reported figure is thought to underestimate the true incidence of HCV.

B. ETIOLOGY. HCV is thought to cause at least 85% of NANBH cases. Hepatitis C is caused by an RNA virus between 30 and 60 nm. The remaining cases of NANBH also may be caused by HCV (but our assays may not be sensitive enough to detect these cases) or by a second virus not yet identified.

C. TRANSMISSION. By percutaneous sexual and perinatal routes. Household and occupational transmission also occurs, but the mechanism is not understood.[6]

1. Because all blood is screened for HBcAb and HBsAg, HCV has become the most frequent form of hepatitis occurring after blood transfusion. Of all blood donors positive for HCV antibody, 90% have an infectious virus in their blood. Discarding this blood eliminates half of all cases of transfusion-associated hepatitis.[7] In addition, if the liver function tests of the donated blood show elevated values, HCV is presumed present and the blood is discarded.

2. No perinatal transmission has occurred after a second-trimester acute infection. Maternal chronic infection and third-trimester acute infection may lead to neonatal infection (45% to 87.5% incidence).[8]

3. Sexual transmission is noted in up to 30% of patients' partners and up to 20% of their children.[9]

D. INCUBATION PERIOD. 18 to 100 days.

E. MATERNAL MORBIDITY. Of all acute infections, 50% progress to chronic liver disease.[8]

F. EVALUATION

1. The clinical illness is similar to that of HBV.

2. Selective screening of high-risk patients is recommended.

3. The presence of HCV-RNA genome or correlated antigen[10] in serum during an infection is a reliable marker, but a polymerase chain reaction is required. (This is not routine in most laboratories, and no test has been developed that detects HCV antigen in serum.) Some university and community laboratories offer an immunoassay that detects anti-HCV antibodies, but these have a 50% false positivity.[8] Hepatitis C antibody (HCAb) is not detected in blood until 3 to 4 months after the acute episode (Fig. 6-3). In the correct clinical setting, when the HCAb assay is negative, elevated liver enzymes may be suggestive of its presence.

G. THERAPEUTIC MANAGEMENT. As with HAV and HBV, management is supportive. ACOG recommends treatment with immunoglobulin (Ig), 0.06 ml/kg, after exposure to HCV (the efficacy of this is unproven, as

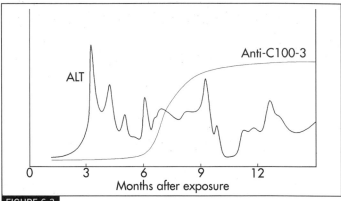

FIGURE 6-3

Graph demonstrates that the rise and fall of this biochemical marker is unrelated to disease activity and clinical infectivity. *ALT,* Alanine aminotransferase; *Anti-C100-3,* the standard anti-C antibody. *(Courtesy Dr. Ted Bader.)*

compared with hepatitis A where it is well proven). This infection is not well studied in pregnancy.

HEPATITIS D VIRUS (DELTA AGENT)

I. BACKGROUND

A. **ETIOLOGY.** Hepatitis D is caused by an RNA virus (or portion of a virus) that requires the presence of HBV for infectivity.

B. **INCIDENCE.** The exact incidence is unknown, but it is less than that of HBV. In the United States, intravenous drug abusers are the principal group at risk. Homosexuals in the United States have not yet acquired the delta agent.

C. **TRANSMISSION, INCUBATION, AND EVALUATION.** The same as for HBV. Commercialized screening for the delta antibody is available. Presence of the delta antibody means that the patient is currently infected. This test should be ordered only if the patient is HBsAg positive (because the delta virus uses HBsAg as its outer coat). Vertical transmission from the mother to the infant is of minor epidemiologic relevance, and thus routine screening of patients who are positive for HBsAg is not recommended.[11] If a patient is known to be positive for the delta antibody, the recommendations for **management of the neonate** are the same as those for neonates who are positive for HBsAg alone.

HEPATITIS E VIRUS (FORMERLY CALLED EPIDEMIC NANBH)

I. BACKGROUND

Hepatitis E is a 32-nm RNA virus that has caused large outbreaks of acute NANBH in Southeast Asia, India, Africa, and Mexico. It is transmitted by fecal-oral means and thus is different from hepatitis C (percutaneous NANBH).

II. CLINICAL PRESENTATION

Hepatitis E is an acute, self-limited disease that is similar to the other enterically transmitted hepatitis, HAV. The outcome is usually benign but with the peculiar feature that pregnant women have had from 20% to 100% case-mortality rate in epidemics (the majority of these have been in Third World countries where increased mortality in all types of hepatitis in pregnancy has been reported). The primary time of fatality has been in the third trimester.

III. DIAGNOSIS

No serologic tests are available. Hepatitis E can be suspected if the patient has traveled in the past 3 months and has a clinical picture of hepatitis A but tests negative for IgM HAV. A stool specimen can be sent to the CDC for confirmation.

IV. IMPLICATIONS

There have been no **de novo** cases of hepatitis E arising in the United States. There have been a number of imported cases, principally from Mexico. Although the CDC has not issued a formal statement, it seems prudent to advise pregnant women not to travel to Southeast Asia, India, Africa, or rural Mexico, particularly during their third trimester.

V. TREATMENT

There is no evidence that immunoglobulins manufactured in the United States will prevent hepatitis E. The best way to avoid it is to avoid contaminated food or water.

HEPATITIS G VIRUS (ALSO KNOWN AS GB VIRUS C [HGV-GBV-C])[12,13]

I. BACKGROUND

A. **ETIOLOGY.** Present in 2% of accepted blood donations in the United States.
B. **TRANSMISSION.** Parenteral. No known risk factors for its transmission.

6

HEPATITIS

II. CLINICAL PRESENTATION

Patients diagnosed with it are asymptomatic. Infected patients have viremia of HGV-GBV-C and an elevated serum ALT which does not differ from controls. The importance of this viremia as a public health concern needs further study.

REFERENCES

1. Dinsmoor MJ: Hepatitis in the obstetric patient, *Infect Obstet* 11(1):77-91, 1997.
2. Duff B: Hepatitis A vaccine: ready for prime time, *Obstet Gynecol* 91:468-471, 1998.
3. Immunization Practices Advisory Committee: Recommendations for protection against viral hepatitis, *MMWR Morb Mortal Wkly Rep* 34:313-335, 1985.
4. Progress in chronic disease prevention, *MMWR Morb Mortal Wkly Rep* 38:507, 1989.
5. American College of Obstetricians and Gynecologists: *Guidelines for hepatitis B virus screening and vaccination during pregnancy.* Committee Opinion No. 78, Jan 1990.
6. Kane MA: Hepatitis viruses and the neonate, *Clin Perinatol* 24(1):181-191, 1997.
7. Platt OS: Transmission of hepatitis C virus: route, dose, and titer, *N Engl J Med* 330(11):784-785, 1994.
8. Esteban JI et al: Evaluation of antibodies to hepatitis C virus in a study of transfusion associated hepatitis, *N Engl J Med* 323(16):1107-1112, 1990.
9. Lynch-Salamon DI, Combs CA: Hepatitis C in obstetrics and gynecology, *Obstet Gynecol* 79(4):621-629, 1992.
10. Alter MJ: The detection, transmission, and outcome of hepatitis C virus infection, *Infect Agents Dis* 2:155-166, 1993.
11. Ohto H et al: Transmission of hepatitis C virus from mothers to infants, *N Engl J Med* 330(11):744-750, 1994.
12. Zanetti AR et al: Perinatal transmission of the hepatitis B virus and the HBV-associated delta agent from mothers to offspring in northen Italy, *J Med Virol* 9(2):139-148, 1982.
13. Zanetti AR et al: Multicenter trial on mother-to-infant transmission of GBV-C virus. The Lombardy Study Group on Vertical/Perinatal Hepatitis Viruses Transmission, *J Med Virol* 54(2):107-112, 1998.

CHRONIC HYPERTENSION

I. BACKGROUND

A. **DEFINITION.** Blood pressure (BP) >140/90 mm Hg on two occasions more than 6 hours apart, before pregnancy (Table 7-1).

1. **Mild:** systolic BP = 140 to 159 mm Hg or diastolic BP = 90 to 109 mm Hg

2. **Severe:** systolic BP >160 mm Hg or diastolic BP >110 mm Hg

B. **INCIDENCE.** Chronic hypertension (HTN) is present in 2% of pregnancies.

C. **ETIOLOGY**

1. The cause of chronic HTN is detailed in Table 7-2.

2. Primary essential HTN accounts for most cases of chronic HTN seen during pregnancy. An intensive workup of HTN need not be performed during pregnancy, but a thorough physical examination must be performed and consultation with an internist must be obtained if concern arises regarding the possibility of secondary HTN.

3. Progesterone's smooth muscle–relaxing effect results in a fall of peripheral vascular resistance (average systolic fall is 5 to 10 mm Hg, average diastolic fall is 10 to 15 mm Hg) during the first 24 weeks of pregnancy (Table 7-1).[1] In 49% of women with mild chronic HTN during pregnancy, the BP was in the normal range.[2] Thus unless the prepregnancy BP is known, women may erroneously be diagnosed as having pregnancy-induced HTN in the third trimester.

D. **PERINATAL MORBIDITY AND MORTALITY.** Intrauterine growth retardation (IUGR) is increased in infants who are born to mothers with HTN. The perinatal mortality is 8% to 15%.

E. **MATERNAL MORBIDITY AND MORTALITY[3]**

1. Of patients with an elevated BP during pregnancy, 30% have essential HTN (not pregnancy-induced HTN).

2. Between 10% and 50% of patients with chronic HTN will develop superimposed pregnancy-induced HTN during their pregnancy.

3. These patients are at risk for abruptio placentae (incidence 0.45% to 10%, depending on the duration and severity of the HTN).

II. EVALUATION

A. **HISTORY.** Inquiries should be made about the following:

1. A family history of HTN

2. Previous HTN treated with medications

3. Current use of medications, particularly monoamine oxidase inhibitors

4. Monoamine oxidase inhibitor intolerance (HTN develops after ingesting foods containing tyramine or cold medications, which include such agents as phenylpropanolamine.)

TABLE 7-1		
CARDIOVASCULAR CHANGES IN PREGNANCY		
Parameter	Amount of Change	Timing
Arterial blood pressures		
Systolic (S)	↓ 4-6 mm Hg	All bottom at 20-24 wk
Diastolic (D)	↓ 8-15 mm Hg	gestation, then rise
Mean*	↓ 6-10 mm Hg	gradually to prepregnancy
		values at term
Heart rate	↑ 12-18 bpm	Early second trimester,
		then stable
Stable volume	↑ 10%-30%	Early second trimester,
		then stable
Cardiac output	↑ 33%-45%	Peaks in early second
		trimester, then stable
		until term†

From Main DM, Main EK: *Obstetrics and gynecology: a pocket reference,* St Louis, 1984, Mosby.

*Mean arterial blood pressure is calculated by the formula $MAP = \dfrac{S + 2D}{3}$.

A more manageable formula is $MAP = D + 1/3(S - D)$.

†The timing of the changes in cardiac output is controversial. Initial studies suggested a gradual rise to a peak at 26 to 28 wk gestation with a fall as term approached. More recent studies indicate an earlier rise in output that remains stable until delivery. The difference may be related to techniques and maternal position.

TABLE 7-2	
ETIOLOGY OF CHRONIC HYPERTENSION	

Primary essential hypertension
Secondary hypertension
  Arterial
    Coarctation of the aorta
    Renal arterial stenosis
  Chronic renal disease
  Neurologic disorders
  Endocrine disorders
    Acromegaly
    Cushing's syndrome
    Conn's syndrome (primary hyperaldosteronism)
    Pheochromocytoma
    Hyperthyroidism
Drug-induced hypertension
  Amphetamines
  Cocaine

5. A history suggestive of a pheochromocytoma (frequent heart palpitations, excessive and inappropriate sweating, anxiety, facial pallor)
6. Frequent previous hospitalizations during pregnancy
7. Primary aldosteronism (polyuria, proximal muscle weakness, and paresthesias, all of which are secondary to hypokalemia)
8. Thyrotoxicosis (fatigue, palpitations, heat intolerance, weight loss, increased frequency of bowel movements)
9. History of systemic lupus erythematosus, diabetes mellitus, pyelonephritis, urinary tract disorders (may result in chronic nephritis)

B. PHYSICAL EXAMINATION. Perform a complete physical examination with specific attention to the following:

1. Examine the **eyes** for findings suggestive of hyperthyroidism. Look for periorbital swelling, exophthalmos chemosis, conjunctival infection, and proptosis. Perform a **funduscopic** eye examination to evaluate for long-standing and accelerated HTN.
2. Palpate the **thyroid gland** for enlargement.
3. Measure the **BP** in the patient's arms bilaterally with the appropriate size cuff, and **listen for bruits. Palpate the femoral arteries** to exclude aortic coarctation.
4. Auscultate the **abdomen** (in early gestations) to rule out a murmur consistent with renal artery stenosis.
5. Examine the patient's **general appearance.** Truncal obesity, plethora, muscle wasting, virilization or hirsutism, and thin skin are suggestive of Cushing's syndrome.
6. Perform a clinical evaluation of the chest, as outlined in Table 7-3.

C. DIAGNOSTIC DATA

1. The **laboratory evaluation**[4] should include the following:
    a. **Urinalysis** to screen for renal disease
    b. **Hematocrit** (Fig. 7-1)
    c. Plasma **potassium** (Hypokalemia, if the patient is not taking diuretics, is suggestive of early hyperaldosteronism; hyperkalemia may suggest renal parenchymal disease.)
    d. Plasma **creatinine** (elevated levels are suggestive of renal parenchymal disease), **calcium,** and **uric acid** levels
    e. Fasting serum **cholesterol** and triglycerides
    f. **One-hour post-Glucola,** if not recently obtained (Glucose intolerance, if accompanied by truncal obesity, plethora, muscle wasting, virilization, or hirsutism and thin skin, is suggestive of Cushing's syndrome.)
    g. **Electrocardiogram (ECG)** (Left ventricular hypertrophy may suggest chronic HTN.)
    h. Consider obtaining a **24-hour urine** collection for protein and creatinine in the presence of severe HTN.
    i. Consider sending **liver enzymes** to provide a baseline evaluation of liver function in the event that the patient develops superimposed preeclampsia.

7

CHRONIC HYPERTENSION

TABLE 7-3

CLINICAL EVALUATION OF THE CHEST

A. Cardiac auscultation*

1. Sounds: First sound is louder with exaggerated splitting; second sound minimally changed; third sound is heard loudly in a majority of women; a fourth sound is heard only occasionally.
2. Murmurs: Early systolic ejection murmur (occasionally midsystolic) develops in more than 90% of women; 18% were grade I, and 82% were grade II. Some (18%) also had a soft diastolic "flow" murmur.

B. Chest x-ray

Diaphragm elevates (approximately 4 cm) with subsequent lateral and anterior displacement of the heart significantly changing the cardiac silhouette. Flaring of ribs is also noted with an increase in the subcostal angle from 68 degrees in early pregnancy to 103 degrees at term.

C. ECG†

A study of 102 women with serial ECGs through pregnancy and postpartum has better defined the normal range. There are no clinically significant changes in cardiac rhythm or in ECG intervals. The QRS amplitude increases slightly. On average there is a mild but significant left axis shift in both QRS and T-wave axis, particularly in the third trimester. However, there is great individual variation with a substantial minority exhibiting axis changes to the right (maximal changes were 40 degrees either direction). Other studies have noted the development of a Q wave in lead III and an increased frequency of ectopic beats (both PAC and PVC).

D. Echocardiogram‡

Serial studies on normal gravidas found progressive left ventricular enlargement (approximately 10% increase in end-diastolic ventricular size). However, shortening characteristics including ejection fraction were not altered. Overall, despite increased heart rate and left ventricular size, ventricular function was well preserved.

From Main DM, Main EK: *Obstetrics and gynecology: a pocket reference,* St Louis, 1984, Mosby.
*From Cutforth R, MacDonald CB: *Am Heart J* 71:741, 1966.
†From Carruth JE et al: *Am Heart J* 102:1075, 1981.
‡From Katz R, Karliner JS, Resnick R: *Circulation* 58:434, 1978.

2. **Antenatal surveillance**
   a. **Ultrasound evaluation**
      (1) Obtain a baseline scan at 16 to 18 weeks' gestation to confirm gestational age.
      (2) Beginning at 26 to 28 weeks' gestation, obtain follow-up scans every 3 to 4 weeks with serial measurements to rule out IUGR.
      (3) If preeclampsia develops, begin serial scans at the time of diagnosis (if before 26 to 28 weeks' gestation).
   b. **Antepartum testing** (see Appendix L)
      (1) Begin testing at 32 to 34 weeks' gestation in patients with uncomplicated HTN.

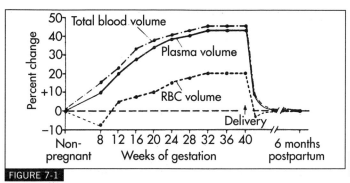

FIGURE 7-1

Circulatory changes in pregnancy. Changes in blood volume, plasma volume, red blood cell (RBC) volume, and cardiac output begin in the first trimester, rise most sharply in the second trimester, and peak early in the third trimester. These curves were constructed from various reports in the literature and illustrate trends in the percent of change from nonpregnant values. It is important to realize that there can be large individual variation. For example, although it is accepted that the average maximal increase in blood volume is between 40% and 50%, individuals have had a reported increase in their volume as little as 20% and as much as 100%. Cardiac output remains elevated during the third trimester if measured in the lateral position. *(From Bonica JJ: Obstetric analgesia and anesthesia, ed 2, Amsterdam, 1980, World Federation of Societies of Anesthesiologists.)*

(2) Begin testing at the time of diagnosis of superimposed preeclampsia or IUGR.
(3) Consider delivery at 38 to 39 weeks' gestation. If the patient's dates are poor, consider amniocentesis to evaluate fetal lung maturity.

III. THERAPEUTIC MANAGEMENT

A. OUTPATIENT MANAGEMENT

1. Generally, BP that is consistently >150/100 requires antihypertensive treatment. Consider home BP monitoring twice daily for all hypertensive patients. Patients with chronic HTN should continue on the same medications they were taking before conception, with the exception of diuretics and angiotensin-converting enzyme inhibitors (e.g., Captopril).
2. **Atenolol** (Tenormin), a β-selective adrenoreceptor blocking agent, is the newest drug of choice. Dosing is usually 50 to 100 mg/d orally and may be increased up to 250 mg/d.
3. Previously, **methyldopa** (Aldomet), whose metabolite stimulates central α-adrenergic receptors, was the drug of choice. It is administered in 250- to 500-mg doses PO every 6 hours. It is still frequently used.

4. **Labetalol** (Normodyne; Trandate) is a combination α-blocker and β-blocker drug that can easily be initiated during pregnancy. The dose is 100 mg orally every 6 to 8 hours to a maximum of 800 mg in 24 hours.

5. **If the patient's BP decreases markedly** during the first or early second trimester, consider lowering the dosage or discontinuing her anti-HTN medication. When BP elevations are noted after 20 weeks' gestation, promptly evaluate the patient for superimposed preeclampsia. In the absence of preeclampsia, consider reinitiating antihypertensive therapy (especially in the presence of diastolic BP >100) versus continued observation until delivery. Base the decision on the severity of the patient's HTN.

6. **The frequency of office visits** correlates with disease severity. Initially, mildly hypertensive patients may be seen as often as patients with uncomplicated pregnancies. Reevaluate the frequency of visits if the patient develops proteinuria or a **sudden rise in BP.** If either proteinuria or BP is severe, evaluate the patient in the labor and delivery unit.

B. **INPATIENT MANAGEMENT**

1. Patients who have been admitted for worsening HTN or superimposed preeclampsia are usually hospitalized for the duration of their pregnancies.

    a. If the gestation is near or at term, deliver the infant. Induce labor if the patient is not in labor and neither a fetal nor maternal indication exists to warrant a cesarean delivery.

    b. If the patient's condition is severe, consider immediate delivery regardless of gestational age. Induce labor if no indication for cesarean delivery is present.

    (1) Refer to Chapter 18 for management of patients with severe preeclampsia.

    (2) In a **hypertensive emergency,**[5,6] consider the following:

    (a) **Hydralazine has traditionally been the drug of choice in an emergency.**

    - The usual dose is 2.5 mg by slow intravenous push. This may be repeated in 5 to 10 minutes if the patient's BP does not decrease. Subsequently, titrate 1 to 2 mg IV over 5 to 10 minutes until a BP of about 150/100 is achieved. Hydralazine requires 20 minutes for its full effect to be manifested. Do *not* bring BP to normotensive levels. If the diastolic BP drops to <90 mm Hg, uteroplacental insufficiency may occur. The dosage may be increased as needed.

    - Alternative medications include the following (Table 7-4):

    (b) **Labetalol:** 20 mg by intravenous push (IVP), then 20 to 80 mg IVP (1 to 2 mg/min) every 10 minutes up to 300 mg. IV administration results in a 7:1 β/α blockade (com-

TABLE 7-4

PHARMACOLOGIC AGENTS FOR HYPERTENSIVE EMERGENCY

Generic Name	Trade Name	Mechanism of Action	Dosage	Onset	Duration of Action	Adverse Effects and Comments
Hydralazine hydrochloride	Apresoline	Arterial vasodilator	5 mg IV, then 5-10 mg IV every 20 min to total 40 mg	1-20 min	3-6 h	Hypotension, fetal distress, tachycardia, headache, nausea, vomiting, local thrombophlebitis; infusion site should be changed after 12 h
Labetalol	Normodyne Trandate	Selective α- and nonselective β-antagonist	20 mg IV, then 20-80 mg IV every 10 min to total 300 mg; titrated IV infusion 1-2 mg/min	5-10 min	3-6 h	Hypotension, heart block, heart failure, bronchospasm, nausea, vomiting, scalp tingling, paradoxic pressor response; may not be effective in patients receiving α- or β-antagonists
Nitroglycerin	Nitrostat IV Tridil Nitro-Bid IV	Relaxation of venous (± arterial) vascular smooth muscle	5 μg/min IV infusion, increase by 5 μg/min every 3-5 min; at 20 μg/min may increase by 10 μg/min	1-2 min	3-5 min	Headache, nausea, vomiting

Continued

7

CHRONIC HYPERTENSION

TABLE 7-4

PHARMACOLOGIC AGENTS FOR HYPERTENSIVE EMERGENCY—cont'd

Generic Name	Trade Name	Mechanism of Action	Dosage	Onset	Duration of Action	Adverse Effects and Comments
Sodium nitroprusside	Nipride Nitropress	Arterial and venous vasodilator	0.25 μg/kg/min IV infusion, increase 0.25 μg/kg/min every 5 min; maximum infusion 10 μg/kg/min	Immediate	2-3 min	Hypotension, nausea, vomiting, apprehension; risk of thiocyanate and cyanide toxicity is increased in renal and hepatitis insufficiency, respectively; levels should be monitored; must shield from light

Modified from Calhoun DA, Oparil S: *N Engl J Med* 323(17):1177-1183, 1990; Dildy GA, Clark SL: *Contemp Ob/Gyn* 38(6):11-22, 1993.

pared to 3:1 with oral administration). An IV infusion may be initiated at 1 to 2 mg/min and subsequently titrated.

(c) **Nitroglycerin**
- 5 μg/min by infusion pump. Increase by 5 μg/min every 3 to 5 minutes up to 20 μg/min and then by 10 μg/min every 3 to 5 minutes.
- Methemoglobinemia (level >3%) may result at high dose (>7 μg/kg/min). This may be treated by infusion of methylene blue, 1 to 2 mg/kg.

(d) **Sodium nitroprusside**
- 0.25 μg/kg/min initially as a continuous IV infusion. Increase by increments of 0.25 μg/kg/min every 5 minutes to a maximum of 10 μg/kg/min.
- Medication is light sensitive; thus cover container with foil. Correct hypovolemia before nitroprusside administration to avoid large arterial pressure drop.
- Although this occurs rarely, cyanide toxicity may occur and produce lactic acidosis, air hunger, or confusion. Venous hyperoxia may occur as a result of reduced cellular extraction of oxygen. Methemoglobinemia may also occur (as with nitroglycerin). Monitor arterial blood gases periodically to detect metabolic acidosis (a marker of developing cyanide toxicity). Avoid prolonged nitroprusside administration.

(e) Place a Foley **catheter** for strict monitoring of intake and output. Central monitoring may be necessary (see Tables 18-1 and 18-2 for indications and normal values of hemodynamic monitoring in pregnancy).

(3) **Monitor the fetus** carefully.

2. Patients in stable condition with gestations remote from term are managed similarly to patients with pregnancy-induced HTN receiving long-term antepartum care (see Chapter 16). Obtain an ECG and an ophthalmic examination.

3. If the patient is discharged home antepartum, do the following:
   a. Instruct her on the use of the BP cuff. Recommend that she purchase a cuff, record her BP every 4 hours during the day, and bring the record to each office visit.
   b. These patients are at an increased risk for placental abruption; thus any vaginal bleeding should be promptly evaluated. Instruct the patient to report any bleeding to you immediately.

REFERENCES

1. Sibai BM: Treatment of hypertension in pregnant women, *Drug Therapy* 335(4):257-265, 1996.
2. Gabbe SG, Niebyl JR, Simpson JL: *Obstetrics: normal and problem pregnancies,* ed 3, New York, 1996, Churchill Livingstone.

CHRONIC HYPERTENSION

7

3. Neerhof MG: Pregnancy in the chronically hypertensive patient, *Clin Perinatol* 24(2):391-406, 1997.
4. Magann EF, Martin JN, Jr: The laboratory evaluation of hypertensive gravidas, *CME Review Article* 50(2):138-144, 1995.
5. Khedun SM et al: Drug management of hypertensive disorders of pregnancy, *Pharmacol Ther* 74(2):221-258, 1997.
6. Calhoun DA, Oparil S: Treatment of hypertensive crisis, *N Engl J Med* 323(17):1177-1183, 1990.

CHRONIC IMMUNOLOGIC THROMBOCYTOPENIA

I. BACKGROUND

A. CHRONIC IMMUNOLOGIC THROMBOCYTOPENIA (ITP). ITP is the antibody-mediated destruction of maternal platelets. This condition may be diagnosed antenatally, or it may be detected by means of a prenatal screening complete blood cell count (CBC) in asymptomatic individuals. It is classified as follows:

1. Patients with an antenatal diagnosis of **ITP**
   a. **Intermediate ITP:** platelet count 50,000 to 100,000/mm^3
   b. **Severe ITP:** platelet count <50,000/mm^3

2. **Gestational (incidental) ITP[1]:** maternal platelet count of <150,000/mm^3

B. INCIDENCE. ITP primarily affects women in their reproductive years. It is the most common autoimmune disease of pregnancy, occurring in 0.01% to 0.02% of pregnancies.

C. PERINATAL MORBIDITY AND MORTALITY

1. Of all infants born to mothers with ITP, 20% to 25% have neonatal thrombocytopenia. Of infants at high risk for neonatal thrombocytopenia, 20% to 26% have severe thrombocytopenia. Ten percent of infants will have platelet counts of <50,000/mm^3; and 5% will have platelet counts of <20,000/mm^3.[2]

2. The perinatal mortality is 6% to 14%, with deaths usually associated with prematurity, intracranial hemorrhage, and shock.

D. MATERNAL MORBIDITY AND MORTALITY. The maternal mortality is 5.5%, and the maternal morbidity from hemorrhage (bleeding requiring transfusion) is 5% to 26%.

E. ETIOLOGY. Immunoglobulin G (IgG) (predominantly IgG1, although frequently associated with IgG3), directed against maternal platelets, binds the platelets, causing them to be cleared by the reticulo-endothelial system. IgG crosses the placenta and may precipitate fetal thrombocytopenia. The instigating factor for the antiplatelet antibody is unknown.

F. DIFFERENTIAL DIAGNOSIS. Before making the diagnosis of **ITP,** the following should be ruled out:

1. The use of medications (quinidine, sulfonamides, heparin, furosemide, aspirin), which may cause thrombocytopenia
2. Disseminated intravascular coagulation
3. Lymphoproliferative disorders (Hodgkin's disease, leukemia, aplastic anemia)
4. Systemic lupus erythematosus
5. Hypersplenism
6. Viral or bacterial infections (especially mononucleosis)

7. Thrombotic thrombocytopenic purpura
8. Hemolytic uremic syndrome
9. Thyroid disease
10. Sarcoidosis
11. Preeclampsia

II. EVALUATION

A. **HISTORY.** In an asymptomatic individual with recently detected ITP, instigating factors of thrombocytopenia (preceding section) should be elicited. The patient should be questioned about her bleeding tendency (antenatal menorrhagia, epistaxis, episodes of gastrointestinal [GI] bleeding, known retinal hemorrhages, joint bleeding, episodes of hematuria). The physician should inquire whether the patient has noticed petechial or purpuric lesions or subconjunctival hemorrhage.

B. **PHYSICAL EXAMINATION.** Perform a thorough physical examination. In patients with **ITP,** the skin may demonstrate petechial and purpuric lesions. During the ocular examination, observe for subconjunctival hemorrhage and retinal hemorrhage (rare). Inspect the patient's gums for bleeding. The remainder of the physical examination is usually within normal limits for pregnancy. Hypertension suggests preeclampsia, whereas splenomegaly and lymphadenopathy suggest infection (particularly mononucleosis), sarcoidosis, systemic lupus erythematosus, or a lymphoproliferative disorder.

C. **DIAGNOSTIC DATA.** Evaluate the results of a CBC with differential and platelet count, platelet-associated IgG (antiplatelet antibody), antinuclear antibody titer, lupus anticoagulant, anticardiolipin, blood cultures, coagulation screen (usually prothrombin time), thyroid function tests, fibrinogen, Venereal Disease Research Laboratory (VDRL) test for syphilis, serum protein electrophoresis, and a bone marrow aspirate.

III. THERAPEUTIC MANAGEMENT

A. **ANTEPARTUM MANAGEMENT**

1. Patients with thrombocytopenia (platelet count $<100,000/mm^3$) are admitted to the hospital when symptoms occur or when the platelet count is of concern to the admitting physician. Platelet count **less than 20,000/mm^3 mandates admission.**

2. Consult a **hematologist** regarding a diagnostic bone marrow biopsy and steroid therapy. **Initiate medical treatment according to the patient's clinical status when her platelet count drops below 50,000.**

   a. **Corticosteroids** are the primary treatment modality.[3]

      (1) Administer prednisone in doses of up to **60 to 100 mg/d** or 1 to 1.5 mg/kg/d (higher doses for platelet counts $<10,000$) until a response is evident. Divided doses appear to be more effective than single daily doses or alternate-day therapy.

      (2) A positive response is evidenced by a rise in the platelet count within 3 weeks and a decreasing incidence of new skin lesions.

(3) Gradually **taper the dose after a favorable response.** In those patients not responding within 3 weeks, consider another mode of therapy.

(4) Steroids decrease antiplatelet antibody production, interfere with antiplatelet antibody interaction with the platelet surface (thus increasing the amount of circulating, unbound antiplatelet antibody), decrease clearance of platelets coated with antiplatelet antibody, and improve abnormal capillary fragility.

(5) The circulating antibody concentration correlates inversely with the fetal platelet count; thus corticosteroids increase the risk of fetal thrombocytopenia.

(6) Additional **side effects** include maternal Cushing's syndrome, psychosis, preeclampsia, fetal adrenal insufficiency, and growth retardation.

b. High-dose **intravenous IgG** (400 mg/kg/d for 5 days) may transiently increase the platelet count. (IV IgG may interfere with the phagocyte Fc receptor–mediated immune clearance, thus allowing an increased number of platelets to circulate in the patient.)

(1) This is second-line therapy[1,5] for those who fail corticosteroid management. IgG is thought to take up to 3 weeks to cross the placenta and positively affect fetal outcome. No evidence of harm exists.

(2) It is hypothesized that IV IgG also blocks the placental Fc receptors for transfer of the antiplatelet antibodies, thus reducing the amount of antibody transferred to the fetus.

(3) After the diagnosis and therapeutic regimen are established and the patient is stable, she may be discharged home. Stress the importance of follow-up platelet counts, avoidance of injections or trauma, and avoidance of using certain drugs (aspirin and nonsteroidal antiinflammatory drugs unless otherwise indicated) to reduce the risk of bleeding.

c. **Splenectomy** is indicated in patients who do not respond to corticosteroids and IV IgG, who have a life-threatening hemorrhage, or who are noncompliant.

(1) A favorable response is usually noted within a few hours after surgery; the optimal response occurs 1 to 3 weeks later.

(2) When the **platelet count rises above 1,000,000/mm³**, acetylsalicylic acid (or a similar product) is recommended to prevent thromboembolism.

d. **Platelet transfusion** may be a temporary lifesaving measure in the presence of hemorrhage. Transfused platelets are destroyed rapidly by antiplatelet antibodies.

e. **Immunosuppressive drugs** (azathioprine, cyclophosphamide, vinca alkaloids) have been administered to patients who do not respond to corticosteroid therapy and splenectomy; however, these medications pose risks to the fetus of intrauterine growth retardation, teratogenicity, and oncogenicity, in addition to adverse maternal side effects. Their use remains experimental.

f. **Plasmapheresis** to remove antiplatelet antibodies may be used as an adjunct to primary treatment or in an emergency when a rapid response is needed.

B. INTRAPARTUM MANAGEMENT

1. Patients in labor are usually not transfused before, during, or after delivery (unless symptomatic).

2. Each unit of platelets is from one donor, representing a **hepatitis C** risk of 3% and an acquired immunodeficiency syndrome (AIDS) risk of 1/250,000. Each unit raises the platelet count by about 10,000/mm^3 in a normal individual; however, in the **ITP** patient the rise may be much less as a result of immune destruction of the transfused platelets.

3. Steroid and intravenous IgG therapy for patients in active labor and with **ITP** is somewhat controversial. **Use of corticosteroids** is usually the primary therapy for patients in active labor.
   a. Proponents state that steroids decrease the incidence and severity of fetal thrombocytopenia.
   b. Opponents state that the opposite effect occurs (see sections IIIA2a[4] and IIIA2a[5]). In patients who continue to bleed despite steroid therapy, IV IgG may be administered.

4. **IV IgG** is transported inconsistently and unpredictably across the placenta. Some studies have suggested that the use of high-dose gamma globulin is safer and more effective than steroids in the treatment of maternal and fetal thrombocytopenia, but experience in pregnancy is limited at this point.

C. DELIVERY MANAGEMENT

1. A maternal platelet count of >50,000/mm^3 at delivery is preferable. Patients with lower counts, especially **<30,000/mm^3, are at high risk for postpartum bleeding complications.** The primary risk of bleeding occurs with lacerations and incisions. **ITP rarely** causes postpartum uterine hemorrhage. Patients with platelet counts of <50,000/mm^3 may be treated either with steroids or with IV IgG.

2. If the patient is taking steroids long term, increase to stress doses (25 mg of Solu-Medrol IV Push or 100 mg of Solu-Cortef IV push).

3. **Neonates with severe ITP may be predisposed to intracranial hemorrhage** if delivered vaginally (with its inherent compression of the fetal cranium). It is important to identify neonates at high risk of thrombocytopenia and to examine their blood for evidence of severe **ITP.**
   a. Mothers with **gestational ITP** who are first diagnosed during pregnancy (incidental and asymptomatic) **are at low risk** of having a fetus with severe neonatal thrombocytopenia.[1,6]
   b. Mothers who carry an antenatal diagnosis of **ITP** but who currently **do not have circulating indirect antiplatelet antibodies** are also at **low risk** of delivering a fetus with severe neonatal thrombocytopenia.
   c. All patients other than those listed previously are candidates for

evaluation of fetal platelet counts.[3,7] Two methods are available, both with inherent risks and benefits. Controversy exists over the need for fetal evaluation. Some advocate that the risk of the procedures is greater than the risk of having a baby damaged by the disease, and thus testing is not justified. If testing is performed, strongly consider cesarean delivery if the fetal platelet count is $<50,000/mm^3$.

(1) **Percutaneous umbilical vein blood sampling**

    (a) Percutaneous umbilical vein blood sampling is the more difficult procedure; however, it is more accurate than fetal scalp blood sampling.

    (b) Schedule the procedure to be performed at 37 to 39 weeks' gestation because it cannot be performed intrapartum.

(2) **Fetal scalp blood sampling.** Drawbacks to the procedure include the following:

    (a) The procedure may not be performed until the cervix is partially dilated and the membranes are ruptured. Intracranial hemorrhage may have occurred before the sampling, although this is considered to be infrequent.

    (b) Significant bleeding may occur from the scalp lesion. Firm pressure usually prevents this.

    (c) If the specimen is contaminated with amniotic fluid, the platelet count may be artificially lowered.

    (d) There is little time to do the procedure and get results.

    (e) Clumping of platelets on the slide commonly occurs, giving erroneous results. If the fetal platelet count is normal on the scalp platelet count, it can be considered reliable; but when the count is $<50,000/mm^3$ at least 50% of the time, it is normal.

d. If a fetal platelet count cannot be determined antenatally in a patient at high risk for fetal thrombocytopenia, consider cesarean delivery.

D. POSTPARTUM MANAGEMENT

1. The intensive medical care initiated antepartum must be continued through the initial postpartum period.

2. Breast milk may contain antiplatelet antibodies; however, these antibodies are destroyed in the infant's intestines and thus are not absorbed in their functional state. Corticosteroids may also be transmitted to the infant through the breast milk.

REFERENCES

1. Samuels P et al: Estimation of the risk of thrombocytopenia in the offspring of pregnant women with presumed immune thrombocytopenic purpura, *N Engl J Med* 323:229-235, 1990.

2. Burrows RF, Kelton JG: Pregnancy in patients with idiopathic thrombocytopenic purpura: assessing the risks for the infant at delivery, *Obstet Gynecol Surv* 48:781-788, 1993.

3. Pillai M: Platelets and pregnancy, *Br J Obstet Gynaecol* 100:201-204, 1993.
4. Sacher RA: ITP in pregnancy and the newborn: introduction, *Blut* 59:124-127, 1989.
5. Fehr J, Hofmann V, Kappeler U: Transient reversal of thrombocytopenia in idiopathic thrombocytopenic purpura by high-dose intravenous gamma globulin, *N Engl J Med* 306(4):1254-1258, 1982.
6. Burrows RF, Kelton JG: Incidentally detected thrombocytopenia in healthy mothers and their infants, *N Engl J Med* 319(3):142-145, 1988.
7. Carolis SD et al: Immune thrombocytopenic purpura and percutaneous umbilical blood sampling: an open question, *Fetal Diagn Ther* 8:154-160, 1993.

SEIZURE DISORDERS

I. BACKGROUND

A. CLASSIFICATION

1. **Generalized**
   a. **Grand mal:** loss of consciousness with symmetric tonic or clonic movements
   b. **Petit mal:** brief lapses of consciousness
2. **Partial:** symptoms of seizures reflect area of brain involvement
3. **Unilateral**
4. **Unclassified**
5. When a seizure disorder occurs during pregnancy, the first cause to consider is **eclampsia.** Treat the patient for eclampsia until this diagnosis is ruled out.

B. INCIDENCE. Seizure disorders, the most common neurologic problems of pregnancy, occur at a rate of 1 in 1000 pregnancies.

1. Of seizures, 75% are idiopathic in cause and 25% are organic.
2. Of women with seizure disorders, 50% will report no change in seizure status during pregnancy.

C. PERINATAL MORBIDITY AND MORTALITY. An increased rate of stillbirths among epileptic women taking anticonvulsant medication has been documented, although the gestational age at which this occurs has not yet been defined. Some researchers have reported a 7% to 10% incidence of low birth weight (less than 2500 g) and a 4% to 11% risk of prematurity.[1-3] Stillbirth and neonatal and perinatal death rates are elevated (double the incidence in the general population).[2,4]

D. MATERNAL MORBIDITY AND MORTALITY. Maternal morbidity and mortality are the same as in uncomplicated pregnancies.[5]

II. EVALUATION

A. HISTORY. Did attacks begin in childhood? If the patient has had a recent seizure, did anyone witness the attack? **Is she currently taking anticonvulsant medications?** Did tongue biting, urinary or fecal incontinence, or a postictal period occur? Is there any history of drug abuse, drug withdrawal, or trauma?

B. PHYSICAL EXAMINATION. In the patient with recent seizures, pay particular attention to blood pressure (BP), skin (for evidence of trauma), tongue (for evidence of tongue biting during seizure), and the neurologic examination (i.e., deep tendon reflexes).

C. DIAGNOSTIC DATA

1. If the patient has had a recent seizure, do the following:
   a. Obtain serum glucose, calcium (Ca^{2+}), magnesium (Mg^{2+}), electrolyte panel, and arterial blood gas levels.
   b. Obtain a medication level if she has been taking anticonvulsants.

2. Exclude the diagnosis of eclampsia before initiating anticonvulsant treatment.

III. THERAPEUTIC MANAGEMENT

A. ANTICONVULSANT MEDICATION

1. If a change in the patient's anticonvulsant medication is needed, consider consultation with a neurologist.
2. **Phenobarbital** is the drug of choice for a noneclamptic seizure disorder in pregnancy. The average dose of phenobarbital is 100 mg two or three times a day, and the therapeutic level is 10 to 20 μg/ml. Measure the patient's blood phenobarbital level after she has been taking the medication for 2 weeks.
3. **Phenytoin sodium** (Dilantin) is also used frequently during pregnancy. The average dose is 400 mg/d in a single or divided dose. Up to 1200 mg/d may be required to maintain a therapeutic blood plasma level of 10 to 20 μg/ml. (See Chapter 18, section IIIB1b3 for further details on evaluating phenytoin levels.)[6]
4. Monitor **plasma drug levels** carefully.
   a. Anticonvulsant levels require monthly monitoring and adjustment of drug dosages as indicated.
   b. Subtherapeutic plasma drug levels in patients taking phenytoin may result from decreased drug absorption and an alternate metabolic pathway.
   c. If seizures continue despite therapeutic medication levels when only one drug (i.e., phenobarbital) is being prescribed, a second drug may be needed.
   d. Anticonvulsant drugs taken during the first trimester double the infant's risk of a **major congenital malformation** (cleft lip, cleft palate, congenital heart disease); however, seizures pose a more serious risk to the mother and the fetus than do anticonvulsant drugs. All medications appear to increase the risk of mental retardation. Some have specific teratogenic effects:
      (1) **Phenytoin** may cause fetal hydantoin syndrome, which consists of craniofacial and limb abnormalities.[7,8]
      (2) **Carbamazepine** (Tegretol) may cause craniofacial defects and fingernail hypoplasia, as well as a 9% incidence of spina bifida.[9]
      (3) **Valproic acid** (Depakene) may result in fetal neural tube defects (15% incidence).[9] Other malformations, such as meningomyelocele and anomalies of the cardiovascular, urogenital, skeletal, and craniofacial regions, have also been documented.[10]
      (4) **Trimethadione** is associated with a high prevalence of mental retardation, growth retardation, and severe birth defects and is thus considered absolutely contraindicated in pregnancy.[11,12]
   e. Patients taking carbamazepine or valproic acid are candidates for prenatal evaluation to rule out neural tube defects. Consider obtaining either of the following:

(1) Maternal serum α-fetoprotein (AFP) and a targeted ultrasound

(2) Amniocentesis for AFP and a targeted ultrasound

B. ANTEPARTUM SURVEILLANCE

1. Ultrasound evaluation

a. Perform an initial scan and fetal echocardiography at 18 to 20 weeks' gestation to rule out anomalies.

b. Assess fetal growth through serial scans starting at 26 to 28 weeks' gestation.

2. Start **antepartum testing** at 34 weeks' gestation unless other factors demonstrate an indication for earlier testing.

3. Advise maternal ingestion of **folate,** 1 mg/d.

4. Consider initiating **vitamin K** supplementation (10 mg IM weekly) starting at 34 weeks' gestation to prevent neonatal coagulopathy (see also section IIIF).[13]

C. MANAGEMENT OF GENERALIZED (TONIC-CLONIC) STATUS EPILEPTICUS IN PREGNANCY (not including eclamptic seizures)[14]

1. Insert an **intravenous** line.

2. Draw blood for ethyl alcohol (ETOH) and anticonvulsant drug levels, glucose, blood urea nitrogen (BUN), electrolytes, serum Ca^{2+}, Mg^{2+}, and CBC with differential.

3. Draw an arterial blood sample for **arterial blood gases;** then start oxygen at a high flow rate (8 L/min) by nasal cannula or face mask.

4. Send a urine sample for a **drug screen** (see Appendix R).

5. Perform an **electrocardiogram (ECG).**

6. Start an IV infusion of normal saline (NS) with B complex. Administer a bolus of 50 ml of 50% glucose, 100 mg thiamine IM.

7. Infuse **diazepam** IV no faster than 5 mg/min until seizures stop (to 40-mg total dose). The duration of diazepam efficacy is only 15 to 20 minutes, and therefore it is used to abort prolonged episodes and to prevent recurrent convulsions while therapeutic brain concentrations of long-acting anticonvulsants are being achieved (Table 9-1).

8. Initiate **phenytoin** IV

a. Infuse no faster than 50 mg/min, to a total of 18 mg/kg of body weight (Table 9-2).

TABLE 9-1

EXAMPLE OF EMERGENCY TREATMENT WITH DIAZEPAM FOR A 60-kg PREGNANT PATIENT IN STATUS EPILEPTICUS

1. Push diazepam **10 mg IV** over **2 min.**
2. If seizures persist, push an additional 10 mg over 2 min.
3. If the patient still does not respond, an additional 20 mg may be used. This provides a **total dose of 40 mg.**
4. **If delivery is imminent,** alert the **pediatrician** (who will be present at the delivery) of the recent diazepam administration—**the infant** will probably be born **depressed** (diazepam has a long half-life).

TABLE 9-2

EXAMPLE OF EMERGENCY TREATMENT WITH PHENYTOIN FOR A 60-kg
PREGNANT PATIENT

1. Push **1 g IV** over **20 min.**
2. Observe for transient hypotension and heart block.

---

    b. If hypotension develops, slow the infusion rate.

    c. Phenytoin, 50 mg/ml in propylene glycol, may be placed in a
       100-ml volume-control set and diluted with NS. Watch the rate of
       infusion carefully.

    d. Alternatively, phenytoin may be injected slowly by IV push (IVP).

    e. Watch for ECG changes:
       (1) Atrial and ventricular conduction depression
       (2) Ventricular fibrillation

  9. If seizures persist, an **IV phenobarbital drip** may be initiated.

    a. Insert an endotracheal tube at this time.

    b. Continue to monitor vital signs.

    c. Administer **phenobarbital,** 20 mg/kg maximum, no faster than
       100 mg/min, until seizures stop or until a loading dose of
       20 mg/kg is given.

10. If seizures continue, institute general anesthesia with **halothane** and
    a neuromuscular junction blocker. If an anesthesiologist is not imme-
    diately available, give 50 to 100 mg of **lidocaine** by IVP, slowly.

    a. If lidocaine is effective, administer an IV drip of 50 to 100 mg di-
       luted in 250 ml of 5% dextrose in water (D_5W) at 1 to 2 mg/min.

    b. If lidocaine has not stopped the seizures within 20 minutes from
       the start of the infusion, administer general anesthesia with
       halothane and a neuromuscular-junction blocker. Continue to mon-
       itor vital signs.

D. MANAGEMENT IN LABOR

1. Patients taking phenobarbital or phenytoin should receive these drugs
    parenterally. The usual dosages for patients with therapeutic levels are
    as follows:

    a. **Phenobarbital,** 60 mg IM or IVP (slow) every 6 to 8 hours

    b. **Dilantin,** 100 mg IVP every 6 to 8 hours (Mix only with NS [will
       precipitate in dextrose].)

2. Monitor drug levels if labor is prolonged.

3. Consider administering vitamin K, 10 mg IM.

E. MANAGEMENT POSTPARTUM. Monitor drug levels frequently when
    the patient is postpartum because of the rapid physiologic changes
    occurring at this time.

F. MANAGEMENT OF THE NEONATE

1. Background

    a. Neonates born to mothers receiving anticonvulsant therapy (espe-
       cially barbiturates and phenytoin) are at increased risk of developing

clinical or subclinical coagulopathy, even in the absence of coagulopathy in their mothers.

b. Factors II, VII, IX, and X values are decreased and factors V and VIII values are normal in affected infants (similar to the abnormality produced by a vitamin K deficiency).

2. Recommendations

a. Consider prophylactic administration of vitamin K to the infant after birth.[1,3,4,13]

b. Measure the prothrombin time (PT) of the cord blood at the time of delivery. If the PT is abnormally low (or clinical evidence of a coagulopathy is present), treat the infant with fresh frozen plasma and IM vitamin K.

REFERENCES

1. Eller DP, Patterson CA, Webb GW: Prescribing in pregnancy: maternal and fetal implications of anticonvulsive therapy during pregnancy, *Obstet Gynecol Clin North Am* 24(3):523-534, 1997.
2. Nelson KB, Ellenberg JH: Maternal seizure disorder outcomes of pregnancy and neurologic abnormalities in children, *Neurology* 32:1247-1254, 1982.
3. Swartjes JM, Van Geijn HP: Pregnancy and epilepsy, *Eur J Obstet Gynecol Reprod Biol* 79:3-11, 1998.
4. Chang S, McAuley JW: The annals of pharmacotherapy: pharmacotherapeutic issues for women of childbearing age with epilepsy, *Ann Pharmacother* 32:794-801, July/Aug 1998.
5. Hiilesmaa VK, Bardy AH, Teramo K: Obstetric outcome in women with epilepsy, *Am J Obstet Gynecol* 152:499-504, 1985.
6. Kochenour NK, Maurice GE, Sawchuk RJ: Phenytoin metabolism in pregnancy, *Obstet Gynecol* 56.577, 1980.
7. Loughnan PM, Gold H, Vance JC: Phenytoin teratogenicity in man, *Lancet* 1:70-72, 1973.
8. Hanson JW, Smith DW: The fetal hydantoin syndrome, *J Pediatr* 87:285-290, 1975.
9. Rosa FW: Spina bifida in infants of women treated with carbamazepine during pregnancy, *N Engl J Med* 324:174-177, 1991.
10. Delgado-Escueta AV, Janz D: Consensus guidelines: preconception counseling, management, and care of the pregnant woman with epilepsy, *Neurology* 42(suppl 5):149-160, 1992.
11. Malone FD, D'Alton ME: Drugs in pregnancy: anticonvulsants, *Semin Perinatol* 21(2):114-123, 1997.
12. Zackai E et al: The fetal trimethadione syndrome, *J Pediatr* 87:280-284, 1975.
13. Yerby MS: Contraception, pregnancy and lactation in women with epilepsy, *Baillieres Clin Neurol* 5(4):887-908, 1996.
14. Roth HL, Drislane FW: Seizures, *Neurol Clin North Am* 16(2):257-284, 1998.

URINARY TRACT INFECTIONS

I. BACKGROUND
A. DEFINITIONS
1. **Asymptomatic bacteriuria (ASB)** is the presence of bacteria in amounts $>10^5$/ml of urine in a patient who is asymptomatic for a urinary tract infection.
   a. **Incidence.** Of women, 2% to 8% have an ASB. This is not increased during pregnancy.
   b. Of pregnant patients with ASB, 20% to 40% will develop acute pyelonephritis if the ASB is not treated.[1,2]
2. **Cystitis** is significant bacteriuria accompanied by urinary urgency, polyuria, and dysuria, without fever or costovertebral angle tenderness.
3. **Pyelonephritis** is the presence of significant bacteriuria in the upper urinary tract, often with symptoms of chills, fever, and sometimes lower urinary tract infection.
   a. **Incidence**
      (1) Pyelonephritis occurs in 1% to 2% of pregnant women.
      (2) Pyelonephritis may be prevented in 60% to 70% of patients by screening for ASB and rendering appropriate treatment.
      (3) Pyelonephritis develops more frequently from an ASB during pregnancy because of urinary stasis in the renal pelvis, which dilates in response to the elevated progesterone during pregnancy or from pressure on the ureters from the gravid uterus.
   b. The **pathogen** is *Escherichia coli* in 85% of patients, whereas the remaining infections are caused by *Klebsiella, Proteus,* enterococcus, staphylococcus, and group D streptococci.
   c. Pyelonephritis is right sided in 85% of patients and left sided in 15%.

II. EVALUATION OF PATIENTS WITH PYELONEPHRITIS
A. **HISTORY.** The patient may complain of dysuria, urinary frequency, back pain, chills, fever, nausea, vomiting, or uterine contractions. Rule out preterm labor in these patients.
B. **PHYSICAL EXAMINATION.** Perform a thorough physical examination. Pay particular attention to the patient's temperature curve and other vital signs, costovertebral angle tenderness, and abdominal examination. (Are uterine contractions appreciated? Is her uterus tender?)
C. **DIAGNOSTIC DATA**
1. Obtain the following:
   a. **Urinalysis** with **culture and sensitivity** (C&S) and Gram's stain of unspun urine. If these studies were previously sent from the office,

the results may be ready for evaluation at the time the patient presents to labor and delivery for evaluation.

    b. **Complete blood cell count (CBC) with differential**

2. Review the patient's prenatal laboratory tests for a previous ASB with a documented C&S to guide current therapy.

D. DIFFERENTIAL DIAGNOSIS. Appendicitis, ruptured ovarian cyst, and cholecystitis. (See Chapter 3 for an evaluation of abdominal pain in pregnancy.)

III. THERAPEUTIC MANAGEMENT OF PATIENTS WITH PYELONEPHRITIS

A. Obtain a catheterized urine sample before treatment is initiated. Do not allow the urine to sit at room temperature. Place the specimen on ice if transport is delayed. Note on the laboratory slip the date and time that the specimen was obtained.

B. If uterine contractions are present, initiate antibiotic treatment promptly and avoid use of tocolytics unless cervical change is documented. The endotoxins released from gram-negative bacteria may stimulate the production of cytokines and prostaglandins and thus cause uterine contractility.[3] Adult respiratory distress syndrome (ARDS) may occur during pyelonephritis[4] and is more frequent with concurrent use of tocolytics.[5]

C. Antibiotic therapy varies according to the specific sensitivity of the causative organisms at your facility and according to the patient's clinical status. The following are detailed suggestions for initiating treatment:

1. The patient who appears hemodynamically stable may be started on cephapirin sodium **(Cefadyl),** 2 g IV piggyback every 6 hours, or **ampicillin,** 2 g IV piggyback every 4 hours.

2. For the patient who appears toxic (high fever, chills, tachycardia), initiate therapy with **ampicillin** (for gram-positive coverage) and **gentamicin** (for gram-negative coverage).

3. Blood cultures rarely add anything to the ability to manage patients because of the following[6]:

    a. The organism can usually be identified by urine culture.

    b. Patients with positive blood cultures have the same outcome as patients with negative blood cultures.

4. Consider obtaining a blood culture in patients with an unexplained heart murmur or risk factors or signs of subacute bacterial endocarditis.[6]

5. After a few days when the patient's condition has stabilized, she is afebrile, and her urine C&S results are obtained, consider discontinuing one of the antibiotics.

D. If results of the C&S warrant or if the patient has not responded to therapy within 48 hours, consider changing antibiotics.

E. Continue intravenous (IV) antibiotics for up to **5 days** or until she is **afebrile for 48 hours,** whichever occurs first. An oral antibiotic may then be initiated to complete a 10-day course. Commonly used oral antibiotics include the following:

1. Cefaclor (Ceclor), 500 mg every 6 hours
2. Nitrofurantoin, 100 mg every 6 hours
3. Ampicillin, 500 mg every 6 hours
4. Others per sensitivity studies

F. If at 72 to 96 hours the patient is still febrile, **a ureteral obstruction** may be present. Obtain a renal ultrasound evaluation to look for renal stones and anomalies (an increased dilation of the calyceal system is noted during antepartum pyelonephritis—this inconsistently resolves after treatment).[6] If a distal ureteral stone cannot be ruled out, obtain a single-shot IV pyelogram.

G. To ensure **adequate hydration,** encourage a large fluid intake (3 to 4 L/d minimum).

H. Place the patient in **semi-Fowler's position** on the side opposite the affected kidney.

I. Obtain a **catheterized urine specimen** for analysis, Gram's stain, and C&S **48 hours after admission.** Before discharge, the patient must have at least a negative Gram's stain, with culture pending, although negative culture results are preferable.

J. Reevaluate the patient in the office within 1 week.

K. If the patient has a **second course of pyelonephritis** during this pregnancy, place her on **antibiotic suppression** (e.g., daily oral nitrofurantoin, 100 mg) after completing a full antibiotic treatment course.[7] Continue the antibiotic suppression until 6 weeks after delivery.

L. Consider obtaining an IV pyelogram **6 weeks after delivery** if the patient had either left-sided pyelonephritis or more than one episode of pyelonephritis
during her pregnancy.

M. Urine cultures should be obtained monthly on all patients with an episode of antepartum pyelonephritis.

10

URINARY TRACT INFECTIONS

REFERENCES

1. American College of Obstetricians and Gynecologists: *Antimicrobial therapy for obstetric patients.* Tech Bull No. 117, Washington, DC, 1988, The College.
2. Romero R et al: Meta-analysis of the relationship between asymptomatic bacteriuria and preterm delivery/low birth weight, *Obstet Gynecol* 73(4):576-582, 1989.
3. Graham JM et al: Uterine contractions after antibiotic therapy for pyelonephritis in pregnancy, *Am J Obstet Gynecol* 168(2):577-580, 1993.
4. Pruett K, Faro S: Pyelonephritis associated with respiratory distress. Part 2, *Obstet Gynecol* 69(3):444-446, 1987.
5. Towers CV et al: Pulmonary injury associated with antepartum pyelonephritis: can patients at risk be identified? *Am J Obstet Gynecol* 164(4):974-980, 1991.
6. Twickler D et al: Renal pelvicalyceal dilation in antepartum pyelonephritis: ultrasonographic findings. Part 1, *Am J Obstet Gynecol* 165(4):1115-1119, 1991.
7. Sandberg T, Brorson JE: Efficacy of long-term antimicrobial prophylaxis after acute pyelonephritis in pregnancy, *Scand J Infect Dis* 23:221-223, 1991.

PART III

Obstetric Complications

HYPEREMESIS GRAVIDARUM

I. BACKGROUND

A. DEFINITION. *Hyperemesis gravidarum* is persistent vomiting unresponsive to outpatient therapy and severe enough to cause acetonuria, dehydration, electrolyte imbalances, or weight loss (or all of these) in the first trimester of pregnancy.

B. INCIDENCE. Hyperemesis gravidarum occurs in 3.5 of 1000 pregnancies.

C. ETIOLOGY

1. Elevated estradiol and human chorionic gonadotropin levels are most likely related to the cause of hyperemesis gravidarum. Various studies have demonstrated higher estradiol levels in women who are nulliparous, heavyset, or in the first trimester of their first pregnancy. Cigarette smoking has been shown to decrease estrogen levels. Human chorionic gonadotropin level is known to be elevated in patients with multiple gestations.

2. The profile of patients with hyperemesis gravidarum includes those who are younger, nulliparous, or heavyset or who have multiple gestations. In addition, patients with hyperemesis gravidarum are less likely to smoke cigarettes and are more likely to be better educated than those who do not have any form of emesis resulting from pregnancy.

D. DIFFERENTIAL DIAGNOSIS. Pancreatitis, hepatitis, cholelithiasis, cholecystitis, peptic ulcer, pneumonia, hyperthyroidism, intestinal or ovarian torsion, volvulus, appendicitis, diabetes mellitus, and brain tumors.

E. PERINATAL MORBIDITY AND MORTALITY

1. Both hyperemesis gravidarum and the less severe nausea and vomiting during pregnancy are associated with good pregnancy outcomes and low spontaneous abortion rates.

2. Antiemetics do not appear to be teratogenic.

3. Patients with true hyperemesis gravidarum with weight loss and electrolyte disturbances have demonstrated a statistically significant increase in intrauterine growth retardation; thus these fetuses should be monitored carefully for appropriate weight gain.[1]

F. MATERNAL MORBIDITY AND MORTALITY. The primary morbidity caused by hyperemesis gravidarum is the need for recurrent hospitalizations. Transient hyperthyroidism[2] may develop, and, although rare, hyperparathyroidism, liver dysfunction,[3] or Wernicke's encephalopathy may develop.[4] Otherwise, maternal morbidity and mortality are unchanged from those of uncomplicated pregnancies.

11

II. EVALUATION

A. HISTORY. Quantify the amount of vomiting and its temporal relation to meals, physical activity, illness, stress, and emotional trauma (desire for pregnancy, response to pregnancy, and support of the patient's husband or partner).

B. PHYSICAL EXAMINATION. A thorough physical examination must be performed to rule out other causes of nausea in pregnancy.

1. Inspect the skin for turgor, the tongue for furrowing, the thyroid gland for enlargement and nodularity, the lungs for evidence of infection, and the abdomen for evidence of peritoneal irritation.

2. If pain or tenderness is present, evaluate its location, radiation, and severity. Gastrointestinal disorders present differently during pregnancy. (See Chapter 3 for further details on evaluating abdominal pain in pregnancy.)

3. Observe the vomitus for color, amount, and consistency. (Is it true vomitus or saliva?)

C. DIAGNOSTIC DATA. Obtain a blood glucose, electrolyte panel, amylase or diastase, complete blood cell count with differential, urinalysis to look for ketones (if present, obtain a serum acetone test) and specific gravity (to evaluate overall fluid status), and a stool Hemoccult.

III. THERAPEUTIC MANAGEMENT

A. OUTPATIENT

1. For patients with mild symptoms and who are not experiencing significant starvation and dehydration, follow instructions in Table 11-1.

2. Patients with **moderate** symptoms, or those who were previously instructed to follow the recommendations in Table 11-1 but now return with persistent symptoms, may be treated pharmacologically.

   a. **IV hydration,** if indicated.

   b. **Antihistamines** such as **promethazine** (Phenergan, category C), 25 mg PO every 4 to 6 hours, and **doxylamine succinate** (Decapryn, Unisom, category B), 25 mg PO at bedtime and in the morning as needed may be prescribed with or without **vitamin B_6,**

TABLE 11-1

DIETARY INSTRUCTIONS FOR PATIENT WITH HYPEREMESIS GRAVIDARUM

Keep a supply of crackers at the bedside, and eat a few of these upon awakening in the morning, before getting out of bed.

Eat approximately six small high-protein meals a day.

Ice chips and liquids (including weak teas and colas) may be taken between meals, but minimize fluid intake with meals.

Avoid substances irritating to the intestinal tract.

Adhere to the preceding recommendations as closely as possible for resolution of nausea.

10 to 50 mg PO daily.[5] Inform the patient that drowsiness may be a side effect of antihistamines.

3. Patients with **persistent symptoms** despite treatment detailed above may be hydrated intravenously (establish an IV line) and prescribed any one of the following three medications:

   a. **Phenothiazines** (dopamine antagonists)

      (1) **Prochlorperazine** (Compazine, category C), 10 mg IM or PO or a 25-mg rectal suppository every 8 hours as needed.

      (2) **Metoclopramide** (Reglan, category B), 10 mg PO after every other meal (for patients adhering to six small meals a day) and at bedtime or as needed.

      (3) Side effects of both these medications include extrapyramidal symptoms (EPS) and primarily dystonic and akathisic reactions.

   b. **Diphenhydramine** (Benadryl, category C), 25 to 50 mg PO every 8 hours, may be used alone or in conjunction with the phenothiazines and may prevent EPS.

B. INPATIENT. Hospitalization is indicated when outpatient management fails or when significant dehydration or electrolyte imbalance exists.

1. Obtain blood and urine samples for any testing not yet run for analysis, as discussed in section IIC above.

2. Establish an intravenous line.

3. Hydrate with a minimum of 1 L of IV crystalloid (such as lactated Ringer's to which specific electrolytes may be added); often 2 L of fluids are required on admittance to hospital to correct electrolyte imbalances.

4. Provide antiemetics (for the obvious as well as sedation), such as:

   a. **Diphenhydramine (Benadryl),** 50 mg every 8 hours PO, IM, or IV. Decrease to 25 mg every 6 hours as indicated by the patient's sedation level. May be used **alone** or **with** any **one** of the following to prevent EPS caused by them:

      (1) **Prochlorperazine,** 10 mg IM or 25-mg suppositories every 6 hours *or*

      (2) **Hydroxyzine pamoate** (Vistaril, category C), 50 mg IM or PO, may be used every 4 hours *or*

      (3) **Droperidol** (Inapsine, category C), a butyrophenone (dopamine antagonist), is more potent than the phenothiazines and has fewer cardiovascular, respiratory, and EPS side effects. It may be administered as follows:

         (a) 2.5 mg IM or IV every 6 hours

         (b) A **continuous infusion** of 25 mg in 500 ml of D_5W (5% dextrose in water) (0.05 mg/ml). Run in a 2.5-mg bolus; then set at 1 mg (20 ml)/h.

   b. **On recovery,** IV antiemetics may be discontinued and oral therapy initiated. **Oral metoclopramide** (10 mg) and **hydroxyzine pamoate** (50 mg) are to be used concurrently, with administration of each one-half hour before every other meal (if the patient is eating six small meals a day) and at bedtime (for a total of four doses of each medication daily). Discontinue droperidol at least 60 minutes before initiating oral antiemetic therapy.

5. Bed rest with privacy is desirable, with dietary restrictions until the patient recovers (usually 24 hours).

6. When nausea resolves, initiate a diet with small frequent meals, as detailed in Table 11-1. Consultation with a dietitian is recommended.

7. If the patient is unable to tolerate any amount of oral intake for several days, **hyperalimentation** may avoid the need for prolonged recurrent hospitalization.

8. A **team approach** to the patient's care is recommended, with involvement of nursing personnel experienced in the care of patients with hyperemesis as well as involvement of dietary and social service personnel. On discharge from the hospital, initiate telephone contact with the patient (at least once before her next office visit) for positive reassurance and encouragement of adherence to the dietary guidelines.

9. The patient is to return to the office within 1 week from discharge. Often a follow-up phone call each of the first few days after discharge can help her transition and prevent rehospitalization.

ACKNOWLEDGMENT

Droperidol administration instructions courtesy of Gerald G. Briggs, B.Pharm., Long Beach Memorial Medical Center, Long Beach, Calif.

REFERENCES

1. Gross S, Librach C, Cecutti A: Maternal weight loss associated with hyperemesis gravidarum: a predictor of fetal outcome, *Am J Obstet Gynecol* 160:906-909, 1989.
2. Goodwin TM, Montoro M, Mestman JH: Transient hyperthyroidism and hyperemesis gravidarum: clinical aspects, *Am J Obstet Gynecol* 167(3):648-652, 1992.
3. Abell TL, Riely CA: Hyperemesis gravidarum, *Gastroenterol Clin North Am* 21(4):835-849, 1992.
4. Bergin PS, Harvey P: Wernicke's encephalopathy and central pontine myelinolysis associated with hyperemesis gravidarum, *BMJ* 350:517-518, 1992.
5. Niebyl JR: Therapeutic drugs in pregnancy: caution is the watchword, *Postgrad Med* 75:165-172, 1984.

INCOMPETENT CERVIX

I. BACKGROUND

A. **DEFINITION.** *Incompetent cervix* is a condition in which the cervix is mechanically inadequate, spontaneously dilating at or beyond 16 weeks' gestation, with a resultant premature pregnancy loss.

B. **INCIDENCE.** Cervical incompetence occurs in 0.05% to 1% of all pregnancies and is responsible for 15% to 20% of second-trimester pregnancy losses.[1]

C. **ETIOLOGY**

1. **Cervical trauma**
   a. Dilation (diagnostic curettage or elective abortion)
   b. Conization
   c. Laceration after a precipitous or operative vaginal delivery
   d. Cervical amputation (archaic treatment for uterine prolapse)

2. **Congenital structure changes**
   a. Associated with uterine anomalies[2]
   b. In utero diethylstilbestrol exposure
   c. Increased cervical muscular composition with resultant decreased inherent cervical resistance

D. **PATHOPHYSIOLOGY.** The region of incompetence is postulated to be the site of cervical resistance,[3] not the cervical isthmus, which is completely distended by 20 weeks' gestation. As the collagen concentration of the cervix declines in proportion to an increase in the muscular content, cervical resistance is lowered and an increase in incompetence is noted.

E. **PERINATAL MORBIDITY AND MORTALITY.** This is related to when a cerclage is placed (prophylactically early in the second trimester, or emergently once dilation occurs). When a cerclage is placed prophylactically, the incidence of preterm deliveries decreases from 40% to 14% and term deliveries increase from 20% to 76%. In emergency cases, perinatal mortality is 42%.[4]

F. **MATERNAL MORBIDITY AND MORTALITY.** Patients undergoing cerclage have a risk of premature rupture of membranes (38%) and chorioamnionitis (6.6%, greatest in those undergoing emergency surgery and those with greater cervical dilation).[5] Cerclage has also rarely been associated with vesicocervical fistula[6] and an increased cesarean delivery rate.[5]

II. ANTENATAL EVALUATION

The following evaluation is for a patient with a prior second-trimester pregnancy loss.

A. **OBSTETRIC HISTORY.** The patient's obstetric history is crucial in diagnosing an incompetent cervix.

1. Inquire whether a **classic** or **nonclassic presentation** for cervical incompetence was present before the spontaneous abortion.

2. The **classic presentation** of a patient with cervical incompetence is a history of one or more spontaneous abortions between 14 and 28 weeks' gestation. In general, the patient has an uneventful pregnancy until the midsecond trimester. At this time, painless cervical effacement and dilation occur, with a watery discharge and bulging of the membranes (creating a vague abdominal or pelvic pressure). Typically, contractions are absent until late in the process. Eventually the membranes rupture, and abortion follows.

3. A **nonclassic presentation** is much more difficult to diagnose accurately. In this case the patient may present with atypical preterm labor. Uterine contractions may be present but occur once every 10 to 15 minutes. The cervix is dilated despite mild uterine activity. In addition, the cervix may appear to fall open despite a gentle examination. Suspicion of cervical incompetence must be high when a patient presents in this manner.

4. Ask the patient about the etiologic factors detailed in section IC1.

B. PHYSICAL EXAMINATION. During the physical examination, inspect the cervix for anomalies and prior trauma.

C. DIAGNOSTIC DATA

1. No objective criteria are available to establish the diagnosis of cervical incompetence in the nonpregnant state. Previously, attempts were made at using hysterosalpingograms and cervical dilators to detect incompetence, but the data were unreliable.

2. More recently, early pregnancy ultrasound has been applied to assist in this diagnosis. Vaginal probe ultrasound may demonstrate widening of the internal cervical os with resultant cervical funneling and cervical shortening, which may not be detected by digital examination.[7,8] The diagnostic value of ultrasound in nonclassic cervical incompetence has been limited.

III. SECOND-TRIMESTER EVALUATION ON PRESENTATION TO EMERGENCY ROOM

A. HISTORY. Inquire about the patient's symptoms.

1. Was her pregnancy uneventful until this time? Has she had any known recent cervical infections? Has she felt contractions? Have her membranes ruptured?

2. Does she have any risk factors (cervical trauma, congenital etiology [listed previously], or a previous episode of a second-trimester loss thought to result from cervical incompetence)?

B. PHYSICAL EXAMINATION. Perform a thorough physical examination. Evaluate the cervix for dilation and effacement. It is difficult to inspect the cervix for anomalies and prior trauma at this time.

C. DIAGNOSTIC DATA

1. Monitor the uterus for contractions.

2. If contractions are present, rule out preterm labor.

IV. THERAPEUTIC MANAGEMENT

Surgery is the primary treatment for an incompetent cervix (Table 12-1).

A. **In a nonpregnant woman** with a strong history of an incompetent cervix, search for an anatomic defect during the **physical examination.** If a substantial defect is present, consider a primary repair (e.g., Lash procedure or cerclage at the uterosacral-cardinal ligaments, as indicated). If no anatomic abnormality is present, prophylactically place a cerclage at 14 to 16 weeks' gestation in the patient's next pregnancy. Also consider a hysterosalpingogram or hysteroscopy to rule out a müllerian fusion defect.

B. In a patient presenting for a **routine prenatal examination in the first trimester** with a history suggestive of an incompetent cervix, consider placing a cerclage prophylactically at 14 to 16 weeks' gestation. Weekly cervical examinations may be performed to assess cervical dilation in the first few weeks of the second trimester, before the planned procedure. The McDonald and Shirodkar techniques are the most commonly performed cerclage procedures in this setting.

C. When cervical incompetence is **diagnosed during pregnancy,** do the following:

1. Place the patient in the **Trendelenburg position** (at least 10 degrees). If the membranes have prolapsed into the vagina, Trendelenburg positioning may allow them to recede back into the uterine cavity.

2. Patients ineligible for cerclage placement or those who refuse the procedure have poor pregnancy outcomes. An abortion often occurs imminently.

3. Placement of a **cervical cerclage** is available to patients without the contraindications listed in section IVC3e. Before cerclage it is recommended that a patient be observed for 12 to 24 hours to rule out preterm labor and occult infection.

  a. A McDonald cerclage is the most commonly used surgical procedure for treatment of cervical incompetence during pregnancy.

  b. Before cerclage placement, obtain cervical cultures for gonorrhea and group B β-streptococcus.

  c. Consider amniocentesis before cerclage (some authors report a 25% to 51.5% prevalence of chorioamnionitis in patients with $\geq$2 cm dilation in the second trimester).[9-11] Organisms commonly isolated include *Ureaplasma urealyticum, Gardnerella vaginalis, Mycoplasma hominis, Candida albicans,* and *Fusobacterium* sp. (NOTE: *U. urealyticum* cannot be seen on Gram's stain.) An amniocentesis may also be performed therapeutically to decompress the bulging bag of water.[9,10]

  d. The optimal time to place a cerclage is between 14 and 16 weeks' gestation. If the gestation is more than 20 weeks, the success rate dramatically decreases.

  e. **Contraindications to cervical cerclage**

TABLE 12-1

TREATMENT MODALITIES FOR THE INCOMPETENT CERVIX

Procedure	Indication	Timing	Notes	Complications
Lash	Anatomic defect caused by cervical trauma	Nonpregnant state	Repair of anatomic defect	Infertility (rarely)
Shirodkar	Cervical incompetence	Nonpregnant or 14-16 weeks' gestation	Placement of a 5-mm Mersilene band at level of internal os; bladder is advanced off the cervix	Hemorrhage, cervical dystocia, PROM, chorioamnionitis, placental abscess, uterine rupture, maternal death
McDonald	Useful when lower uterine segment is significantly effaced	Nonpregnant or 14-16 weeks' gestation	Placement of a 5-mm Mersilene band or other permanent suture in a purse-string fashion high on the cervix	Hemorrhage, cervical dystocia, PROM, chorioamnionitis, placental abscess, uterine rupture, maternal death
Uterosacral-cardinal ligament cerclage	Amputated or congenitally short cervix; subacute cervicitis; previous failed Shirodkar or McDonald cerclage	Nonpregnant	Intraabdominal and vaginal procedures are possible; cesarean delivery is mandatory	Hemorrhage, cervical dystocia, PROM, chorioamnionitis, placental abscess, uterine rupture, maternal death
Hefner	Well-developed lower uterine segment with minimal cervix remaining	Late diagnosis of incompetence	Mattress or U sutures	Hemorrhage, cervical dystocia, PROM, chorioamnionitis, placental abscess, uterine rupture, maternal death

PROM, Premature rupture of membrane.

(1) Hyperirritability of the uterus, with bulging membranes
(2) Cervical dilation >4 cm
(3) Fetal malformation or demise
(4) Premature rupture of fetal membranes (PROM)
f. **Complications of emergency cervical cerclage**
   (1) PROM (1% to 9%)
   (2) Chorioamnionitis (1% to 7%): the risk of PROM and chorioam-
       nionitis for an elective cerclage at the beginning of the second
       trimester is less than 1%. The risk increases as the pregnancy
       progresses. When the cervix is dilated more than 3 cm with pro-
       lapsed membranes, a 30% risk of rupture of the membranes or
       chorioamnionitis (or both) is present.
   (3) Preterm labor
   (4) Cervical laceration or amputation: may occur during the proce-
       dure or at delivery. A band of scar tissue may form on the cervix
       at the site of the suture, resulting in either failure to progress or
       a cervical laceration.
   (5) Bladder injury (rare)
g. In addition to the standard **surgical technique** of cerclage placement, consider the following:
   (1) **Spinal conduction anesthesia** (to prevent maternal straining)
   (2) **Filling the bladder** via a Foley catheter with approximately 500
       to 1000 ml of normal saline or sterile water (to assist in elevat-
       ing the membranes off the cervix)[10,12]
   (3) **Antibiotic prophylaxis** of chorioamnionitis (especially for gesta-
       tions beyond 18 weeks) for 2 to 3 days after the cerclage place-
       ment (e.g., ampicillin, 2 g, intravenous piggyback every 6 hours
       for 3 days)[10]
   (4) Administration of **indomethacin** (Indocin), 50 mg (orally or rec-
       tally) before the procedure and 25 mg every 6 hours for one or
       two additional doses after the procedure (to block the
       prostaglandins that will be released during the procedure)
h. **Postoperative care**
   (1) It is important that the patient is at bed rest for 24 hours and is
       observed for increased uterine activity.
   (2) The patient is to have pelvic rest for the remainder of her preg-
       nancy, with limited physical activity and frequent rest periods
       each day.
   (3) If increased uterine activity occurs, consider tocolysis, depending
       on the gestational age of the fetus.
   (4) The patient should be seen in the office weekly.
   (5) Instruct the patient of the early signs and symptoms of
       chorioamnionitis. Have her monitor her temperature each day
       and return immediately to the office or hospital if any signs of
       infection develop.

12

INCOMPETENT CERVIX

(6) Remove the cerclage if she subsequently prematurely ruptures her chorioamniotic membranes.[13]

(7) Remove the cerclage electively at 37 weeks' gestation in the office if her antepartum course has not required earlier removal.

(8) Provide preterm labor education, including precautions.

i. **Success.** It is difficult to define the true success of a cerclage because data concerning the recurrence rate of cervical incompetence are lacking. It is stated that 80% to 90% of pregnancies in which a cerclage is placed have resulted in live, viable births. Eighty-five percent of patients with one previous preterm birth and 70% with two preterm births will deliver at term.

REFERENCES

1. Gabbe SG, Niebyl JR, Simpson JL: *Obstetrics: normal and problem pregnancies,* ed 2, New York, 1991, Churchill Livingstone.

2. Seidman DS et al: The role of cervical cerclage in the management of uterine anomalies, *Surg Gynecol Obstet* 173:384-386, 1991.

3. Jewelewicz R: Incompetent cervix: pathogenesis, diagnosis and treatment, *Semin Perinatol* 15(2):156-161, 1991.

4. Chryssikopoulos DB et al: Cervical incompetence: a 24 year review, *Int J Gynecol Obstet* 26:245-253, 1988.

5. Treadwell MC, Bronsteen RA, Bottoms SF: Prognostic factors and complication rates for cervical cerclage: a review of 482 cases, *Am J Obstet Gynecol* 165(3):555-558, 1991.

6. Golomb J et al: Conservative treatment of a vesicocervical fistula resulting from Shirodkar cervical cerclage, *J Urol* 149:833-834, 1993.

7. McGregor J: Preterm birth, premature rupture of membranes, and cervical incompetence, *Curr Opin Obstet Gynecol* 4:37-42, 1992.

8. Hyricak H et al: Cervical incompetence: preliminary evaluation with MR imaging, *Radiology* 174:821-826, 1990.

9. Romero R et al: Infection and labor. VIII. Microbial invasion of the amniotic cavity in patients with suspected cervical incompetence: prevalence and clinical significance. Part 1, *Am J Obstet Gynecol* 167(4):1086-1091, 1992.

10. Goodlin RC: Surgical treatment of patients with hour glass shaped or ruptured membranes prior to the twenty-fifth week of gestation, *Surg Gynecol Obstet* 165:410-412, 1987.

11. Goodlin RC: Cervical incompetence, hourglass membranes and amniocentesis, *Obstet Gynecol* 54:748-750, 1979.

12. Scheerer LJ et al: A new technique for reduction of prolapsed fetal membranes for emergency cervical cerclage, *Obstet Gynecol* 74:408-410, 1989.

13. Yeast JD, Garite TJ: The role of cervical cerclage in the management of preterm premature rupture of membranes, *Am J Obstet Gynecol* 158:106-110, 1988.

ISOIMMUNIZATION IN PREGNANCY

I. BACKGROUND

A. **DEFINITION.** *Isoimmunization* is the development of maternal antibodies against any fetal blood group antigen that is not possessed by the mother and is inherited from the father or is present during a blood transfusion. The degree of antigenicity and the amount of antibody formed determine the level of reaction against the fetus.

13

1. *Erythroblastosis fetalis (EBF)* is the fetal condition caused by destruction of the fetal red blood cells (RBCs), which results in anemia, jaundice, and an increased amount of erythroblasts in the bloodstream.

2. *Hydrops fetalis* is the severe form of EBF.

B. **PATHOPHYSIOLOGY.** Incompatible RBCs entering the maternal circulation from a previous or current fetus (at the time of delivery or, less often, spontaneously or with obstetric procedures) cause an isoimmunization in the mother. The transmission of these antibodies to the fetus then results in **hemolysis** of the fetal blood cells and results in anemia and hyperbilirubinemia. **Hyperbilirubinemia** is not significant to the fetus at any time because the mother's liver clears the excess bilirubin across the placenta and only becomes significant after birth. The **anemia** can be significant to the fetus, particularly when the results of that anemia include decreased colloid osmotic pressure and high output cardiac failure, both of which can lead to hydrops fetalis. The other contributing pathophysiologic explanation for hydrops fetalis in these fetuses is the **low serum albumin** that results from the extramedullary hematopoiesis in the liver. (This process reduces the liver's ability to produce albumin.)

C. **INCIDENCE.** Anti-D (also known as *Rh*) immunization is the most common cause of EBF in white Americans, African Americans, American Indians, and American Hispanics, with 15%, 5% to 8%, less than 3%, and 5% to 10%, respectively, D negative. Asian races originally were entirely D positive. Indoeurasians have a 2% incidence of D-negative status. A D-negative woman has a 70% chance of producing a D-positive fetus with a known D-positive partner. Of pregnancies in the white and black populations, respectively, 10% and 5% are D incompatible, but sufficient fetomaternal hemorrhage to cause an antibody response occurs in less than 20% of incompatible pregnancies.[1] Because of the widespread use of D immunoglobulin, the incidence of D sensitization is dramatically lower than in previous decades. Other factors are now responsible for an increasing proportion of hemolytic disease in the newborn (Table 13-1).

TABLE 13-1		
ANTIBODIES CAUSING HEMOLYTIC DISEASE IN THE NEWBORN*		
Blood Group System	Antigens Related to Hemolytic Disease	Severity of Hemolytic Disease
CDE	D	Mild to severe
	C	Mild to moderate
	c	Mild to severe
	E	Mild to severe
	e	Mild to moderate
Lewis		Not a proven cause of hemolytic disease of the newborn
I		Not a proven cause of hemolytic disease of the newborn
Kell	K	Mild to severe with hydrops fetalis
	k	Mild to severe
Duffy	Fya	Mild to severe with hydrops fetalis
	Fyb	Not a cause of hemolytic disease of the newborn
Kidd	Jka	Mild to severe
	Jkb	Mild to severe
MNSs	M	Mild to severe
	N	Mild
	S	Mild to severe
	s	Mild to severe
Lutheran	Lua	Mild
	Lub	Mild
Diego	Dia	Mild to severe
	Dib	Mild to severe
Xg	Xga	Mild
P	PP1Pk (Tja)	Mild to severe
Public	Yta	Moderate to severe
	Ytb	Mild
	Lan	Mild
	Ena	Moderate
	Ge	Mild
	Jra	Mild
	Coa	Severe
Private	Coa-b	Mild
	Batty	Mild
	Becker	Mild
	Berrens	Mild
	Evans	Mild
	Gonzale	Mild
	Good	Severe

Continued

TABLE 13-1		
ANTIBODIES CAUSING HEMOLYTIC DISEASE IN THE NEWBORN*—cont'd		
Blood Group System	Antigens Related to Hemolytic Disease	Severity of Hemolytic Disease
Private—cont'd	Heibel	Moderate
	Hunt	Mild
	Jobbins	Mild
	Radin	Moderate
	Rm	Mild
	Ven	Mild
	Wright-a	Severe
	Wright-b	Mild
	Zd	Moderate

From American College of Obstetricians and Gynecologists: *Management of isoimmunization in pregnancy.* Tech Bull No. 148, Washington, DC, 1990, The College.
*Note that conditions listed as being mild can only be treated like ABO incompatibility. Patients with all other conditions should be monitored as if they were sensitized to D.

1. In the CDE (e.g., rhesus) system, after D, the C antigen causes the most severe EBF. The Lewis antibodies are the most frequently encountered antibodies other than D. These are **cold agglutinins,** predominantly **IgM,** and are poorly expressed on fetal erythrocytes and therefore **not** a cause of EBF.
2. **Kell** antibodies may be caused by a prior transfusion and can cause severe fetal hemolytic disease. Ninety percent of men are Kell negative; thus the chance for Kell to cause a reaction in a fetus is unlikely. Less common antigens that can cause EBF include **Duffy, Kidd, MNSs, Lutheran, Diego, Xg, Public,** and **Private.** Atypical antibodies are present in approximately 2% of women,[2,3] but only a small portion of these can trigger fetal hemolytic disease.
3. ABO incompatibilities are present in 20% to 25% of all pregnancies, and this accounts for 60% of cases of newborn hemolytic disease.[4,5] Less than 1% of cases require exchange transfusion.[5] Often moderate anemia and mild to moderate neonatal hyperbilirubinemia are manifest within the first 24 hours after birth. ABO incompatibility most commonly occurs when the mother has blood type O and the infant has A or B.[4] This is likely to recur in subsequent pregnancies.
D. **ETIOLOGY.** Isoimmunization may occur in response to a fetomaternal bleed (in which a sufficient number of fetal erythrocytes enter the maternal circulation) or to a blood transfusion. The amount of fetal blood necessary to immunize the mother is thought to be 0.1 ml, although larger amounts are more likely to be associated with subsequent hemolytic disease.

E. **DIFFERENTIAL DIAGNOSIS.** When fetal hydrops is diagnosed by
ultrasound, it may be a result of erythrocyte antibodies (e.g., D
immunization) or a variety of other causes. When it is not caused by
erythrocyte antibodies, it is called *non*immune hydrops fetalis (NIHF).
The incidence of NIHF is between 1 in 2500 and 1 in 3500 births.[6,7]
NIHF is caused by chromosomal abnormalities in approximately 25%
of patients and by multiple anomalies (often including a cardiac defect)
in 18% of patients.[1] Fetal cardiac arrhythmias (e.g., supraventricular
tachycardia) are also a cause of NIHF. Table 13-2 provides methods of
diagnosis of various causes of NIHF.

F. **PERINATAL MORBIDITY AND MORTALITY.** Fetal hemolytic disease is
usually as, or more, severe in each subsequent pregnancy. Hemolysis
and hydrops usually develop at the same time or earlier in subsequent
pregnancies. Perinatal survival rates in severe D isoimmunization are
now more than 80% because of technologic advancements in
transfusion techniques and neonatal intensive care.[4,5]

G. **MATERNAL MORBIDITY AND MORTALITY** Are not higher than that of
the general pregnant population.

TABLE 13-2

EVALUATION OF NONIMMUNE HYDROPS FETALIS

Test	Possible Diagnosis
Maternal studies	
Complete blood count	α-Thalassemia carrier
Kleihauer-Betke test	Fetomaternal hemorrhage
TORCH screen, RPR	Congenital infections
Medical history	Hereditary diseases, metabolic diseases, infections, medications
Fetal studies (amniocentesis/cordocentesis)	
Karyotype	Chromosomal abnormalities
Hematocrit	Fetal anemia (e.g., from fetomaternal hemorrhage)
Viral cultures	Cytomegalovirus, herpes simplex virus, parvovirus, other viruses
Total plasma IgM	Congenital infections
Hemoglobin electrophoresis	α-Thalassemia
Specific metabolic tests	Metabolic disorders
Fetal sonography	Anomalies, tumors, cardiac arrhythmias

From Gabbe SG, Niebyl JR, Simpson JL: *Obstetrics: normal and problem pregnancies*, ed 2, New York, 1991, Churchill Livingstone.
TORCH, Toxoplasmosis, rubella, cytomegalovirus, and herpes simplex (infection); *RPR*, rapid plasma reagin (test for syphilis); *IgM*, immunoglobulin M.

II. EVALUATION

A. HISTORY

1. An obstetric history of a stillbirth caused by fetal hydrops or a hydropic fetus, with or without stillbirth, indicates a need for immune evaluation. Some women with known Rh-negative status may not have received D immunoglobulin in a previous pregnancy because of the following[8]:
   a. The patient's blood type was not available early in pregnancy when bleeding or a miscarriage occurred.
   b. D immunoglobulin was either not ordered or not given.
   c. An inadequate dosage of D immunoglobulin was given.
   d. The patient refused D immunoglobulin.
   e. The mother's, baby's, or father's blood was mistyped.
   f. Clerical inaccuracies occurred.

2. A positive D^u test signifies that the mother carries a variant of the D antigen and practically is treated as D Rh positive. Likewise, D^u-negative status is equivalent to D Rh negative.

B. EXAMINATION.
The maternal examination is usually unremarkable other than that fundal height is possibly greater than expected for a given gestational age if polyhydramnios (representing early hydrops) is present. Ultrasound evaluation may demonstrate additional signs of EBF (see section IIC4).

C. DIAGNOSTIC DATA

1. A prenatal blood type and antibody screen detects the presence of an antibody that may cause hemolytic disease. Subsequently, the paternal antigen status and zygosity must be determined. (If this cannot be determined, assume the baby is antigen positive.)

2. Patients who are sensitized to antigens other than D that are known to cause moderate to severe hemolytic disease should be managed in a manner similar to that recommended for D isoimmunization. Kell, however, is an exception because amniotic fluid analysis fails to correlate with the degree of fetal anemia. A Kell-sensitized patient requires more aggressive fetal assessment than that detailed in section IIC3-6.

3. **Maternal antibody titers**
   a. Titers <1:16 for anti-D throughout an initial immunized gestation represent a fetus at minimal risk. (If EBF is present, it is usually mild.) Subsequent immunized pregnancies with this titer may be at higher risk. Critical titers for other RBC antibodies are not as well established.
   b. Starting at 16 to 18 weeks' gestation, titers need to be obtained every 2 to 4 weeks. Serum from the previous titer should be preserved and used as a control during subsequent testings to correct for interassay variance. In patients who require amniocentesis, repeat titers are unnecessary.

4. Sonograms are an accurate method of evaluating serious EBF-related fetal deterioration.[9,10] Ultrasonographic changes may not be found in mild, moderately affected fetuses.

a. Patients who have low titers (1:4 or 1:8) may be checked with an occasional ultrasound to ensure a healthy fetus (rarely would hydramnios or hydrops develop).

b. Patients who have higher titers or those who had a previously sensitized pregnancy may be observed with ultrasound in conjunction with amniotic fluid analysis for ΔOD_{450} (optical density at 450 nm) (detailed in section IIC5) to assess fetal status. When the fetus is moderately to severely affected, changes such as polyhydramnios, pericardial effusion, and cardiomegaly can be seen. When severe EBF is present, ultrasound is useful in monitoring the fetal status by evaluating the resolution or progression of various indicators of EBF. The ultrasonic signs of EBF include the following:

   (1) **Placental thickening** to >50 mm in moderate or severe EBF. A homogeneous texture may be present.

   (2) **Polyhydramnios** (amniotic fluid index [AFI] >24 cm) is inconsistently seen with mildly or moderately affected infants. When polyhydramnios is present, it is usually associated with hydrops fetalis and thus a poor prognosis.

   (3) **Pericardial effusion** is one of the earliest markers of EBF.

   (4) **Cardiac size** may increase as a result of congestive heart failure with severe EBF. A heart or thoracic circumference ratio more than 0.5 is considered cardiomegaly.

   (5) **Ascites** indicates severe EBF.

   (6) **Hepatosplenomegaly** occurs as a result of the increased erythropoiesis in an Rh-sensitized fetus.

   (7) Edema of scalp and other skin occurs.

5. Amniotic fluid analysis allows for more detailed assessment of fetal status. Destruction of fetal RBCs leads to a bilirubin by-product. Bilirubin may be excreted by pulmonary tracheal secretions and may diffuse across fetal membranes. In 1961 Liley demonstrated the correlation between amniotic fluid bilirubin concentration and fetal outcome. Amniotic fluid is processed spectrophotometrically so that the observed absorption in optical density at 450 nm (ΔOD_{450}) (Fig. 13-1) is plotted in relation to gestational age on a Liley graph (Fig. 13-2). Meconium and RBCs (or their porphyrin breakdown products) will alter the 450-nm analysis but can be overcome with chloroform extraction of the amniotic fluid. The Liley graph is excellent at depicting degrees of sensitization in gestations past 26 weeks.

6. Before 26 weeks' gestation or D sensitization with a heterozygous father, the physician may want to consider percutaneous umbilical cord blood sampling (PUBS) at the time of the initial study to determine the fetal blood type. Documentation of fetal D-negative status prevents the mother from undergoing further studies. The recent introduction of amniotic fluid analysis of Rh (D) status using polymerase chain reaction (PCR) may soon replace the need for PUBS for fetal Rh typing.

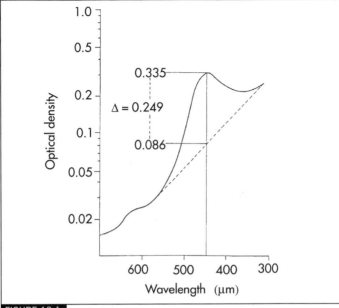

FIGURE 13-1

Spectrophotometric scan of amniotic fluid taken from an Rh-sensitized pregnancy with fetal hydrops. The heavy solid line represents the actual spectrophotometric scan of the bilirubin-containing fluid. The interrupted line illustrates the predicted scan result if fluid bilirubin levels remained constant. The difference between the optical density at the peak of the heavy solid line at 450 nm and the interrupted line at 450 nm is the OD_{450}. *(From Gabbe SG, Niebyl JR, Simpson JL: Obstetrics: normal and problem pregnancies, ed 2, New York, 1991, Churchill Livingstone.)*

III. THERAPEUTIC MANAGEMENT[8]

A. In patients with an uncomplicated obstetric history and an initial titer of 1:16 found after 26 weeks' gestation, the physician performs amniocentesis and charts the ΔOD_{450} of fluid on the Liley graph.

1. Maintenance of ΔOD_{450} in Liley **zone I** is reassuring that the fetus who is either Rh negative or Rh positive has mild hemolytic disease, at worst.

2. A ΔOD_{450} in Liley **mid zone II** distinguishes a fetus at moderate to severe risk. Infants in this category who have documented pulmonary maturity require delivery. For infants in this area of the Liley graph who are <32 weeks' gestation consider accelerating lung maturity (see Appendix M) prior to delivery. Method of delivery for infants in this category is based on the ΔOD_{450} trend, previous obstetric history, antepartum fetal evaluation by biophysical profiles, heart rate testings, pulmonary maturity, and maternal cervical status (Bishop score).

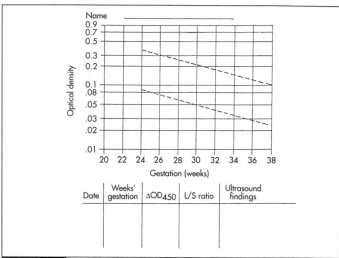

FIGURE 13-2

Liley graph used at the University of Utah Medical Center. *L/S,* Lecithin-sphingomyelin. *(From Gabbe SG, Niebyl JR, Simpson JL: Obstetrics: normal and problem pregnancies, ed 2, New York, 1991, Churchill Livingstone.)*

3. **Upper zone II** ΔOD_{450} values need to be confirmed by PUBS or repeat amniocentesis within 1 week of obtaining this upper zone II result.

4. **Zone III** values or ultrasound-detected hydrops mandates the consideration of intrauterine blood transfusion[11] versus delivery; gestational age, fetal condition, and perinatal or neonatal team preferences determine the treatment plan.

B. Patients with **poor obstetric histories** or with **titers >1:16** before 26 weeks' gestation need an ultrasound evaluation. Strongly consider consulting a perinatologist for patient management. In severely affected infants the physician should consider PUBS to evaluate fetal hematocrit and antigen status, especially if the father is heterozygous for the particular antigen.

1. If **anemia** is detected, transfusion may be performed intravascularly at the time of the initial PUBS. Table 13-3 provides normal second-trimester fetal hematologic values.

2. In the **absence of anemia,** history and ultrasound findings dictate the timing of follow-up diagnostic studies (Fig. 13-3).

C. A **severely anemic** fetus in the second or third trimester is a candidate for an intrauterine transfusion. Because of rapid technological advancements, intraperitoneal transfusions are now primarily performed percutaneously directly into the umbilical cord. Transfusions may be initiated

TABLE 13-3

HEMATOLOGIC VALUES FOR NORMAL FETUSES*

Hematologic Value	Gestational Age (wk)					
	15	16-17	18-20	21-22	23-25	26-30
Hgb (g/dl)	10.9 ± 0.7	12.5 ± 0.8	11.48 ± 0.78	12.29 ± 0.89	12.4 ± 0.77	13.36 ± 1.18
RBC (×10⁹/L)	2.43 ± 0.26	2.68 ± 0.21	2.66 ± 0.29	2.97 ± 0.27	3.06 ± 0.27	3.52 ± 0.32
MCV (±1)	143 ± 8	143 ± 12	133.9 ± 8.83	130 ± 6.17	126.2 ± 6.23	118.2 ± 5.7

From American College of Obstetricians and Gynecologists: *Management of isoimmunization in pregnancy.* Tech Bull No. 148, Washington, DC, 1990, The College.

Hgb, Hemoglobin; *RBC,* red blood cell; *MCV,* mean corpuscular volume.

*Values are for normal fetuses from 15 to 30 wk of estimated gestational age.

13

ISOIMMUNIZATION IN PREGNANCY

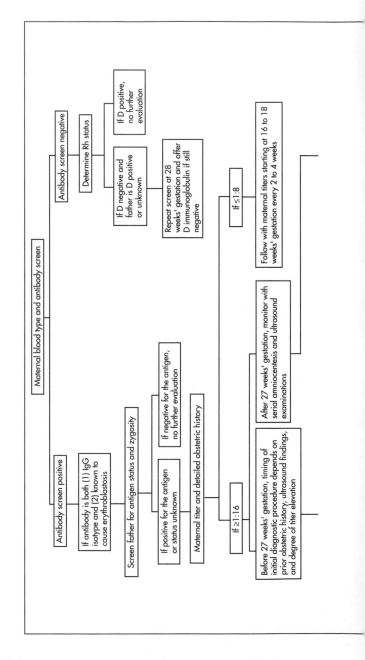

Maternal blood type and antibody screen

Antibody screen positive

If antibody is both (1) IgG isotype and (2) known to cause erythroblastosis

Screen father for antigen status and zygosity

If positive for the antigen or status unknown

If negative for the antigen, no further evaluation

Maternal titer and detailed obstetric history

If ≥1:16

Before 27 weeks' gestation, timing of initial diagnostic procedure depends on prior obstetric history, ultrasound findings, and degree of titer elevation

After 27 weeks' gestation, monitor with serial amniocentesis and ultrasound examinations

If ≤1:8

Follow with maternal titers starting at 16 to 18 weeks' gestation every 2 to 4 weeks

Antibody screen negative

Determine Rh status

If D negative and father is D positive or unknown

If D positive, no further evaluation

Repeat screen at 28 weeks' gestation and offer D immunoglobulin if still negative

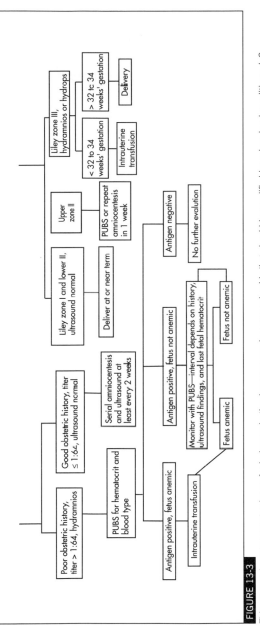

ISOIMMUNIZATION IN PREGNANCY

FIGURE 13-3

This proposed management scheme for isoimmunization in pregnancy is a general guide that should be modified based on local conditions. *IgG,* Immunoglobulin G; *PUBS,* percutaneous umbilical blood sampling. *(From American College of Obstetricians and Gynecologists: Management of isoimmunization in pregnancy. Tech Bull No. 148, Washington, DC, 1990, The College.)*

as early as 18 weeks' gestation. Intravascular transfusion has significantly improved survival rates of all anemic fetuses, especially those severely affected (86.1% perinatal survival rate and 43% were hydropic at initial transfusion).[10]

IV. PREVENTION OF D ISOIMMUNIZATION[8]

A. To reduce the fetal morbidity and mortality of D hemolytic disease, the physician needs to **identify** women at **risk** and must administer D immunoglobulin appropriately.

B. **Prenatal testing** for ABO and rhesus blood type is indicated during each pregnancy. Women who are D negative with a negative antibody screen require a repeat antibody screen at 28 weeks' gestation. Women who have a negative antibody screen at 28 weeks' gestation are appropriate candidates for the administration of D immunoglobulin.

C. **Abortion** (whether induced or spontaneous) and ectopic pregnancy lead to D sensitization in 4% to 5% of susceptible women. A dose of 50 μg of D immunoglobulin is thought to prevent sensitization before 13 weeks' gestation; 300 μg is given for later pregnancies. The immunoglobulin needs to be administered within 72 hours of initial bleeding.

D. **Chorionic villus sampling** may cause fetal-to-maternal bleeding; thus it is recommended that 50 μg of D immunoglobulin be administered at the time of sampling.

E. **Amniocentesis** may result in D sensitization. First- and second-trimester procedures require the administration of 300 μg of D immunoglobulin to D-negative, unsensitized patients (unless they are covered by a previous administration), and then routine antepartum and postpartum prophylaxis is administered. If delivery is planned to follow third-trimester amniocentesis within 48 hours, immunoglobulin may be withheld until after delivery, when the newborn's blood type is analyzed. All other D-negative, unsensitized women undergoing third-trimester amniocentesis need 300 μg of D immunoglobulin. When delivery of an Rh-positive infant occurs within 21 days of administration of D immunoglobulin, the indirect Coombs' test needs to be performed. If the test remains positive, adequate immunoglobulin remains. If the test is negative and if excessive fetal-to-maternal bleeding occurred at delivery, additional immunoglobulin is needed. Occasionally a baby will have a positive direct Coombs' test as a result of Rh immunoglobulin (Ig) transferred transplacentally.

F. **PUBS** in a known D-negative, unsensitized individual requires analysis of fetal blood type. If the blood type is D positive (or cannot be analyzed), administer 300 μg of D immunoglobulin.

G. **Antepartum bleeding** in a D-negative, unsensitized woman necessitates administration of D immunoglobulin. Consider obtaining a Kleihauer-Betke or rosette test to determine the amount of fetal-to-maternal bleeding. If more than 15 ml of fetal cells has entered the maternal circulation, additional D immunoglobulin is needed. Consider obtaining an indirect Coombs' test 72 hours after the administration of immunoglobulin to evaluate the presence of excess D immunoglobulin.

1. A 20-μg dose of D immunoglobulin provides protection against approximately 1 ml of packed D-positive RBCs (300 μg protects against 15 ml of fetal blood cells).

2. Situations in which **testing might be indicated** include the following:

   a. Abruptio placentae

   b. Placenta previa

   c. Intrauterine manipulation (e.g., delivery of twins)

   d. Manual extraction of placenta

H. Delivery is the most common cause of D isoimmunization. When a D-negative, unsensitized woman gives birth to a D-positive or D^u-positive infant, she needs D immunoglobulin to prevent sensitization. In a mother whose only blood type testing occurs at delivery (none antepartum), fetal cells in the mother's blood may produce a false-positive test for the D^u factor; thus these women who test D^u positive may need D immunoglobulin.

I. Transfused blood products should always be matched for D status. The D antigen is restricted to RBC membranes; thus only transfusion of RBCs should theoretically be of concern in a transfusion. However, platelets and granulocytes can theoretically be contaminated with RBCs. If D-positive cells are accidentally transfused, 20 μg of D immunoglobulin is needed to block 1 ml of D-positive packed RBCs.

J. The human immunodeficiency virus (HIV) transmission risk for plasma-derived products such as D immunoglobulin is estimated to be minimal. All plasma has been tested for HIV since 1985, and the fractionation process used in preparing D immunoglobulin removes HIV particles.

13

ISOIMMUNIZATION IN PREGNANCY

REFERENCES

1. Gabbe SG, Niebyl JR, Simpson JL: *Obstetrics: normal and problem pregnancies,* ed 2, New York, 1991, Churchill Livingstone.

2. Queenan JT et al: Irregular antibodies in the obstetric patient, *Obstet Gynecol* 34:767, 1969.

3. Polesky HF: Blood group antibodies in prenatal sera, *Minn Med* 50:601, 1967.

4. Consensus conference on anti-D prophylaxis transfusion, *Royal College of Physicians of Edinburgh, Royal College of Obstetricians and Gynecologists* 38:97-99, 1998.

5. Zipursky A et al: The transplacental passage of fetal red blood cells and the pathogenesis of Rh immunization during pregnancy, *Lancet* 2:489, 1963.

6. Hutchinson AA et al: Nonimmunologic hydrops fetalis: a review of 61 cases, *Obstet Gynecol* 59:347, 1982.

7. Maidman JE et al: Prenatal diagnosis and management of non-immunologic hydrops fetalis, *Obstet Gynecol* 56:571, 1980.

8. American College of Obstetricians and Gynecologists: *Prevention of D isoimmunization,* Washington, DC, 1990, The College.

9. Gurevich P et al: The role of the fetal immune system in the pathogenesis of RhD-hemolytic disease of newborns, *Hum Antibodies Hybridomas* 8(2):76-89, 1997.
10. Chitkara U et al: The role of sonography in assessing severity of fetal anemia in Rh- and Kell-isoimmunized pregnancies. Part 1, *Am J Obstet Gynecol* 71:393-398, 1988.
11. Bowman JM, Manning FA: Intrauterine fetal transfusions: Winnipeg, 1982, *Obstet Gynecol* 61:201, 1983.

GROUP B STREPTOCOCCAL INFECTIONS

I. BACKGROUND

A. **DEFINITION.** Group B streptococcus (GBS) is a common and important cause of life-threatening perinatal infection (early- and late-onset neonatal sepsis, pneumonia, meningitis).[1] Maternal infection may also occur. Maternal and perinatal GBS infections are, in part, preventable.

1. **Early-onset** infection is caused by transmission of GBS from the mother to the fetus and occurs most commonly during parturition. Transplacental transmission occurs but is uncommon. Intraamniotic colonization with GBS may cause intrauterine sepsis in patients with preterm labor or premature rupture of fetal membranes (PROM). This vertical transmission results in early-onset GBS sepsis. Early onset (<7 days) is commonly apparent within 6 hours of birth (but may occur within 24 hours) and represents up to 70% of all neonatal GBS infections. Findings of early-onset neonatal sepsis include respiratory distress, hyperthermia or hypothermia, hypotension, and shock.

2. **Late-onset** GBS sepsis usually results from postnatal acquisition of the bacteria. Late-onset infection is apparent after 7 days of life and represents up to 30% of all neonatal GBS infections (i.e., most commonly meningitis, arthritis, or pneumonia).

B. **INCIDENCE.** Asymptomatic vaginal and rectal GBS colonization is present in 15% to 40% of pregnant women.[2-5] Before the initiation of GBS prevention protocols, data showed that 12,000 neonatal GBS infections occurred each year in the United States; 50% to 70% of these were a result of maternal-baby transmission at delivery, and the remainder were a result of delayed infections subsequent to delivery.[6] Rates are now lower in geographic areas where prevention protocols are widespread.[7]

1. **Early-onset** GBS sepsis will develop in 1/1000 to 3/1000 live-born infants (10/1000 to 30/1000 infants born to mothers carrying GBS when no GBS prevention protocol is used). When risk factors such as PROM, premature delivery, chorioamnionitis, or a previously infected infant are present, 40/1000 infants develop early-onset GBS sepsis when no prevention is undertaken. These numbers decrease by more than 50% in the presence of a prevention protocol.

2. **Late-onset** neonatal infection occurs in 0.5/1000 to 1/1000 live births. This number is not affected by GBS prevention protocols.

C. **ETIOLOGY.** GBS colonization of the maternal rectum, vagina, cervix, or urinary tract accounts for 50% to 70% of neonatal infections (the remainder may be acquired from hospital or community sources). GBS bacteriuria has a prevalence rate of 2.5% in women during their second and third trimesters.[8] Data indicate an infant GBS colonization rate of 87/1000.[7] Infants born to mothers with GBS bacteriuria had 2.54 greater odds of becoming colonized themselves if their mothers had a high versus low GBS colony count.[9] Vaginal colonization may appear intermittently, whereas anorectal carriage is more constant because of higher inocula in the lower gastrointestinal tract. The infant can be infected or colonized while inhaling or swallowing vaginal bacteria. Various toxins are produced by some GBS, causing pulmonary architecture destruction, pulmonary vascular spasm, pulmonary hypertension, myocardial depression, and shock.[8-13]

D. PERINATAL MORBIDITY AND MORTALITY. When GBS prevention is not enacted, infants who weigh >2500 g have a 10/1000 live birth infection rate, with a 20% or less case fatality rate for all (this approaches 90% for very-low-birth-weight infants).[14]

1. Infants born to colonized mothers with risk factors have as high as a 25% chance of developing GBS infection (Table 14-1).[15,16] Infants born to mothers with GBS colonization, but without risk factors, have a 0.5% or less risk of developing infection. Infants with no risk factors for infection account for 33% of infant GBS infections and 10% of GBS mortality.[6]

2. Antepartum screening with selective intrapartum prophylaxis of GBS carriers prevents 48% of neonatal infection.[7,17] Empiric intrapartum treatment reduces GBS neonatal infection by more than 50%.[18] Antiseptic disinfection of the vagina during labor with chlorhexidine has been shown to reduce early neonatal morbidity from GBS.[19]

E. MATERNAL MORBIDITY AND MORTALITY. Includes chorioamnionitis, endomyometritis, bacteremia, and urinary tract infection. Maternal puerperal infection may be in the range of 13/1000 deliveries (95% are cesarean births).[20] Cesarean delivery after initiation of labor or ruptured membranes dramatically increases a woman's risk for postpartum endomyometritis.[20,21] Low levels of serum antibody to capsular antigens of GBS and maternal diabetes are factors for maternal

TABLE 14-1
MATERNAL RISK FACTORS FOR NEONATAL GBS INFECTION

Maternal GBS colonization, in addition to one of the following:
1. Preterm labor (<37 wk)
2. Preterm premature rupture of membranes (<37 wk)
3. Prolonged rupture of membranes (>18 h) at term
4. Multiple gestation
5. Birth of a previous child affected by GBS infection
6. Maternal fever during labor

GBS infection.[22] Chorioamnionitis, endomyometritis, and sepsis risks are decreased with intrapartum chemoprophylaxis.[23]

II. EVALUATION

A. HISTORY. Usually (>2/3) mothers will not experience GBS infection despite fetal involvement.

1. PROM, preterm labor, urinary tract infection resulting from GBS, multiple gestation, and fever in labor may be present. Women with urinary tract GBS colonization are possibly at slightly increased risk of preterm delivery caused by preterm labor and PROM.

2. Patients with clinical chorioamnionitis or postpartum endometritis in a previous pregnancy should be suspected for GBS carriage. Diabetes and multiple gestation may increase the risk of GBS perinatal infection.

B. EXAMINATION. Examination of the mother should be directed in response to her presenting symptoms. Dysuria and frequency indicate a need to rule out cystitis and pyelonephritis (see Chapter 10). Patients with fever before or during labor need to be evaluated for chorioamnionitis (see Chapter 15), and those with preterm labor need an appropriate work-up for various etiologies of preterm labor, including GBS colonization of the cervix, as do patients with preterm PROM (see Chapter 17).

C. DIAGNOSTIC DATA. Culture of the lower vagina, rectum, and urine (as appropriate) is the most sensitive method for detecting GBS. Selective broth media increase culture sensitivities from 50% to 100%.[1] Most laboratories provide Culturettes with a nonselective transport medium (i.e., Amies) to transport swabs to their facility, which might cause false-negative results.[7] Rapid diagnostic tests using latex agglutination or enzyme-linked immunosorbent assay (ELISA) are commercially available and may provide results in less than 1 hour. These rapid antigen ELISA tests are less sensitive and have a higher false-positive rate (>50%) than selective media cultures.[24,25] The rapid antigen tests are most sensitive at identifying heavily colonized patients.[24]

III. THERAPEUTIC MANAGEMENT

A. Patients with GBS chorioamnionitis or a fever of unknown origin during labor require antibiotic therapy (e.g., penicillin G [Na^+ or K^+ salt], 2 million units every 4 hours; or ampicillin, 2 g intravenous piggyback [IVPB], then 1 g every 4 hours[26]; in penicillin-allergic patients, use erythromycin, 500 mg IVPB every 6 hours, or clindamycin, 900 mg IVPB every 8 hours). Prompt delivery is indicated.

B. Cystitis requires a full course of outpatient antibiotic therapy (penicillin VK, 500 mg every 6 hours for 7 days), whereas pyelonephritis requires initial hospital management as detailed in Chapter 10.

C. Preterm labor, if associated with GBS vaginal colonization, requires an initial 48 hours of intravenous antibiotics (see section IIIA for antibiotic and dosing requirements). After 48 hours repeat the culture (while the

14

STREPTOCOCCAL INFECTIONS

patient continues on IV antibiotics) to evaluate for bacterial suppression. When the results return, discontinue treatment if negative. If the culture is positive, continue IV therapy for an additional 5 to 7 days.[7]

D. Postpartum GBS endomyometritis should be treated until the patient is afebrile and free of symptoms for at least 24 hours (i.e., the same treatment as for chorioamnionitis).

IV. PREVENTION

A. Intrapartum chemoprophylaxis for women at high risk of developing maternal or neonatal GBS (women who are colonized or who have unknown genital GBS status) is recommended by the U.S. Centers for Disease Control and Prevention (CDC) and the American College of Obstetricians and Gynecologists.[27]

B. Throughout pregnancy, no one site of genitourinary or intestinal carriage is more predictive than another of perinatal infection. A positive culture site at one time in pregnancy may later become negative and vice versa. Concurrent testing of the lower vagina and rectum late in the second trimester demonstrates a 96% predictive value for GBS colonization at delivery.[1] If more than 5 weeks pass from a previous negative culture, it should be repeated before delivery.

C. Treatment of a GBS urinary infection or asymptomatic bacteriuria (ASB) is indicated at the time of culture. Treatment of GBS urinary tract colonization may reduce the frequency of preterm labor and PROM.[28]

D. It is strongly recommended that all hospitals adopt **a prevention policy.** This policy may be either screening based or risk based.[7]

1. Screening-based prevention policy
   (a) Treat women with any one of the following:
   - Previous GBS-infected infant
   - GBS bacteriuria in current pregnancy
   - Preterm labor
   (b) For all other women, a vaginal or rectal culture is to be obtained between 35 and 37 weeks' gestation. Women with a positive culture are to be treated in labor, as early as possible.

2. Risk-based prevention policy
   (a) No screening cultures are done for GBS.
   (b) Intrapartum antibiotics are given for patients listed in Table 14-1.[29]
   (c) The primary limitation of this policy is that symptomatic colonized women at term are not identified; 30% to 50% of early-onset GBS sepsis occurs in children born to mothers without risk factors.[30]

3. Antibiotic choice
   (a) **Penicillin G** is recommended by the CDC as a physician's first choice because GBS are universally sensitive to penicillin and it has a narrower coverage spectrum.
   (b) **Ampicillin** is recommended as one's second choice. Use of ampicillin for GBS chemoprophylaxis appears to be linked to increasing bacterial ampicillin resistance.[31]

(c) In penicillin-allergic patients who do not have a history of an immediate hypersensitivity, consider using **a cephalosporin** such as **Ancef.**

(d) For those penicillin-allergic patients who it is known will have an immediate hypersensitivity reaction, use **clindamycin** or **erythromycin.** Fifteen percent of GBS cultures are resistant to clindamycin,[32] and 21% are resistant to erythromycin.[33] Thus carefully monitor for sepsis in infants born to GBS-positive mothers treated with these medications.

4. **Initiation of antibiotics** is recommended **on admission** of a **high-risk patient in active labor.** Studies have shown that when a mother with GBS receives her first antibiotic dose more than 4 hours before delivery, infant GBS colonization is 1.2%. When the first dose was administered between 2 and 4 hours before delivery, 2.9% of infants become colonized, and when the interval was within 1 hour before delivery, 46% were colonized.[34]

5. **Elective cesarean** delivery at term before labor and ruptured membranes probably does *not* require chemoprophylaxis of GBS-colonized women. This recommendation is based on a recently completed 10-year prospective study of 3590 elective cesarean deliveries in which approximately 15% (539) of mothers were positive for GBS.[35] No transmission of GBS to infants occurred.

6. Recommendations for care of patients with **preterm labor** and **preterm PROM** may be found in Chapters 17 and 16, respectively. If the initial GBS culture in these patients is negative the likelihood it would become positive in the following 5 weeks is 5%, and thus it is unnecessary to repeat within this time interval. If a patient has a recently obtained negative culture and she subsequently undergoes preterm labor, she does not require chemoprophylaxis.

7. Women with a negative GBS culture late in the third trimester who have prolonged rupture of membranes (ROM) without clinical signs of infection do not require chemoprophylaxis.

8. When a clinical risk factor is present but GBS results are unavailable, give empiric antibiotic chemoprophylaxis.

E. A vaccine for prevention of neonatal GBS sepsis is currently being studied.[36]

14

GROUP B STREPTOCOCCAL INFECTIONS

REFERENCES

1. Committee on Infectious Diseases and Committee on Fetus and Newborn: Prevention of group B streptococcal (GBS) infection disease: a public health perspective, *MMWR Morb Mortal Wkly Rep* 45(RR-7):1-24, 1996.

2. Gardner SE et al: Failure of penicillin to eradicate group B streptococcal colonization in the pregnant woman: a couple study, *Am J Obstet Gynecol* 135:1062-1065, 1979.

3. Anthony BF et al: Genital and intestinal carriage of group B streptococci during pregnancy, *J Infect Dis* 143:761-766, 1981.

4. Allardice JG et al: Perinatal group B streptococcal colonization and infection, *Am J Obstet Gynecol* 142:617-620, 1992.

5. Vaginal Infections and Prematurity Study Group et al: The epidemiology of group B streptococcal colonization in pregnancy, *Obstet Gynecol* 77:604-610, 1991.

6. Katz V: Management of group B streptococcal disease in pregnancy, *Clin Obstet Gynecol* 36(4):832-842, 1993.

7. Hager DW et al: Prevention of perinatal group B streptococcal infection: current controversies, *Clin Commentary* 96(1):141, 2000.

8. Molter M et al: Rupture of fetal membranes and premature delivery associated with group B streptococci in urine of pregnant women, *Lancet* 2:69-70, 1984.

9. Regan JA et al: Colonization with group B streptococci in pregnancy and adverse outcome: VIP Study Group, *Am J Obstet Gynecol* 174:1354-1360, 1996.

10. Katz VL, Bowes WA Jr: Perinatal group B streptococcal infections across intact amniotic membranes, *J Reprod Med* 33:445-449, 1988.

11. Peevy KJ et al: Myocardial dysfunction in group B streptococcal shock, *Pediatr Res* 19:511-513, 1985.

12. Gibson RL, Truog WE, Redding GJ: Hypoxic pulmonary vasoconstriction during and after infusion of group B streptococcus in neonatal piglets, *Am Rev Respir Dis* 137:774-778, 1988.

13. Rubens CE et al: Pathophysiology and histopathology of group B streptococcal sepsis in *Macaca nemestrina* primates induced after intraamniotic inoculation: evidence for bacterial cellular invasion, *J Infect Dis* 164:320-330, 1991.

14. Baker CJ, Edwards MS: Group B streptococcal infections. In Remington J, Klein JO, editors: *Infectious diseases of the fetus and newborn infant,* Philadelphia, 1990, Saunders.

15. Boyer KM, Gotoff SP: Antimicrobial prophylaxis of neonatal group B streptococcal sepsis, *Clin Perinatol* 15:831-850, 1988.

16. Boyer KM, Gotoff SP: Prevention of early-onset neonatal group B streptococcal disease with selective intrapartum chemoprophylaxis, *N Engl J Med* 314:1665-1669, 1986.

17. Mohle-Boetani JC et al: Comparison of prevention strategies for neonatal group B streptococcal infection, *JAMA* 270(12):1442-1447, 1993.

18. Katz VL et al: Group B streptococci: results of a protocol of antepartum screening and intrapartum treatment, *Am J Obstet Gynecol* 170(2):521-525, 1994.

19. Burman LG et al: Prevention of excess neonatal morbidity associated with group B streptococci by vaginal chlorhexidine disinfection during labour, *Lancet* 340(8811):65-69, 1992.

20. Faro S: Group B beta-hemolytic streptococci and puerperal infections, *Am J Obstet Gynecol* 139:686-689, 1981.

21. Minkoff HL et al: Vaginal colonization with group B beta-hemolytic streptococcus as a risk factor for post-cesarean section febrile morbidity, *Am J Obstet Gynecol* 142:992-995, 1982.

22. Baker CJ: Summary of the workshop on perinatal infections due to group B streptococcus, *J Infect Dis* 136:137-152, 1977.

23. Greenspoon JS, Wilcox JG, Kirschbaum TH: Group B streptococcus: the effectiveness of screening and chemoprophylaxis, *Review* 46(8):499-508, 1991.

24. Yancy MK et al: Assessment of rapid identification tests for genital carriage of group B streptococci, *Obstet Gynecol* 80:1038-1047, 1992.

25. Hagay ZJ et al: Evaluation of two rapid tests for detection of maternal endocervical group B streptococcus: enzyme-linked immunosorbent assay and gram stain, *Obstet Gynecol* 82(1):84-87, 1993.

26. Boyer KM, Gotoff SP: Prevention of early-onset neonatal group B streptococcal disease with selective intrapartum chemoprophylaxis, *N Engl J Med* 314:1665, 1985.

27. American College of Obstetricians and Gynecologists: *Group B streptococcal infections in pregnancy.* Tech Bull No. 173, Washington, DC, 1996, The College.

28. Thomsen AC, Morup L, Hansen KB: Antibiotic elimination of group-B streptococci in urine in prevention of preterm labour, *Lancet* 1:591-593, 1987.

29. Yancey MK et al: The accuracy of late antenatal screening cultures in predicting genital group B streptococcal colonization at delivery, *Obstet Gynecol* 88:811-815, 1996.

30. Rosenstein N, Schuchat A: Neonatal GBS Disease Study Group. Opportunities for prevention of perinatal group B streptococcal disease: a multi-state surveillance analysis, *Obstet Gynecol* 90:901-906, 1997.

31. Towers CV et al: Potential consequences of widespread antepartal use of ampicillin, *Am J Obstet Gynecol* 1979(7):879-883, 1998.

32. Pearlman MD, Pierson CL, Faix RG: Frequent resistance of clinical group B streptococci isolates to clindamycin and erythomycin, *Obstet Gynecol* 92:258-261, 1998.

33. Rouse DJ et al: Antibiotic susceptibility profile of group B streptococcus acquired vertically, *Obstet Gynecol* 92:931-934, 1998.

34. deCueto M et al: Timing of intrapartum ampicillin and prevention of vertical transmission of group B streptococci, *Obstet Gynecol* 91:112-114, 1998.

35. Ramus RM, McIntire DD, Wendel CD: Antibiotic chemoprophylaxis for group B streptococci is not necessary in elective cesarean section at term, *Society for Perinatal Obstetricians,* San Francisco, 277, 1998 (abstract).

36. Coleman RT, Sherer DM, Maniscalco WM: Prevention of neonatal group B streptococcal infections: advances in maternal vaccine development, *Obstet Gynecol* 80(2):301-308, 1992.

GROUP B STREPTOCOCCAL INFECTIONS

CHORIOAMNIONITIS

A. DEFINITION
1. *Clinical chorioamnionitis* is a clinical syndrome of intraamniotic infection associated with acute inflammation of the fetal membranes that is clinically manifested before delivery by fever and other signs of infection (including uterine tenderness, maternal and fetal tachycardia, and uterine contractions).
2. By convention, if the clinical syndrome resolves within the first 24 hours after delivery, chorioamnionitis is the only diagnosis; however, if the fever, uterine tenderness, and other signs of infection persist beyond this time, the patient now has the additional complication of **endometritis** or **endomyometritis.**

B. INCIDENCE. Clinical (vs. histologic) chorioamnionitis occurs in 0.5% to 2% of all pregnancies[1] and in 3% to 25% of patients with premature rupture of fetal membranes (PROM) lasting longer than 24 hours.

C. ETIOLOGY. Infection ascends transplacentally either through intact or (more commonly) ruptured membranes or descends from the abdominal cavity through the fallopian tubes (rare). Table 15-1 lists commonly identified microbial agents.[2] It has been found that upper genital tract colonization with bacterial vaginosis organisms may precede conception. For most pregnancies, this has no effect. In a few patients, however, a chronic fetal inflammatory response takes place that may in turn cause both preterm delivery and neonatal morbidity.[3]

D. PERINATAL MORBIDITY AND MORTALITY. In the presence of chorioamnionitis, sepsis occurs in 2% to 5% of preterm fetuses or neonates. Fetal sepsis can be reduced significantly if antibiotics are administered before birth.[4] Of the preterm infants who become infected, approximately 5% will have serious infectious complications. Perinatal death may also be increased.[5,6]

E. MATERNAL MORBIDITY AND MORTALITY. Maternal complications include preterm labor[7] and endometritis.[5] If sepsis occurs, any of its sequelae may result, such as acute respiratory distress syndrome, renal failure, disseminated intravascular coagulation, and shock.

F. RISK FACTORS. Include lower reproductive tract infection,[8] amniocentesis, PROM, repetitive vaginal examinations, and internal fetal heart rate monitoring.

A. HISTORY. Elicit information regarding membrane rupture, recent and repetitive vaginal examinations, and amniocentesis because the most common route of infection, before or after PROM, is transvaginally. Patients with a history of bacterial vaginosis[9] (*Gardnerella vaginalis,*

15

TABLE 15-1		
DISTRIBUTION OF MICROBES IN 408 CASES OF INTRAAMNIOTIC INFECTION		
Microbe	No.	%
Group B streptococci	60	15
Enterococci	22	5
Escherichia coli	33	8
Gardnerella vaginalis	99	24
Other aerobic gram-negative rods	21	5
Peptostreptococci	38	9
Bacteroides bivius	120	29
Fusobacterium species	23	6
Bacillus fragilis	14	3
Mycoplasma hominis	125	31
Ureaplasma urealyticum	193	47

From Gibbs RS, Duff P: *Am J Obstet Gynecol* 164(5):1317-1326, 1991.

anaerobic bacteria, *Mycoplasma hominis*) *and* gonorrhea have an increased incidence of chorioamnionitis.[8]

B. PHYSICAL EXAMINATION

1. Maternal fever is seen in most patients with clinical chorioamnionitis.
2. About one fifth demonstrate foul-smelling amniotic fluid.
3. Uterine tenderness is noted in a minority of patients.
4. A thorough fever work-up should be conducted for all patients with suspected chorioamnionitis so that the potential causes of febrile morbidity are not missed. Rule out other sources of infection, such as the upper respiratory tract, urinary tract, and abdomen (see Chapter 3).

C. DIAGNOSTIC DATA

1. In the presence of ruptured membranes, the diagnosis of chorioamnionitis is made in the presence of fever (≥37.8°C) and one or more of the following (Table 15-2)[2]:
   a. Uterine tenderness
   b. White blood cell count >15,000 or left shift
   c. Fetal tachycardia (>160 bpm)
   d. Maternal tachycardia (>100 bpm)
   e. Foul-smelling vaginal effluent
2. In patients with intact membranes and an unexplained fever (especially in the presence of preterm labor), amniocentesis may be necessary to confirm the diagnosis. In the presence of clinically apparent chorioamnionitis, amniocentesis should reveal both leukocytes and bacteria to be consistent with the diagnosis. Gram's stain may show microorganisms. Aerobic and anaerobic cultures should be done. Affirm VP III DNA probe testing for *Gardnerella vaginalis* may be performed if this organism is of concern and the equipment is available (45-minute turnaround time, 95% sensitivity, and 99% specificity make it extremely valuable).[5]

TABLE 15-2

FREQUENCY OF POSITIVE CRITERIA FOR INTRAAMNIOTIC INFECTION

Criterion	Frequency (%)
Intrapartum fever >37.8°C	100
Maternal tachycardia >100 bpm	20-80
Fetal tachycardia >160 bpm	40-70
White blood cell count (mm³)	
>15,000	70-90
>20,000	3-10
Foul amniotic fluid	5-22
Uterine tenderness	4-25

From Newton ER: *Clin Obstet Gynecol* 36(4):795-808, 1993.

15

CHORIOAMNIONITIS

3. In patients at term who are in labor, fluid may be withdrawn from an intrauterine pressure catheter and sent to the laboratory for Gram's staining (this aids in early confirmation of the diagnosis and in identifying the causative organism) and culture. (The initial aliquot should be discarded to reduce contamination.)

4. Vaginal and cervical cultures are of little help in the evaluation of chorioamnionitis.

III. THERAPEUTIC MANAGEMENT

A. PREVENTION

1. After membrane rupture, avoid sterile digital vaginal examinations and use speculum or possibly ultrasound examination to assess the status of the cervix when necessary until the patient is in active labor.

2. See Chapter 16, section IV.

B. The basic management of chorioamnionitis includes delivery of the infant and the administration of antibiotics. There is no place for expectant management; after the diagnosis is made, delivery must be expedited regardless of gestational age.

C. The route of delivery should not be affected by the diagnosis of chorioamnionitis. If the patient is otherwise a candidate for vaginal delivery and is not in labor, labor is induced. If she is in labor, cesarean delivery is reserved for the usual obstetric indications and the duration of labor allowed is not altered.

D. The presence of clinical chorioamnionitis increases the risk of dysfunctional labor and cesarean delivery.

E. After the diagnosis of chorioamnionitis is made, antibiotics should be started promptly. Antibiotic choices vary, but reasonable choices include combinations of (1) an aminoglycoside (e.g., gentamicin) and **ampicillin,** (2) ampicillin with sulbactam (Unasyn), or (3) a second-generation cephalosporin (e.g., cefoxitin or cefotetan). Clindamycin can be added to the aminoglycoside and ampicillin regimen if a severe anaerobic infection is suspected.

F. In the presence of chorioamnionitis and maternal fever the fetus is commonly tachycardic. This is not indicative of fetal distress of itself and is not an indication for cesarean delivery.

G. After delivery, antibiotics are generally continued for at least 24 hours. Many patients will defervesce immediately postpartum, and antibiotics can be discontinued completely in these patients at 24 hours. If the fever persists after delivery, the patient should have antibiotics continued as in patients with endometritis.

REFERENCES

1. Newton ER: Chorioamnionitis and intraamniotic infection, *Clin Obstet Gynecol* 36(4):795-808, 1993.
2. Gibbs RS, Duff P: Progress in pathogenesis and management of clinical intraamniotic infection. I, *Am J Obstet Gynecol* 164(5):1317-1326, 1991.
3. Iams JD: *Controversies in infectious disease.* ACOG 48th annual clinical meeting postgraduate course: San Francisco, May 2000.
4. Yoder PR et al: A prospective, controlled study of maternal and perinatal outcome after intra-amniotic infection at term, *Am J Obstet Gynecol* 145(6):695-701, 1983.
5. Garite TJ, Freeman RK: Chorioamnionitis in the preterm gestation, *Am J Obstet Gynecol* 59:539-545, 1982.
6. Maberry MC, Gilstrap LC III: Intrapartum antibiotic therapy for suspected intraamniotic infection: impact on the fetus and neonate, *Clin Obstet Gynecol* 34(2):345-351, 1991.
7. Skoll MA, Moretti ML, Sibai BM: The incidence of positive amniotic fluid cultures in patients with preterm labor with intact membranes, *Am J Obstet Gynecol* 161:813-816, 1989.
8. Gibbs RS: Chorioamnionitis and bacterial vaginosis. II, *Obstet Gynecol* 169(2):460-462, 1988.
9. Master et al: *Abstract C-165.* 98th general meeting of the American Society of Perinatal Obstetricians, p 5, 1998.

PREMATURE RUPTURE
OF THE FETAL MEMBRANES

I. BACKGROUND

A. DEFINITION. Premature rupture of fetal membranes (PROM), probably better termed *prelabor rupture of membranes (ROM),* is the spontaneous rupture of the chorioamniotic membrane at any time before the onset of labor. The definition does not denote gestational age.

1. **Preterm PROM (PPROM, pPROM)** is rupture before 37 weeks' gestation.

2. Prolonged ROM is rupture for more than 24 hours.

B. INCIDENCE. PROM complicates 10% of pregnancies,[1] and PPROM occurs in 1% to 3% of pregnancies[2,3] and accounts for 30% to 60% of preterm deliveries when elective preterm deliveries, twin gestations, and stillbirths before labor are excluded.[4]

C. ETIOLOGY

1. The cause of PROM is usually unknown. At term, PROM may be a physiologic event. PROM is associated with a decrease in collagen fibers in membranes. Microbial invasion may weaken the membranes[2] and may cause rupture.[5,6] It is uncertain whether there is an association between weekly term antepartum cervical examinations and PROM.[7]

2. PROM is often thought to result from an occult chorioamnionitis.[8] Sources of infection causing PPROM include the following:
   a. Endocervical colonization by group B streptococcus (GBS)[9-11]
   b. Cervical *Chlamydia trachomatis* infection[12-14] or gonorrhea[15]
   c. Vaginal trichomoniasis, *Bacteroides,* and *Ureaplasma* infections[16]
   d. Bacterial vaginosis (BV)[9]

3. Less common possible causes include the following:
   a. Polyhydramnios
   b. Incompetent cervix
   c. Amniocentesis
   d. Trauma (rare)
   e. Multiple gestation
   f. Placental abruption
   g. Placenta previa
   h. Genetic abnormalities

II. PERINATAL AND MATERNAL MORBIDITY

A. Labor usually follows PROM within a relatively short time (at term, 70% within 24 hours and 95% within 72 hours).[17] If PPROM occurs, **premature labor and delivery** constitute the most common complication (50% within 1 week and 72% within 2 weeks)[3] with resultant perinatal mortality of 43.5% at 25 to 28 weeks' gestation, 11.3% at 29 to 32 weeks' gestation, and 4.5% at 33 to 34 weeks' gestation.[18,19]

Respiratory distress syndrome is inversely related to age at delivery, not to length or timing of PPROM.[20,21]

B. Infection, either maternal (chorioamnionitis) or fetal (e.g., sepsis or pneumonia), may occur as a result of ascending vaginal infection after PROM or if an occult intraamniotic infection preceded the ROM. This risk, however, is considered less significant than with the risk of preterm delivery, especially in early gestational ages (≤33 weeks).[22]

C. Umbilical cord compression may result from oligohydramnios resulting from PROM. This may occur antepartum or intrapartum and, if severe, may result in asphyxia or fetal death.

D. Abruptio placentae occurs more frequently in the presence of PROM.

E. FETAL DEFORMATION SYNDROME may occur in the very premature gestation with prolonged ROM and marked oligohydramnios. This includes intrauterine growth retardation, pulmonary hypoplasia (vascularization of the lungs occurs between 19 and 28 weeks' gestation),[23] and limb and face deformities resulting from compression.

III. PATIENT EVALUATION

A. HISTORY. A typical history includes a gush of fluid from the vagina with subsequent continued leakage. A consistent history correctly identifies the diagnosis more than 90% of the time.

B. PHYSICAL EXAMINATION

1. Avoid direct digital examination of the cervix in patients not in apparent active labor. Digital cervical examination dramatically increases the risk of infection and decreases the latency period.[24]

2. Diagnosis

   a. In patients with a history suggestive of PROM, the diagnosis is confirmed by **sterile speculum examination,** at which at least two of the following criteria are noted:

   (1) **Pooling.** A pool of fluid is visible in the posterior fornix.

   (2) **Phenaphthazine** (Nitrazine). Yellow Nitrazine paper turns **dark blue** in the presence of alkaline amniotic fluid.

   (3) **Ferning.** A smear of fluid from the vaginal fornix creates a typical fern pattern if amniotic fluid is present.

   (4) **Oligohydramnios.** Ultrasound showing little or no amniotic fluid is consistent with PROM.

   b. Evaluate the patient to **rule out infection,** specifically chorioamnionitis and cervicitis or vaginitis.

   (1) Findings of chorioamnionitis include the following (see Chapter 15 for further details):

   (a) Fever

   (b) Tender uterus

   (c) Foul-smelling amniotic fluid leaking from the vagina

   (d) Fetal tachycardia

   (e) Leukocytosis

(2) Consider amniocentesis (successful in 45% to 75% of PROM patients[3] to further identify a fetus at risk, especially if suggestive but not definitive signs are present). Obtain fluid for Gram's stain (NOTE: mycoplasma is not visible by this study), white blood cell count (WBC), and glucose level (obtain additional fluid for pulmonary maturity studies if desired). Factors suggestive of chorioamnionitis in patients with PROM include the following[25]:

    (a) Gram's stain, microorganisms identified (23.8% sensitivity; 98.5% specificity)

    (b) WBC count $\geq 30/mm^3$ (57.1% sensitivity; 77.9% specificity)

    (c) Glucose <10 mg/dl (57.1% sensitivity; 73.5% specificity)

(3) Findings of lower reproductive tract infection include purulent discharge at the cervix or vagina. Whether or not these findings are present, consider obtaining a vaginal swab and testing for BV, *Trichomonas,* GBS, *Bacteroides,* and *Ureaplasma.* Affirm VP III DNA probe testing is the preferred method of evaluation for BV and *Trichomonas* if available because of its significantly higher sensitivity and specificity than wet mount and at least equal sensitivity and specificity but more rapid turnaround time than culture. GBS isolation will require culturettes to be transported and grown in a selective transport medium. Standard aerobic and anaerobic cultures may be performed for other organisms of concern.[26-30] Treatment for common organisms includes erythromycin or clindamycin (300 mg orally three times daily for 7 days) for cervicitis. Metronidazole (500 mg orally twice daily for 7 days) is treatment for trichomoniasis and bacterial vaginosis.

c. **Rule out fetal distress**

  (1) **Prolonged fetal monitoring** (12 to 24 hours) in labor and delivery is recommended on admission to the hospital.

  (2) Follow with a **daily nonstress test (NST)** to rule out cord compression and fetal sepsis if the patient is placed on expectant management.

d. Evaluate the **gestational age** and **fetal maturity.**

  (1) Carefully review the patient's dating criteria.

  (2) Obtain ultrasound biometry. A low biophysical profile (BPP) may suggest impending fetal infection, but a reactive NST is all that is needed for fetal well-being. The BPP should be reserved for nonreactive fetuses.

  (3) If the gestational age is <33 weeks, consider obtaining fetal lung maturity testing by the following methods:

    (a) Amniocentesis (lecithin/sphingomyelin ratio or other tests)

    (b) Fluid collection from the vagina: can be reliably tested for phosphatidyglycerol (PG) and possibly fluorescent polarization

16

PREMATURE RUPTURE OF THE FETAL MEMBRANES

IV. THERAPEUTIC MANAGEMENT

A. OVERVIEW

1. Management of PROM continues to be debated, and approaches vary among institutions. Fetal well-being must remain the primary concern. It is important to note that the incidence of maternal and neonatal infection increases with the duration of ruptured membranes.[9] In term gestations there is an increased risk of infection as the duration of ruptured membranes becomes prolonged.

2. Two variables enter into the basic management decision of whether to deliver immediately or to await the spontaneous onset of labor:
   a. Gestational age
   b. Increased likelihood of cesarean delivery with induction of labor by oxytocin but not with prostaglandin E_2[31]

B. OPTIONS FOR MANAGEMENT OF GESTATIONS ≥36 WEEKS

1. **Active management.** Begin prostaglandin E_2 (gel or suppository) or oxytocin induction on admission. Consider amnioinfusion if indicated clinically.

2. **Expectant management.** Await the spontaneous onset of labor, and intervene sooner only for clinical infection, fetal distress, or other obstetric indications.

3. **Other options**
   a. **Sequenced active management.** Allow a reasonable time (6 to 24 hours) for spontaneous labor, and then begin induction if labor does not ensue.
   b. Administer preinduction prostaglandin followed by **induction** with oxytocin.

C. OPTIONS FOR MANAGEMENT OF A PRETERM GESTATION (<36 WEEKS' GESTATION)

1. Most physicians use some form of **expectant management** in preterm gestations awaiting spontaneous labor and deliver sooner only for fetal distress, infection, or other obstetric indications. Most patients remain hospitalized from initial rupture until delivery. Fetal surveillance to assess fetal well-being may consist of either nonstress or biophysical testing.[3]

2. Variations
   a. **Tocolysis.** Some use tocolytics for preterm labor in PROM, but evidence of benefit is lacking.
   b. **Corticosteroids.** Corticosteroid use in PPROM is no longer controversial.
      (1) Studies show the benefit of steroid use in reducing the newborn's risk of respiratory distress syndrome, intraventricular hemorrhage, and necrotizing enterocolitis.[32-39]
      (2) Limit the use of corticosteroids primarily to patients who are at <32 weeks' gestation, where the additional benefit of reducing intraventricular hemorrhage may be realized.[40]

c. **Thyrotropin-releasing hormone (TRH)** is no longer used to accelerate fetal pulmonary maturity because of recent studies demonstrating no benefit and possible harm to the fetus.

d. **Antibiotics** have been used to prolong the latency period and decrease the incidence of infectious complications.

(1) Erythromycin, clindamycin, and ampicillin have been shown in studies to prolong the latency period.[41-45]

(2) Infectious complications, including neonatal infection and sepsis and maternal chorioamnionitis, are decreased in some studies with the use of ampicillin or penicillin[41] and unchanged in others when erythromycin is used.[42-44,46,47] (This has not been studied for clindamycin.)

e. **Selective active management**

(1) Delivery for patients with amniotic fluid testing indicating fetal maturity

(2) Delivery for patients with amniotic fluid (derived by amniocentesis) demonstrating interleukin-6 (if clinically available) or microorganisms on Gram's stain (NOTE: *Mycoplasma* is not detected by Gram's stain [no cell wall]). Consider delivery for patients with amniotic fluid WBC count $\geq 30/mm^3$ or glucose <10 mg/dl on amniocentesis-derived amniotic fluid if additional clinical factors suggest chorioamnionitis.

REFERENCES

1. Romero R, Ghidini A: Premature rupture of membranes: relevance and frequency, *Contemp Obstet Gynecol*, pp 33-44, May 1993.

2. Gibbs RS, Eschenbach DA: Use of antibiotics to prevent preterm birth, *Am J Obstet Gynecol* 177:375-380, 1997.

3. Hanley ML, Vintzileos AM: Biophysical testing in premature rupture of membranes, *Semin Perinatol* 20(5):418-425, 1996.

4. Lewis R, Mercer BM: Selected issues in premature rupture of the membranes: herpes, cerclage, twins, tocolysis, and hospitalization, *Semin Perinatol* 20(5):451-461, 1996.

5. Lavery JP, Miller CE: The viscoelastic nature of chorioamniotic membranes, *Obstet Gynecol* 50:467, 1977.

6. Lavery JP, Miller CE: Deformation and creep in the human chorioamniotic sac, *Am J Obstet Gynecol* 134:366, 1979.

7. McDuffie RS et al: Effect of routine weekly cervical examinations at term on premature rupture of the membranes: a randomized controlled trial, *Obstet Gynecol* 79(2):219-222, 1992.

8. Romero R et al: The relationship between spontaneous rupture of membranes, labor, and microbial invasion of the amniotic cavity and amniotic fluid concentrations of prostaglandins and thromboxane B_2 in term pregnancy. I, *Am J Obstet Gynecol* 168(6):1654-1668, 1993.

9. McGregor JA, French JI, Seo K: Premature rupture of membranes and bacterial vaginosis. II, *Am J Obstet Gynecol* 169(2):463-466, 1993.

16

PREMATURE RUPTURE OF THE FETAL MEMBRANES

10. McDonald H, Vigneswaran R, O'Loughlin JA: Streptococcus colonization and preterm labor, *Aust NZ Obstet Gynaecol* 29:291, 1989.

11. Newton ER, Clark M: Group B streptococcus and preterm rupture of membranes, *Obstet Gynecol* 71:198, 1988.

12. Sweet RL et al: *Chlamydia trachomatis* infection and pregnancy outcome, *Obstet Gynecol* 156:824, 1987.

13. Harrison HR et al: Clinical *Chlamydia trachomatis* and mycoplasmal infections in pregnancy, *JAMA* 250:1721, 1983.

14. Alger LS et al: The association of *Chlamydia trachomatis, Neisseria gonorrhoeae* and Group B streptococcus with preterm rupture of the membranes and pregnancy outcome, *Am J Obstet Gynecol* 159:397, 1988.

15. Edwards LE et al: Gonorrhea in pregnancy, *Am J Obstet Gynecol* 132:637, 1978.

16. Minkoff H et al: Risk factors for prematurity and premature rupture of membranes: a prospective study of the vaginal flora in pregnancy, *Am J Obstet Gynecol* 150:965, 1984.

17. Johnson JWC et al: Premature rupture of the membranes and prolonged latency, *Obstet Gynecol* 57:547, 1981.

18. Morales WJ, Talley T: Premature rupture of membranes at <25 weeks: a management dilemma, *Am J Obstet Gynecol* 168(2):503-508, 1993.

19. Johnson JWC et al: Premature rupture of the membranes and prolonged latency, *Obstet Gynecol* 57:547, 1981.

20. Jones MD et al: Failure of association of premature rupture of membranes with respiratory distress syndrome, *N Engl J Med* 292:1253, 1975.

21. Hallak M, Bottoms SF: Accelerated pulmonary maturation from preterm premature rupture of membranes: a myth, *Am J Obstet Gynecol* 169(4):1045-1050, 1993.

22. Daikoku NH et al: Premature rupture of membranes and spontaneous preterm labor: maternal endometrial risks, *Obstet Gynecol* 59:13, 1982.

23. D'Alton M et al: Serial thoracic versus abdominal circumference ratios for the prediction of pulmonary hypoplasia in premature rupture of the membranes remote from term, *Am J Obstet Gynecol* 166(2):658-664, 1992.

24. Lewis DF et al: Effects of digital vaginal examinations on latency period in preterm premature rupture of membranes, *Obstet Gynecol* 80(4):630-634, 1992.

25. Romero R et al: A comparative study of the diagnostic performance of amniotic fluid glucose, white blood cell count, interleukin-6, and Gram stain in the detection of microbial invasion in patients with preterm premature rupture of membranes, *Am J Obstet Gynecol* 169(4):839-851, 1993.

26. Hillier SL et al: *Evaluation of Affirm VP Microbial Identification for* Gardnerella vaginalis *and* Trichomonas vaginalis. Presented at General Meeting of the American Society of Microbiology, Jan 1994, p 5.

27. Ferris DG: Office laboratory diagnosis of vaginitis (by certified lab techs), *J Fam Pract,* Dec 1995.

28. Briselden AM, Hillier SL: Evaluation of Affirm VP Microbial Identification Test for *Gardnerella vaginalis* and *Trichomonas vaginalis, J Clin Microb* 32:148-152, 1994.

29. Draper D et al: *Improved diagnosis of symptomatic* Trichomonas vaginalis *(TV) infections in women by the AFFIRM VP III identification test.* Presented at IDSOG, Aug 4-7, 1993, p 16.

30. Genova E et al: Evaluation of rapid DNA probe test for detection of TV in vaginal specimens (abstract), *ICAAC,* Oct 1992.

31. Meikle SF et al: A retrospective review of the efficacy and safety of prostaglandin E$_2$ with premature rupture of the membranes at term, *Obstet Gynecol* 80(1):76-79, 1992.

32. Morales WJ et al: Use of ampicillin and corticosteroids in premature rupture of membranes: a randomized study, *Obstet Gynecol* 73:721, 1989.

33. Crowley P, Chalmeres I, Keiroc MJNC: Effects of corticosteroid treatment before preterm delivery: an overview of evidence from controlled trials, *Obstet Gynecol* 97:25, 1990.

34. Block MF, Kling OR, Crosby WA: Antenatal glucocorticoid for the prevention of respiratory distress syndrome in the premature infant, *Obstet Gynecol* 50:186, 1977.

35. Collaborative Group on Antenatal Steroid Therapy: Effect of dexamethasone administration on the prevention of respiratory distress syndrome, *Am J Obstet Gynecol* 141:276, 1981.

36. Garite TJ et al: Prospective randomized study of corticosteroids in the management of premature rupture of the membranes and premature gestation, *Am J Obstet Gynecol* 141:508, 1981.

37. Iams JD et al: Management of preterm prematurely ruptured membranes: a prospective randomized comparison of observation versus use of steroids and timed delivery, *Am J Obstet Gynecol* 151:31, 1985.

38. Nelson LH et al: Premature rupture of membranes: a prospective randomized evaluation of steroids, latent phase and expectant management, *Obstet Gynecol* 66:58, 1985.

39. Committee on Obstetric Practice: Antenatal corticosteroid therapy for fetal maturation, *presentation of American College of Obstetrics and Gynecology* p 147, Dec 1994.

40. National Institutes of Health Consensus Development Panel on the Effect of Corticosteroids for Fetal Maturation on Perinatal Outcomes: Effect of corticosteroids for fetal maturation on perinatal outcomes, *JAMA* 273(5):413-418, 1995.

41. Owen J, Groome LJ, Hauth JC: Randomized trial of prophylactic antibiotic therapy after preterm amnion rupture, *Am J Obstet Gynecol* 169(4):976-981, 1993.

42. McGregor JA, French JI, Seo K: Antimicrobial therapy in preterm premature rupture of membranes: results of a prospective double blind placebo controlled trial of erythromycin, *Am J Obstet Gynecol* 165:632, 1991.

43. Greenberg RT, Hankins GD: Antibiotic therapy in preterm premature rupture of membranes, *Clin Obstet Gynecol* 34:742, 1991.

44. Ernest JM, Givner LB: A prospective, randomized, placebo-controlled trial of penicillin in preterm premature rupture of membranes, *Am J Obstet Gynecol* 170(2):516-520, 1994.

45. McGregor JA, French JI, Seo K: Adjunctive clindamycin therapy for preterm labor: results of a double blind placebo controlled trial, *Am J Obstet Gynecol* 165:867, 1991.

46. Johnston MM et al: Antibiotic therapy in preterm premature rupture of membranes: a randomized, prospective, double-blind trial, *Am J Obstet Gynecol* 163:743, 1990.

47. Amon E et al: Ampicillin prophylaxis in preterm premature rupture of the membranes: a prospective randomized study, *Am J Obstet Gynecol* 159:539, 1998.

PRETERM LABOR

I. BACKGROUND

A. DEFINITION. Preterm labor (PTL) is frequent contractions (i.e., $\geq$10/h) in the presence of cervical effacement or dilation and eventual preterm (<38 weeks' gestation) birth.

B. INCIDENCE. PTL occurs in 7% to 8% of all pregnancies.[1] Identification of patients at highest risk of PTL has been attempted by many authors. The greatest predictive value comes from whether the patient had a prior preterm birth. The recurrence rate is 25% to 50%.

C. ETIOLOGY. The etiology is presumed to be multivalent, with many cases having combined factors and including the following:

1. Premature rupture of fetal membranes (PROM): 38% (most of these have evidence of infection)
2. Vaginitis (noted in up to 85% of preterm deliveries)[2]
3. Abruption or placenta previa: 15%
4. Deciduitis/choramnionitis: 13% to 33%[3]
5. Short cervix: 10%

D. PERINATAL MORBIDITY AND MORTALITY. PTL accounts for 50% to 75% of perinatal morbidity and mortality, if delivery occurs. Respiratory distress syndrome (RDS) and subsequent bronchopulmonary dysplasia may occur.[4] Premature infants have less glycogen and fat stores than term infants and thus are unable to stabilize their blood sugar levels and temperatures as well as term infants. In addition, their lower levels of clotting factors and fragile epidura increase their risk of subependymal venous bleeding. Cerebral autoregulation is compromised by periods of unstable circulation, which may cause intracerebral hypertension and intraventricular hemorrhage.[5]

E. MATERNAL MORBIDITY AND MORTALITY. The same as that noted in uncomplicated pregnancies unless tocolytics are used. See specific side effects for each tocolytic later in this chapter (section III).

F. RISK FACTORS. The risk factors for PTL may be divided into major and minor categories (Table 17-1). These categories, however, are not very useful. As previously stated, the most important risk factor is a prior preterm birth.

II. EVALUATION

A. HISTORY

1. The patient often complains of low back pain, pelvic pressure, vaginal discharge, loose stools, spotting, and menstrual-like cramps. Inquire as to the duration of the symptoms present.
2. Identify precipitating factors, such as trauma, emesis, integrated genitourinary tract infection, and PROM.

TABLE 17-1

MAJOR AND MINOR RISK FACTORS IN PREDICTION OF SPONTANEOUS PRETERM LABOR*

MAJOR RISK FACTORS

Multiple gestation

Diethylstilbestrol

Hydramnios

Uterine anomaly

Cervix dilated >1 cm at 32 weeks' gestation

Second-trimester abortion × 2

Previous preterm delivery

Previous preterm labor term delivery

Abdominal surgery during pregnancy

History of cone biopsy

Cervical shortening <1 cm at 32 weeks' gestation

Uterine irritability

Cocaine abuse

MINOR RISK FACTORS

Febrile illness

Bleeding after 12 weeks' gestation

History of pyelonephritis

Cigarettes—more than 10/day

Second-trimester abortion × 1

More than two first-trimester abortions

From Creasy RK, Resnik R: *Maternal-fetal medicine,* ed 3, Philadelphia, 1994, Saunders.
*Presence of one or more major factors or two or more minor factors places patient in risk group.

B. **PHYSICAL EXAMINATION.** On admission a thorough physical examination is mandatory. When taking vital signs, pay particular attention to the patient's temperature and blood pressure. During the abdominal examination, assess uterine contractions and tenderness. A cervical examination is important to assess the effect of labor on the cervix. Inspect the fetal heart rate monitor tracing and uterine tocodynamometry.

C. **DIAGNOSTIC DATA**

1. Obtain a **complete blood cell count** with **differential,** platelets, and a serum fibrinogen level if the patient is bleeding.

2. **Urinalysis** (consider obtaining it by bladder catheterization) and urine culture and sensitivity are needed.

3. **Culture the cervix** for *Neisseria gonorrhoeae* and *Chlamydia trachomatis.*[3] Visually evaluate for evidence of cervicitis or vaginitis or both. Consider swabbing the vagina and testing for bacterial vaginosis (BV), *Trichomonas,* group B streptococcus (GBS), *Bacteroides,* and *Ureaplasma.* Affirm VP III DNA probe testing is the preferred method of evaluation for BV and *Trichomonas* if available. DNA probe testing for these

organisms has a significantly higher sensitivity and specificity than wet mount and at least an equal sensitivity and specificity but more rapid turnaround time than culture. GBS isolation will require specific culturettes to be transported and then grown in a selective transport medium. Standard aerobic and anaerobic cultures may be performed for other organisms of concern.[6-10]

4. Perform an **ultrasound** of the fetus to confirm gestational age and to rule out obvious anomalies.

5. **Consider performing an amniocentesis** in the following situations:

   a. If chorioamnionitis is strongly suspected or if labor does not stop easily with tocolytic agents, send fluid for Gram's stain, culture, white blood cell count ($\geq 50/mm^3$ indicates probable infection), and glucose (≤ 14 mg/dl is suggestive of infection).[11] The most common organisms associated with occult intraamniotic infection in PTL are as follows[3]:

      (1) *Ureaplasma urealyticum*

      (2) *Mycoplasma hominis*

      (3) *Trichomonas vaginalis*

      (4) *Bacteroides* species

      (5) *Chlamydia trachomatis*

      (6) Group B streptococcus

      (7) *Neisseria gonorrhoeae*

      (8) *Treponema pallidum*

      (9) *Gardnerella vaginalis*

   b. In gestations between 32 and 34 weeks, determine lung maturity.

III. THERAPEUTIC MANAGEMENT

Most practitioners treat PTL between 25 and 34 weeks' gestation and individualize treatment beyond 34 weeks (studies suggest a probable lack of direct cost benefit for treating PTL beyond 34 weeks' gestation). It is imperative to establish an accurate diagnosis of PTL and, once established, to initiate tocolytic therapy in a timely fashion.

A. **TOCOLYSIS.** In the U.S. Food and Drug Administration (FDA) Statement on Tocolytics,* the FDA states that the use of approved drugs for nonlabeled indications may be entirely appropriate, based on medical advances extensively reported in the medical literature.[12]

   The appropriateness or the legality of prescribing approved drugs for uses not included in their official labeling is sometimes a cause of concern and confusion among practitioners. Under the federal Food, Drug, and Cosmetic (FD&C) Act, a drug approved for marketing may be labeled, promoted, and advertised by the manufacturer only for those uses for which the drug's safety and effectiveness have been established and that the FDA has approved.

---

*From Gabbe SG, Niebyl JR, Simpson JL: *Obstetrics: normal and problem pregnancies,* ed 2, New York, 1991, Churchill Livingstone.

The FD&C Act does not, however, limit the manner in which a physician may use an approved drug. Once a product has been approved for marketing, a physician may prescribe it for uses or in treatment regimens or patient populations that are not included in approved labeling. Such "unapproved" or, more precisely, "off label" uses may be appropriate and rational in certain circumstances (and may in fact reflect approaches to drug therapy that have been extensively reported in medical literature).

Before such advances can be added to the approved labeling, data substantiating the effectiveness of a new use or regimen must be sub-

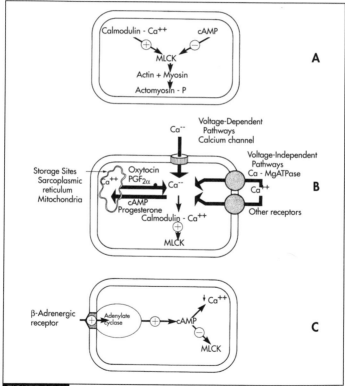

FIGURE 17-1

Control of myometrial contractility. Myosin light chain kinase (MLCK) is the key enzyme. See text details. *PGF$_{2\alpha}$,* Prostaglandin F$_{2\alpha}$; *ATPase,* adenosinetriphosphatase; *cAMP,* cyclic adenosinemonophosphate. *(From Gabbe SG, Niebyl JR, Simpson JL: Obstetrics: normal and problem pregnancies, ed 2, New York, 1991, Churchill Livingstone.)*

mitted by the manufacturer to the FDA for evaluation. This may take time and, without the initiative of the drug manufacturer whose product is involved, may never occur. For that reason, accepted medical practice often includes drug use that is not reflected in approved drug labeling.

B. **BETA-MIMETIC ADMINISTRATION GUIDELINES.** It is important to note that intravenous tocolytics have limited proven effectiveness. Their real use appears to be to "buy time" to allow other medications (e.g., antibiotics, steroids, thyrotropin-releasing hormone) to take effect.

1. **Clinical criteria**
   a. Beta-mimetic tocolytics are commonly used for the management of PTL. Figure 17-1 demonstrates the effect of beta-mimetics at the cellular level. Figure 17-2 demonstrates the chemical structure of epinephrine and β-agonist drugs currently in use in the United States.
   b. Table 17-2 summarizes the use of beta-mimetics and magnesium sulfate for PTL.

2. **Contraindications**
   a. **Absolute** contraindications to the administration of beta-mimetic agents are as follows:
      (1) Maternal cardiac disease (structural, ischemic, or arrhythmic)
      (2) Eclampsia or preeclampsia
      (3) Significant antepartum hemorrhage of any cause

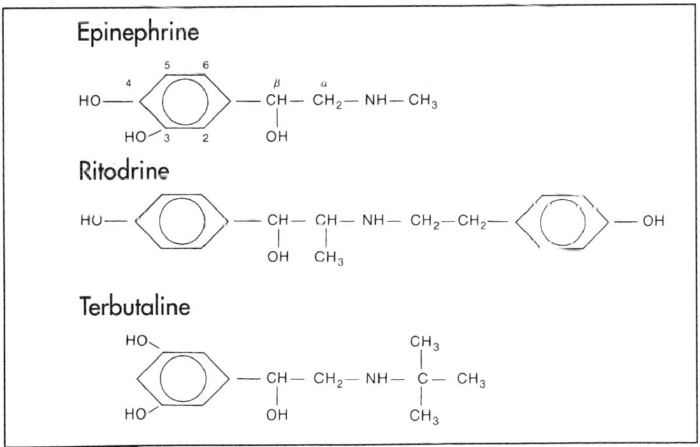

FIGURE 17-2

Structure of epinephrine and β-agonist drugs currently used in the United States. β_2 activity appears to depend on large alkyl substitution on the amino group while maintaining hydroxyl groups at the 3 or 5 position on the benzene ring. *(From Gabbe SG, Niebyl JR, Simpson JL: Obstetrics: normal and problem pregancies, ed 2, New York, 1991, Churchill Livingstone.)*

TABLE 17-2

SUMMARY OF TOCOLYTIC USE FOR PRETERM LABOR

Medication	Contraindication	IV	Doses (IM or SC)	PO
Magnesium sulfate	Severe cardiac disease	4 g loading dose, then 2-3 g/h until labor stops	10 g IM (5 g into each buttock) in addition to 4 g IV; follow with 5 g IM q4h	1 g magnesium gluconate PO q2-4h
Ritodrine (Yutopar)	Absolute: severe cardiac disease Use only with extreme caution in: Hyperthyroidism Hypertension Diabetes Anemia Multiple pregnancy Mild cardiac disease	Initial dose: 50-100 μg/min; increase by 50 μg every 10 min until labor stops or unacceptable side effects develop (maximum dose, 350 μg/min); once labor stops, maintain IV dose for 12 h	None	10 mg PO 30 min before stopping IV, then 10 mg PO q2h or 20 mg PO q4h for 24 h; if stable, may decrease to 10-20 mg q4-6h; maximum dose, 120 mg/d
Terbutaline (Bricanyl, Brethine)	Same as above	Initial dose: 2-5 μg/min; increase by 2-5 μg/min every 20 min until labor stops or maximum dose of 20 μg/min is reached; monitor K^+ levels	250 μg SC q4-6h	5 mg q4-8h or 2.5 mg PO q2-4h

Indomethacin	Use only with every immature gestation in which standard tocolysis has failed Absolute Rule out salicylate sensitivity Peptic ulcer disease Oligohydramnios	None	None	50 mg PO, or PR, then 25 mg PO q4h (premedicate with 1 g sucralfate PO before each oral dose) for maximum q48h
Nifedipine (Procardia)	Absolute Concurrent $MgSO_4$ Sick sinus syndrome Second- or third-degree arterio-ventricular block Shock Congestive heart failure	None	None	30 mg PO or SL, then 20 mg PO q8h to maximum of 10 mg q3h

IV, Intravenously; *IM*, intramuscularly; *SC*, subcutaneously; *PO*, orally; *PR*, per rectum; *SL*, sublingually.

(4) Clinical chorioamnionitis

(5) Fetal mortality or anomaly incompatible with uterine existence

(6) Significant fetal growth retardation

(7) Uncontrolled maternal diabetes mellitus

(8) Maternal medical conditions that would be seriously affected by the pharmacologic properties of the β-adrenergic agonists, such as hyperthyroidism, uncontrolled hypertension, or hypovolemia

(9) Any obstetric or medical condition that contraindicates prolongation of pregnancy

b. Conditions of increased risk and relative contraindications include the following:

(1) Multiple gestation

(2) PROM

(3) Febrile patient

(4) Maternal diabetes (controlled)

(5) Maternal chronic hypertension

(6) Patients receiving potassium-depleting diuretics (consider adding a potassium replacement)

(7) History of severe migraine headaches

C. PHYSIOLOGIC EFFECTS OF β-ADRENERGIC STIMULATION

1. The **maternal physiologic effects of β_1- and β_2-receptor-mediated stimulation** are detailed in Table 17-3.

2. The **fetal response** is detailed in Table 17-4.

3. Ritodrine follow-up studies demonstrate no significant differences in growth, neurologic evaluation, and psychometric testing in 7- to 9-year-old children exposed and unexposed to the medication.[13]

TABLE 17-3

MATERNAL PHYSIOLOGIC EFFECTS OF β-ADRENERGIC RECEPTOR STIMULATION

β_1-Receptor Mediated	β_2-Receptor Mediated
Cardiac	Smooth muscle
↑ Heart rate	↓ Uterine activity
↑ Stroke volume	↓ Bronchiolar tone
	↓ Vascular tone
	↓ Intestinal motility
Renal	Renal
↑ Renal blood flow	↑ Renin
	↑ Aldosterone
Metabolic	Metabolic
↑ Lipolysis (↑ ketones)	↑ Insulin
↓ HCO_3	↑ Glycogen release (↑ glucose)
↑ Intracellular K^+	↑ Skeletal muscle lactate

TABLE 17-4

FETAL RESPONSE TO β-ADRENERGIC RECEPTOR STIMULATION

Cardiac
  ↑ Heart rate
Smooth muscle
  ↓ Vascular tone
Metabolic
  ↑ Serum glucose during medication administration: subsequent rebound
    hypoglycemia may occur
  ↓ Calcium

D. TOCOLYTIC-RELATED PULMONARY EDEMA
1. Recommendations to avoid beta-mimetic, tocolytic-related pulmonary edema during IV administration of beta-mimetics include the following:
   a. Restrict fluid intake to 2.5 L/d (total IV and oral).
   b. Limit the salt content of fluids; avoid saline and lactated Ringer's solutions.
   c. Restrict the total dose and length of IV beta-mimetic therapy.
   d. Respect contraindications to beta-mimetic use.
   e. Monitor the patient's intake and output.
2. Predisposing factors for pulmonary edema when beta-mimetic tocolytics are taken are detailed in Table 17-5.

E. IV THERAPY
1. **Ritodrine (Yutopar)**
   a. **Preparation.** Add 150 mg ritodrine (3 ampules) to 500 ml 5% dextrose in water (D_5W) (0.3 mg/ml). The final concentration is such that each 10 ml/h delivers 50 μg/min.
   b. **Administration**[14]
      (1) The initial rate of the infusion is 50 to 100 μg/min. The rate is increased by increments of 50 μg every 10 minutes until one of the following occurs:
         (a) Uterine relaxation
         (b) Unacceptable side effects
         (c) Maximum rate of 350 μg/min is reached
      (2) Administer ritodrine according to Table 17-6.
      (3) Generally the infusion should be continued for at least 12 hours after uterine contractions cease.

2. **Terbutaline sulfate**
   a. **Preparation**
      (1) Add 7.5 mg (7.5 ampules) to 500 ml D_5W (0.15 mg/ml).
      (2) The final concentration is such that each 10 ml/h delivers 2.5 μg/min.

TABLE 17-5

PULMONARY EDEMA AND BETA-MIMETIC TOCOLYTIC THERAPY: PREDISPOSING FACTORS

UNDERLYING PREDISPOSING FACTORS IN NORMAL PREGNANCY

↑ Intravascular volume

↓ Peripheral vascular resistance

↓ Blood viscosity

↑ Heart rate

↓ Plasma colloid osmotic pressure

↑ Pulmonary vascular permeability (?)

Intrapartum volume shifts

ADDITIVE EFFECTS OF BETA-MIMETIC THERAPY

Further expansion of intravascular volume

Further ↓ in peripheral vascular resistance

Further ↓ in blood viscosity

Further ↑ in heart rate

Further ↓ in plasma colloid osmotic pressure

Further ↑ in pulmonary vascular permeability (?)

EXTRA PREDISPOSING MEDICAL OR TREATMENT FACTORS

Twins

Injudicious fluid management

Heart rate >130 bpm

Treatment >24 h

Unsuspected heart lesions (e.g., mitral stenosis)

Amnionitis

Hypertension

Glucocorticoids (?)

TABLE 17-6

RITODRINE ADMINISTRATION* (CONCENTRATION: 150 mg/500 ml D_5W)

Rate (ml/h)	Delivers (μg/min)
20	100
30	150
40	200
50	250
60	300
70	350

From Pharmaceutical Protocol, Long Beach Memorial Medical Center, 1990.

*All infusions must be regulated by an infusion pump.

   b. **Administration**[14]
      (1) Begin the infusion at 2.5 μg/min.
      (2) Increase the infusion by 2.5 μg/min every 20 minutes to a max-
          imum of 17.5 to 20 μg/min until uterine relaxation or marked
          side effects occur.
      (3) Continue the infusion for at least 12 hours after uterine contrac-
          tions cease.

3. **Patient evaluation during IV therapy**
   a. **Clinical.** Because cardiovascular responses are common and more
      pronounced during IV administration of ritodrine, cardiovascular ef-
      fects (including maternal pulse rate and blood pressure and fetal
      heart rate) should be closely monitored. Care should be exercised
      for maternal signs and symptoms of pulmonary edema. Occult car-
      diac disease may be unmasked with the use of ritodrine or ter-
      butaline.
   b. **Diagnostic data**
      (1) Serum electrolytes, especially potassium, should be monitored
          during ritodrine therapy.
      (2) Blood glucose should be monitored during ritodrine or ter-
          butaline therapy in diabetic patients.
   c. **Adverse reactions** to ritodrine and terbutaline include alterations in
      maternal blood pressure, tachycardia, a transient elevation of blood
      sugar and insulin levels, a reduction in serum potassium, tremor,
      nausea, vomiting, headache, erythema, nervousness, restlessness,
      emotional upset, and anxiety. The severity of the symptoms may de-
      termine if the medications should be discontinued.

F. **ORAL THERAPY.** Proof of efficacy for decreasing preterm deliveries is
   lacking for oral tocolytics, although oral tocolytics have been shown to
   decrease recurrent episodes of preterm contractions.

1. **Ritodrine or terbutaline**
   a. Give one tablet (ritodrine, 10 mg, or terbutaline, 2.5 mg) approxi-
      mately 30 minutes before the termination of IV tocolytic therapy.
      (1) The usual dosage schedule for oral maintenance is one tablet
          every 2 hours if tolerated.
      (2) The total daily dose of ritodrine or terbutaline should not exceed
          120 mg of ritodrine or 30 mg of terbutaline.
   b. Night doses should be held unless the patient awakens. If she does
      wake during the night, do the following:
      (1) Check her pulse.
      (2) A dose may be given if the criteria for the pulse rate are met and
          it has been at least 2 hours since the previous dose was given.

2. **Patient evaluation during oral tocolytic therapy**
   a. Check the patient's pulse before each dose is given. Subsequent
      doses should be given only if her pulse is at or below 115 bpm.
      (1) If her pulse exceeds 115 bpm, recheck it in 30 to 60 minutes.
          Administer the dose when her pulse rate drops to ≤115 bpm.

      (2) A new dosing schedule should be initiated at any time doses are held.

      (3) If it becomes necessary to hold two or more consecutive doses, the physician should be notified.

  b. If continued therapy is required on an outpatient basis, the patient should be instructed on how to take her pulse. Discuss a course of action with her in the event that her pulse rate exceeds 115 bpm.

G. SUBCUTANEOUS INFUSION OF TERBUTALINE.[15,16] Evidence of efficacy in reducing preterm births is lacking.

1. Benefits over oral terbutaline. Subcutaneous dosing minimizes the total terbutaline dose required, with subsequent reduction of side effects and tachyphylaxis.

2. Administration

  a. Dosing may be started at a basal rate of 0.05 ml/h.

  b. Boluses of medication may be scheduled for periods of peak uterine activity.

3. Consult your local subcutaneous pump specialist if this route of administration is desired.

4. The cost of this method of medication administration is much greater than with oral tablets.

H. MAGNESIUM SULFATE TOCOLYSIS

1. Contraindications to tocolysis (Table 17-7)

2. Mechanism of action. The mechanism by which magnesium sulfate ($MgSO_4$) reduces uterine activity remains unknown. Most likely, $MgSO_4$ competes with calcium at either the motor end plate, thus reducing excitation of the muscle, or the cellular membrane, where depolarization occurs.

3. Administration

  a. **IV** administration of $MgSO_4$

      (1) **Loading dose:** 4 to 6 g administered during a period of 20 minutes

      (2) **Maintenance dosage:** 2 to 3 g/h titrated according to the patient's deep tendon reflexes (DTRs) and serum magnesium level (The dosage may be reduced after uterine quiescence.)

TABLE 17-7

CONTRAINDICATIONS TO TOCOLYSIS

Cervical dilation >4 cm

Ruptured membranes

Intrauterine infection

Severe intrauterine growth retardation

Clinically significant bleeding

Fetal anomalies incompatible with life

(3) **Sample orders**
   (a) Administer 50 g MgSO$_4$ in 1 L dextrose in 5% lactated Ringer's solution (D$_5$LR).
   (b) Infuse 4 g (80 ml) over 20 minutes (loading dose).
   (c) Then infuse 2 g/h (40 ml/h).
   (d) Fluid is restricted to 100 ml/h (total intake).
   (e) IV: lactated Ringer's solution is alternated with D$_5$LR at a rate appropriate for fluid restriction.
   (f) Nothing should be taken by mouth except ice chips.
   (g) Input and output are strictly monitored.
   (h) In-and-out catheterization or Foley catheterization placement is used as needed.
   (i) Obtain a Mg^{2+} level 2 hours after load and then every 4 hours.

b. **Intramuscular** administration may be used when the continuous IV route is not possible.
   (1) **Loading dose.** Administer 5 g in a 50% solution (equally with dextrose in water) in each buttock (a total of 10 g) in addition to 4 g in 250 ml D$_5$W infused intravenously over 20 minutes.
   (2) **Maintenance dose.** Administer 5 g in a 50% solution every 4 hours. Before administration, examine DTRs, respiratory rates, and urinary output (UO).

c. **Oral magnesium gluconate**[17]
   (1) Administer 1 g oral magnesium gluconate (54 mg elemental magnesium) every 2 to 4 hours.
   (2) A preliminary study by Martin et al.[17] suggested that this therapy may be as effective an oral tocolytic as β-agonists.

4. **Patient evaluation during IV therapy**
   a. **Adverse reactions** may include nausea, flushing, drowsiness, blurred vision, chest discomfort, difficulty breathing, respiratory arrest, and death (Table 17-8).[18]
   b. **Evaluate** the patient approximately 2 hours after the loading dose is given and then every 4 to 6 hours depending on the patient's status and magnesium infusion rate (Table 17-9).
   c. In case of **magnesium sulfate** toxicity, administer 1 g **calcium gluconate** intravenously by slow push over 3 minutes.
   d. A clinical evaluation of the patient should be performed every hour.
      (1) **Respirations**
         (a) Maintain respirations at a minimum of **12/min.**
         (b) A diminished respiratory rate may indicate magnesium toxicity.
         (c) If respirations are depressed, consider discontinuing magnesium therapy.
      (2) **Urine output**
         (a) Urine output (UO) should be at least **30 ml/h.**
         (b) A decreased UO may result in a high serum magnesium level.

TABLE 17-8

MATERNAL AND FETAL SIDE EFFECTS OF MAGNESIUM SULFATE

	Maternal	Fetal/Neonatal
Metabolic	↑ Serum magnesium	↑ Serum magnesium
	↓ Calcium—usually within lower limits of normal; after administration for several days may become symptomatically low	↓ Serum calcium
	↑ Parathyroid hormone	No change in parathyroid hormone or calcitonin
	No change in calcitonin or phosphorus	
Cardiovascular	Transient decrease in systolic and diastolic blood pressure	No change in fetal heart rate
	↓ Respiratory rate	
	No change in pulse or temperature	
	Slight increase in uterine blood flow in sheep	
Pulmonary	Pulmonary edema reported in cases also treated with corticosteroids	
Toxic	Cardiac arrest	
	Respiratory arrest	
	NOTE: Absent patellar reflexes may represent impending toxicity rather than therapeutic level; need to monitor serum magnesium levels	

From Main DM, Main EK: *Obstetrics and gynecology: a pocket reference,* St Louis, 1984, Mosby.

TABLE 17-9

EFFECT OF MAGNESIUM SULFATE THERAPY

Magnesium Level	Physiologic Effect
4-7 mEq/L (5-8 mg/dl)	Therapeutic range
8-10 mEq/L (9-12 mg/dl)	Loss of deep tendon reflexes
13-15 mEq/L (16-18 mg/dl)	Respiratory arrest
15-20 mEq/L (18-25 mg/dl)	Heart block, cardiac conduction defects (peaked T waves, prolonged PR and QRS intervals)
20-25 mEq/L (25-30 mg/dl)	Cardiac arrest

    (3) DTRs should be present.
    (4) Immediately obtain a serum magnesium level if DTRs are lost, the respiratory rate decreases, or the UO drops below 30 ml/h.
  e. **Diagnostic data**
    (1) Evaluate the serum creatinine level on initiation of magnesium tocolysis because magnesium is excreted by the kidneys.

(2) Consider obtaining a serum magnesium level 2 hours after the loading dose and then every 4 to 6 hours, depending on the patient's status.

I. TOCOLYSIS AND MISCELLANEOUS MEDICATIONS

1. Indomethacin

a. **Mechanism of action.** Indomethacin acts by inhibiting prostaglandin synthesis at the cyclooxygenase pathway. Prostaglandins are part of the final pathway of uterine smooth muscle contraction.

b. **Indication.** Because of the serious fetal side effects, indomethacin should be used only with immature gestations in which standard tocolysis failed. Use of indomethacin is not recommended after 34 weeks' gestation.

c. **Contraindications**

(1) Maternal

  (a) Peptic ulcer disease

  (b) History of salicylate sensitivity

(2) Obstetric

  (a) See Table 17-7

  (b) Oligohydramnios

d. **Administration**

(1) **Loading dose**

  (a) Premedicate the patient with 1 g sucralfate (Carafate) 30 minutes before all oral doses of indomethacin.

  (b) Administer 50 mg orally or rectally by suppository.

(2) **Maintenance dosing** is accomplished by administering 25 mg orally every 4 hours, preceded 30 minutes earlier by sucralfate.

(3) **The duration of therapy** is usually only 24 to 48 hours.[19] If contractions have not subsided by this time, a second course of indomethacin may be given.

e. **Patient evaluation**

(1) **Diagnostic data.** A fetal ultrasound must be performed before administration of this medication to ensure that the amniotic fluid volume is sufficient.

(2) **Adverse reactions** include the following:

  (a) Oligohydramnios[20,21]

  (b) Intrauterine constriction of the ductus arteriosus (not described in fetuses treated for less than 48 hours)[22]

  (c) Neonatal pulmonary hypertension (not described in fetuses treated for less than 48 hours)

  (d) Possible increase of necrotizing enterocolitis (20% vs. 9% in incidence in low–birth-weight infants when the mother received ≥48 hours of indomethacin and delivery occurred within 24 hours of exposure)[23]

  (e) Renal insufficiency (fetal)[24]

(f) Possible increased incidence of fetal grade II to IV intracranial hemorrhage[25,26]

2. **Calcium channel blockers (nifedipine)**
   a. **Mechanism of action.** Calcium channel blockers prevent calcium entry into the cell, thus inhibiting smooth muscle contraction. Nifedipine is a long-acting vasodilator.
   b. **Contraindications**
      (1) See Table 17-7
      (2) Sick sinus syndrome
      (3) Second- or third-degree atrioventricular block
      (4) Shock
      (5) Congestive heart failure
   c. **Administration**
      (1) A single loading dose of 30 mg orally[1] or sublingually (or 10 mg given by these routes hourly for three total doses) may be followed by 10 to 20 mg orally every 8 hours up to a maximum of 10 mg orally every 3 hours.
      (2) Ninety percent of the medication is absorbed when ingested orally or sublingually.
   d. The **onset of action** is 20 minutes when ingested orally (with a peak effect in 1 to 2 hours) and 3 minutes when taken sublingually (peak effect in 10 minutes).
   e. The initial **half-life** is 2.5 to 3 hours.
   f. **Adverse reactions** are uncommon, occurring in less than 10% of patients.
      (1) Fatigue
      (2) Headache
      (3) Dizziness
      (4) Skin rash
      (5) Peripheral edema
   g. If the patient is taking digoxin concurrently, the serum level may rise.
   h. Avoid using nifedipine and $MgSO_4$ concurrently.

J. GROUP B β-STREPTOCOCCUS PREVENTION

1. Treat all patients with antibiotics directed toward group B β-streptococcus until culture results return. Intravenous antibiotics are preferred over those given orally. Of the following regimens, use the one most compatible with your community bacterial resistance patterns.
   a. IV penicillin G (2 million units IV every 4 hours)
   b. Ampicillin (2 g intravenous piggyback [IVPB] every 4 hours)
   c. Erythromycin (if the patient is allergic to penicillin) 500 mg IV every 6 hours.
2. If the culture fails to grow group B β-streptococcus, discontinue antibiotic therapy.
3. If the culture grows group B β-streptococcus or if the patient has a history of group B streptococcus, continue the IV antibiotics started on ad-

mission until patient has had 7 days of penicillin or ampicillin treatment or 10 days of erythromycin. Obtain another vaginal specimen for culture after treatment is completed.

4. If the cervical culture is positive for **gonorrhea,** treat per recommendations from the Centers for Disease Control and Prevention (see Appendix Q) and subsequently reculture (or test for cure).

5. Use steroids to accelerate fetal lung maturity (see Appendix M).[27] The National Institutes of Health currently recommend that all patients at risk of preterm delivery between 24 and 34 weeks' gestation receive betamethasone or dexamethasone.

K. Before transfer to the floor for antepartum patients and before discharge from the hospital, the patient will have undergone tocolysis and may be taking an oral tocolytic agent (e.g., terbutaline).

L. The patient is assessed daily while she is still on the floor for antepartum patients. As her disease becomes more stable, her activity is liberalized.

1. **First day.** Strict bed rest is usually prescribed. The patient should have uterine monitoring twice daily while hospitalized. If five or more contractions per hour are present, the patient requires evaluation and possible treatment (or both).

2. **Second day.** The patient is given bathroom privileges only. If rare or no uterine contractions occur, the patient's condition is considered to be stable.

3. **When the patient is discharged,** the physician should consider giving the patient an oral tocolytic agent. Patients with greater cervical dilation are usually observed for 1 or 2 days longer than those with minimal cervical change.

M. **Weekly office visits** with cervical examinations are recommended. In the presence of recurring uterine contractions or further cervical change, send the patient to labor and delivery for monitoring and care.

N. **Consider** daily phone nurse surveillance and possibly home uterine contraction monitoring (unproven benefit).

IV. PREVENTION

Many prematurity prevention programs are established throughout the United States. Most programs use a screening tool to evaluate risk factors at 8 to 15 weeks' gestation and again at 24 to 28 weeks' gestation. Patients scoring at risk for premature delivery are then enrolled in the program, which usually has the following components[29-31]:

A. Education of patient and family about premature delivery and its prevention

B. Increased intensity of contact with the primary care provider

C. Consideration of daily patient contact with the primary care provider or health care providers (studies suggest that this is as effective as home uterine activity monitoring by tocodynamometry)[32-35]

REFERENCES

1. Smith CS, Woodland MB: Clinical comparison of oral nifedipine and subcutaneous terbutaline for initial tocolysis, *Obstet Gynecol Surv* 49:168-170, 1994.

2. McGregor J: Personal communication, Sept 1995.

3. Gibbs RS et al: A review of premature birth and subclinical infection, *Am J Obstet Gynecol* 166(5):1515-1528, 1992.

4. Northway WH: An introduction to bronchopulmonary dysplasia, *Clin Perinatol* 19(3):489-495, 1992.

5. Fujimura M et al: Clinical events relating to intraventricular hemorrhage in the newborn, *Arch Dis Child* 54:409, 1979.

6. Hillier SL et al: *Evaluation of Affirm VP Microbial Identification for* Gardnerella vaginalis *and* Trichomonas vaginalis. Presented at General Meeting of the American Society of Microbiology, Jan 1944.

7. Ferris DG: Office laboratory diagnosis of vaginitis (by certified lab techs), *J Fam Pract,* Dec 1995.

8. Briselden AM, Hillier SL: Evaluation of Affirm VP Microbial Identification Test for *Gardnerella vaginalis* and *Trichomonas vaginalis, J Clin Microb* 32:148-152, 1994.

9. Draper D et al: *Improved diagnosis of symptomatic* Trichomonas vaginalis *(TV) infections in women by the Affirm VP III identification test.* Presented at IDSOG, Aug 4-7, 1993.

10. Genova E et al: Evaluation of rapid DNA probe test for detection of TV in vaginal specimens (abstract), *ICAAC,* Oct 1992.

11. Romero R et al: The diagnostic and prognostic value of amniotic fluid white blood cell count, glucose, interleukin-6, and Gram stain in patients with preterm labor and intact membranes, *Am J Obstet Gynecol* 169(4):805-816, 1993.

12. Use of approved drugs for unlabeled indications, *FDA Drug Bull* 12(1):4, 1982.

13. Polowczyk D et al: Evaluation of seven- to nine-year-old children exposed to ritodrine in utero, *Obstet Gynecol* 64:485-488, 1984.

14. Caritis SN et al: A double-blind study comparing ritodrine and terbutaline in the treatment of preterm labor, *Am J Obstet Gynecol* 150:7, 1984.

15. Lam F: *The scientific rationale for low-dose terbutaline pump therapy in the management of premature labor: is β2-adrenoreceptor desensitization by down regulation the cause of tocolytic breakthrough?* Presented to the Department of Ob/Gyn at the University of California, Irvine, 1988.

16. Lam F et al: *Use of subcutaneous terbutaline pump for long-term tocolysis.* Presented to the Department of Ob/Gyn at the University of California, Irvine, 1988.

17. Martin RW et al: Comparison of oral ritodrine and magnesium gluconate for ambulatory tocolysis, *Am J Obstet Gynecol* 158(6, pt 1):1440-1445, 1988.

18. Wilkins I et al: Efficacy and side effects of magnesium sulfate and ritodrine as tocolytic agents, *Am J Obstet Gynecol* 159:685-689, 1988.

19. Gabbe SG, Niebyl JR, Simpson JL: *Obstetrics: normal and problem pregnancies,* New York, 1986, Churchill Livingstone.

20. De Wit W, Van Mourik I, Wiesenhaan PF: Prolonged maternal indomethacin therapy associated with oligohydramnios: case reports, *Br J Obstet Gynaecol* 95:303-305, 1988.

21. Hickok DE et al: The association between decreased amniotic fluid volume and treatment with nonsteroidal anti-inflammatory agents for preterm labor, *Am J Obstet Gynecol* 160(6):1525-1531, 1989.

22. Moise KJ Jr et al: Indomethacin in the treatment of preterm labor, *N Engl J Med* 19:327-331, 1988.
23. Major CA et al: Tocolysis with indomethacin increases the incidence of necrotizing enterocolitis in the low–birth-weight neonate. 1, *Am J Obstet Gynecol* 170(1):102-106, 1994.
24. Gloor JM, Muchant DG, Norling LL: Prenatal maternal indomethacin use resulting in prolonged neonatal renal insufficiency, *J Perinatol* 13(6):425-427, 1993.
25. Norton ME et al: Neonatal complications after the administration of indomethacin for preterm labor, *Obstet Gynecol Surv* 49:312-314, 1994.
26. Norton ME et al: Neonatal complications after the administration of indomethacin for preterm labor, *N Engl J Med* 329(22):1602-1607, 1993.
27. Maher JE et al: The effect of corticosteroid therapy in the very premature infant, *Am J Obstet Gynecol* 170(3):869-873, 1994.
28. National Institutes of Health Consensus Development Conference Statement: effect of corticosteroids for fetal maturation on perinatal outcomes: February 28-March 2, 1994, *Am J Obstet Gynecol,* 173(1):246-252, 1995.
29. Fangman JJ et al: Prematurity prevention programs: an analysis of successes and failures, *Am J Obstet Gynecol* 170(3):744-750, 1994.
30. Mamelle N, Munoz F: Occupational working conditions and preterm birth: a reliable scoring system, *Am J Epidemiol* 126(1):150-152, 1987.
31. Ross MG et al: The West Los Angeles preterm birth prevention project. II. Cost-effectiveness analysis of high-risk pregnancy interventions, *Obstet Gynecol* 83(4):506-512, 1994.
32. Iams JD, Johnson FF, O'Shaughnessy RW: A prospective random trial of home uterine monitoring in pregnancies at increased risk of preterm labor, *Am J Obstet Gynecol* 157:638, 1987.
33. Iams JD, Johnson FF, O'Shaughnessy RW: A prospective random trial of home uterine monitoring in pregnancies at increased risk of preterm labor, *Am J Obstet Gynecol* 159:595, 1988.
34. Porto M, Nageotle MP, Hill O: *The role of home uterine activity monitoring in the prevention of preterm birth* (unpublished study).
35. Porto M: Home uterine activity monitoring: essential tool or expensive accessory? *Contemp Ob/Gyn,* pp 114-119, 1990.

17

PRETERM LABOR

PREGNANCY-INDUCED HYPERTENSION AND PREECLAMPSIA

I. BACKGROUND

A. DEFINITIONS[1]

1. **Mild pregnancy-induced hypertension (PIH).** Blood pressure (BP) >140/90 mm Hg (or a 30 mm Hg rise in systolic BP or a 15-mm Hg rise in diastolic BP measured on two occasions 6 hours apart) or a mean arterial BP of 105 mm Hg (or an increase of 20 mm Hg), occurring for the first time during pregnancy.

2. **Mild preeclampsia.** PIH in addition to **proteinuria or edema or both.**
   a. **Proteinuria** is the excretion of ≥0.3 g of protein per liter of urine in a 24-hour specimen or 0.1 g/L in a random specimen.
   b. **Edema** is diagnosed by one of the following:
      (1) Clinically evident swelling, nonresponsive to 12 hours of bed rest
      (2) A weight gain of 5 pounds or more in the preceding week

3. **Severe preeclampsia** is the presence of a BP of 160/110 (on two occasions 6 hours apart with the patient at bed rest on her left side) in addition to any of the following, occurring for the first time during pregnancy:
   a. **Proteinuria** of ≥5 g in 24 hours (or ≥3 g on a qualitative examination)
   b. **Oliguria** ≤500 ml/24 h
   c. **Cerebral** or **visual disturbances**
   d. **Epigastric pain**
   e. **Hemolysis, elevated liver enzymes, and low platelet count (HELLP) syndrome.** The diagnosis of HELLP is suggested by the following:
      (1) *H*emolysis (abnormal peripheral smear, lactic dehydrogenase >600 IU/L, bilirubin ≥1.2 mg/dl)
      (2) *E*levated *l*iver enzymes (aspartate aminotransferase [AST]; serum glutamate oxaloacetate transaminase [SGOT]) >72 IU/L and lactic dehydrogenase >600 IU/L
      (3) *L*ow *p*latelets (platelet count <100,000/mm^3). The differential diagnosis for HELLP includes idiopathic thrombocytopenic purpura, thrombotic thrombocytopenic purpura, hemolytic uremic syndrome, cholecystitis, hepatitis (viral), acute fatty liver of pregnancy, pyelonephritis, pyelolithiasis, glomerulonephritis, and gastroenteritis.
   f. **Pulmonary edema** or cyanosis

18

155

4. **Eclampsia** is the occurrence of seizures in a preeclamptic patient that cannot be attributed to other causes.
5. The term *PIH* is used throughout the remainder of this chapter to refer to PIH and its related disorders (preeclampsia and eclampsia).

B. **INCIDENCE**
1. PIH occurs in 4% to 7%[2] of all pregnancies (the increased incidence in primigravidas may reach 20%). Eclampsia is rare.[3]
2. PIH is more frequent in primigravidas, patients in lower socioeconomic groups, patients with multiple gestations, and patients with previous severe preeclampsia.
3. The prevalence of PIH increases near term, and the disease usually resolves by 6 weeks postpartum.

C. **ETIOLOGY.** The exact cause of PIH is unknown, but theories include uteroplacental ischemia, disseminated intravascular coagulation, poor nutrition, and immunologic disturbances. Research over the past decade has demonstrated an increase in vasoactive thromboxane A_2 and endothelia in preeclamptic women.[4]

D. **RISK FACTORS FOR PIH**
1. Multiple gestations
2. Hydramnios
3. Diabetes mellitus
4. History of chronic hypertension (HTN) (25% to 30% of patients with chronic HTN develop PIH)
5. Family history of PIH
6. Personal history of PIH (22% recurrence incidence for preeclampsia)[3,5]
7. Vascular disease
8. Hydatidiform mole (suggested by the onset of PIH in the second trimester)
9. Obesity[5]

E. **PERINATAL MORBIDITY AND MORTALITY**
1. Abruptio placentae, which is increased in preeclamptic and eclamptic patients, results in a perinatal mortality of 460/1000 when it occurs in the presence of PIH. HELLP syndrome is associated with a 34% perinatal mortality, with 72% preterm births.[6]
2. Prematurity, intrauterine growth retardation, uteroplacental insufficiency, and hypoxic episodes during eclamptic seizures also place the fetus at greater risk of morbidity and mortality. Infants delivering between 26 and 32 weeks' gestation (only 10% of all pregnancies complicated by preeclampsia) have a 56% incidence of respiratory distress syndrome (vs. 31% in deliveries caused by preterm labor).[7]

F. **MATERNAL MORBIDITY AND MORTALITY**
1. PIH is considered one of the leading causes of maternal morbidity.
2. Mothers with preeclampsia are at increased risk for the following complications:
   a. Placental abruption
   b. Vascular damage to all organ systems

    c. Thrombocytopenia

    d. Disseminated intravascular coagulation (DIC)

3. The previously mentioned complications are further increased with HELLP syndrome (DIC, 21%; abruption, 16%; renal failure, 8%; pulmonary edema, 6%; subcapsular liver hematoma, 1%; retinal detachment, 1%; blood transfusion, 55%).[8]

4. Mortality in patients with preeclampsia is unchanged from that seen in patients with uncomplicated pregnancies; however, it is increased in patients with eclampsia and with HELLP syndrome (1% to 13%).[6,8]

II. EVALUATION

A. HISTORY. Inquire about the presence of risk factors for PIH (i.e., diabetes mellitus, previous chronic HTN, renal disease, vascular disease). Ask the patient if she has noticed swelling of her face and extremities (i.e., are her rings or shoes [or both] tighter?) and inquire about neurologic signs (i.e., headaches, tinnitus).

B. PHYSICAL EXAMINATION. Perform a complete physical examination. Measure the patient's blood pressure (BP; with the correct size cuff) with the patient in a left lateral decubitus position and the cuff on the superior portion of the arm. In patients with possible **PIH,** be sure to examine for face, hand, and pretibial edema. A funduscopic examination is important for evidence of chronic **HTN.** Palpate the abdomen for any tenderness or pain.

C. DIAGNOSTIC DATA

1. Obtain a **urinalysis.** First examine the urine dipstick in the emergency room. If ≥1 g protein is present, send a specimen obtained by bladder catheterization to the laboratory for evaluation. Proteinuria indicates renal involvement.

2. Send a **complete blood cell count (CBC) with platelet count** (an elevated hemoglobin and hematocrit indicate hemoconcentration; thrombocytopenia indicates platelet consumption). Abnormal prothrombin time (PT), partial thromboplastin time (PTT), and fibrinogen are not noted unless thrombocytopenia is present.[9]

3. An **AST** or an **ALT** can identify hepatic involvement.

4. **Uric acid, creatinine,** and **blood urea nitrogen (BUN)** indicate the degree of renal involvement.

5. Consider obtaining a **24-hour urine collection** for protein and creatinine to examine renal function (calculate the creatinine clearance) and proteinuria (≥300 mg/24 h is significant). Others have proposed that a 4-hour creatinine clearance test be obtained with the patient resting on her side and receiving adequate hydration.[10]

6. If the patient's fundal height is lagging, obtain an ultrasound to rule out fetal growth retardation, and consider obtaining Doppler flow studies of the umbilical arteries if the technology is available.[11,12]

PREGNANCY-INDUCED HYPERTENSION

18

III. THERAPEUTIC MANAGEMENT (FIG. 18-1)

A. LONG-TERM ANTEPARTUM CARE

1. Preterm patients with mild disease are kept on bed rest (with bathroom privileges), preferably in the left lateral decubitus position. Consider performing an amniocentesis near term to assess fetal lung maturity. Plan the delivery according to the results of lung maturity testing.

2. **Outpatient management** of PIH may be considered in patients with a BP in the range of 140/90 mm Hg that improves with bed rest if the patient has no additional signs of preeclampsia. Home management may include the following[13,14]:
   a. Education of the patient and family on the disease process and related symptoms
   b. Fetal movement counts
   c. BP monitoring every 4 hours during the day
   d. Weight recorded daily
   e. Examination of the urine dipstick every morning for protein; twice weekly antepartum surveillance (nonstress test [NST]) with frequent amniotic fluid assessment
   f. Visits to the primary care physician weekly for full evaluation
   g. Hospital admission for worsening status

3. **Inpatient management** should include the following patient care:
   a. BP monitoring every 4 hours during the day
   b. Daily evaluation of patellar reflexes
   c. Weight recorded daily
   d. Examination of the urine dipstick every morning for protein
   e. CBC, creatinine, and AST twice weekly
   f. Fetal movement counts to be performed by the patient (provide instruction)
   g. NST performed twice weekly with weekly amniotic fluid index
   h. Notify physician of any patient complaints of the following:
      (1) Persistent occipital headache
      (2) Visual symptoms
      (3) Epigastric pain

4. Once hospitalized, these patients usually remain inpatients for the duration of their pregnancy unless they qualify for outpatient management as detailed previously. If the **PIH** worsens, consider delivery. For persistent diastolic BPs >110, consider administration of an antihypertensive in addition to delivery.

5. Consider weekly administration of steroids and thyrotropin-releasing hormone (TRH), if available, to facilitate fetal surfactant production.

6. In patients with severe preeclampsia, consider immediate puerperal uterine curettage. This has been shown to accelerate recovery from preeclampsia without significant complications.[15]

B. Severe preeclampsia and eclampsia warrant immediate delivery regardless of gestational age.

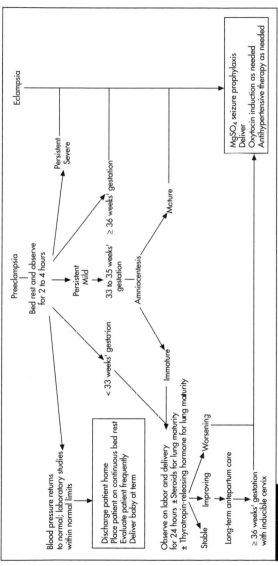

PREGNANCY-INDUCED HYPERTENSION

FIGURE 18-1

Management of preeclampsia and eclampsia.

18

1. **Seizure prophylaxis**
    a. Magnesium sulfate ($MgSO_4$) is commonly used in the United States to prevent eclamptic seizures. Initiate $MgSO_4$ therapy with a 4- to 6-g load over 20 minutes followed by 2 g/h.[16] Refer to Chapter 17 for details of $MgSO_4$ side effects and patient management guidelines. $MgSO_4$ causes vasodilation in vessels distal to the middle cerebral artery and thus is thought to exert antiseizure activity by reducing cerebral ischemia.[17]
    b. **Dilantin** (phenytoin) is commonly used in other countries as eclamptic seizure prophylaxis.[18,19]
        (1) The **loading dose** is based on the patient's weight (10 mg/kg). Phenytoin may be diluted in normal saline and piggybacked into the mainline intravenously (IV). The dose is run at a rate no greater than 50 mg/min.
        (2) A **second bolus** (5 mg/kg) is given 2 hours after the load.
        (3) **Phenytoin levels** need to be checked approximately 6 hours and 12 hours after the second bolus (therapeutic range is 10 to 20 μg/ml; to be routinely drawn immediately before a scheduled dose is given). The measured phenytoin level represents the combined bound and unbound fractions of phenytoin, whereas the therapeutic effect of this drug is based on only the unbound portion (usually 10%). When serum albumin is low, the unbound fraction of phenytoin is correspondingly increased. To correct for a low albumin level, use the following formula:

        $$C_{normal} = \frac{C_{observed}}{0.9 \times (\text{albumin concentration}) + 0.1}$$

        C_{normal} = Phenytoin concentration that would have been observed had the patient's albumin concentration been normal

        $C_{observed}$ = Measured phenytoin concentration

        This equation assumes that the unbound fraction is 0.1 when the albumin is normal.
        (4) **Maintenance doses** are administered initially 12 hours after the second bolus and then every 8 to 12 hours based on serum levels. The dose is 200 mg orally or IV and is to be continued for 3 to 5 days.
        (5) **Adverse reactions** include the following:
            (a) Bradycardia and heart block
            (b) Ataxia, slurred speech, nystagmus, mental confusion, and decreased coordination
            (c) Nausea, vomiting, and constipation
            (d) Local irritation, inflammation, and tenderness at the injection site
2. Use continuous fetal and uterine monitoring.

3. Consider placement of a central line for fluid management (Tables 18-1 and 18-2).
4. Place a Foley catheter for accurate measurement of urinary output.
5. Induce delivery if the patient is not in labor and no fetal or maternal indications for an operative delivery are present.
6. Administer **hydralazine** (Apresoline) in a dose of 2.5 mg by intravenous push (IVP) (slowly) if the diastolic BP is persistently more than 105 to 110.
   a. The usual dose is 2.5 mg by slow intravenous push (IVP). This may be repeated in 5 to 10 minutes if the patient's BP does not decrease. Subsequently, titrate 1 to 2 mg IV for 5 to 10 minutes until a BP of about 150/100 is achieved. Hydralazine requires 20 minutes for its full effect to be manifested. Do *not* bring the BP to normotensive levels. If the diastolic BP drops to <90 mm Hg, uteroplacental insufficiency may occur. The dosage may be increased as needed.
   b. Alternative medications include labetalol, nitroglycerin, and sodium nitroprusside. See Chapter 7, section IIIB, and Table 7-4 for administration guidelines and side effects.[20,21]

TABLE 18-1

NORMAL RESTING HEMODYNAMIC VALUES

	Nonpregnant*	Pregnant
Pressure measurements		
Central venous (M)	1-10 mm Hg	No change
(superior vena cava)		
Right atrium (M)	0-8 mm Hg	No change
Right ventricle (Sys)	15-30 mm Hg	No sig. change†
(ED)	0-8 mm Hg	No sig. change†
Pulmonary artery (Sys)	15-30 mm Hg	No sig. change†
(ED)	3-12 mm Hg	No sig. change†
(M)	9-16 mm Hg	No sig. change†
Pulmonary artery wedge (M)	3-10 mm Hg	No sig. change†
(and left atrium)		
Left ventricle (Sys)	100-140 mm Hg	No sig. change†
(ED)	3-12 mm Hg	No sig. change†
Flow and resistances		
Cardiac output	4.0-7.0 L/min	↑ 30%-45%
Cardiac index	2.8-4.2 L/min/m²	↑ 30%-45%
Total systemic resistance	770-1500 dyn-s/cm³	↓ ~25%
Pulmonary vascular resistance	20-120 dyn-s/cm³	↓ ~25%

From Main DM, Main EK: *Obstetrics and gynecology: a pocket reference*, St Louis, 1984, Mosby.
M, Mean; *Sys*, systolic; *ED*, end diastolic.
*Normal nonpregnant data from Barry WH, Grossman W. In Braunwald E, editor: *Heart disease: a textbook of cardiovascular medicine,* vol 1, Philadelphia, 1980, Saunders.
†While normal ranges have not been established by formal studies, available data indicate these values are not significantly changed by pregnancy.

TABLE 18-2

PULMONARY ARTERY WEDGE PRESSURES

Aliases: Pulmonary wedge pressure, pulmonary capiliary wedge pressure, and pulmonary artery occlusion pressure.

Provides information on (1) level of pulmonary venous pressure, which is a major determinant of pulmonary congestion; (2) left ventricular filling pressure, which allows estimation of cardiac performance. Therefore wedge pressures can predict pulmonary edema with reasonable accuracy *given normal colloid osmotic pressure and normal pulmonary vascular permeability.*

Advantages over central venous pressure monitoring

1. More complete cardiovascular information.
2. CVP inaccurately monitors cardiac performance in patients with myocardial infarction, peritonitis, ischemic ST-T electrocardiogram (ECG) changes, other cardiorespiratory diseases, and severe preeclampsia.

Suggested indications in obstetrics and gynecology

1. Surgery and/or labor and delivery of a patient with New York Heart Association class 3 or 4 cardiac disease.
2. Aortic outflow tract obstruction during delivery.
3. Hypovolemic shock secondary to severe intrapartum blood loss or severe postpartum hemorrhage not responsive to initial fluid therapy.
4. Septic shock requiring volume resuscitation or the use of vasopressor agents.
5. Severe preeclampsia and eclampsia complicated by oliguria, pulmonary edema, or hypovolemia secondary to hemorrhage.
6. Suspected amniotic fluid embolus with vascular collapse.
7. Cardiac failure with suspected pulmonary edema.
8. Intraoperative and postoperative monitoring of fluid therapy in gynecologic oncology patients undergoing radical surgery.

From Main DM, Main EK: *Obstetrics and gynecology: a pocket reference,* St Louis, 1984, Mosby. General references: Cotton DB, Benedetti TJ: *Obstet Gynecol* 56:641, 1980; Pace NL: *Anesthesiology* 47:455, 1977.

7. **Laboratory assessment** during labor and immediately postpartum (until patient status improves) consists of the following:
   a. Check urine protein level with every void or every 2 hours if the Foley catheter is in place.
   b. Assess CBC with platelets every 6 hours if the patient's hemodynamic status is unstable; otherwise daily until hemodynamic status is stable and reassuring.
   c. Assess AST or ALT or both every 6 hours if liver status is unstable; otherwise daily until liver status is normal and stable.
   d. Assess creatinine and BUN levels every 6 hours if renal function is unstable; otherwise daily until renal function is normal and stable.
   e. Consider obtaining a **bleeding time** if an epidural or cesarean delivery is anticipated because platelet function is often poor in patients with preeclampsia.

8. If **HELLP** is present, continue with the above plan of management and labor induction.
   a. Monitor CBC and platelet count.
   b. If the hematocrit drops to 20% to 25%, consider transfusion of packed red blood cells.
   c. If the platelet count drops to <20,000/mm^3 consider transfusion of 6 to 10 U of platelets.
   d. Attempt volume expansion (after central venous pressure [CVP] line is placed if indicated) with crystalloids and 5% to 25% albumin.
   e. Additional factors that might be required include the following:
      (1) Antithrombotic agents: low-dose aspirin, heparin, dipyridamole, antithrombin III, and prostacyclin infusions
      (2) Immunosuppressive agents (e.g., steroids [see Chapter 8, section IIIC2])
      (3) Fresh frozen plasma infusions, exchange plasmapheresis, and rarely dialysis
9. Patient status usually reaches a nadir approximately 24 to 36 hours after delivery with subsequent steady improvement.
10. If preeclampsia (including HELLP syndrome) or eclampsia develops postpartum, treat the patient with an antiseizure medication, as detailed above, in the hospital for at least 24 hours and until she is stable. Additional medical management is dictated by patient status.

C. PREVENTION. Studies over the past decade have focused on various methods of preventing preeclampsia. Most experts currently recommend no prophylaxis for healthy low-risk pregnant women.

1. Low-dose aspirin (60 to 100 mg/d) decreases the incidence of preeclampsia but results in a sevenfold rise in the incidence of placental abruption.[2,22,23] Further research is in progress.
2. Calcium supplementation (2 g/d) beginning at 20 weeks' gestation resulted in a lower incidence of all hypertensive disorders of pregnancy.[24]
3. Ingesting fish oil in 6-g capsules three times per day results in a decrease in thromboxane A$_2$ synthesis[25] but clinically has not demonstrated a reduction in preeclampsia.
4. Zinc and magnesium have been studied but have not yet been shown to reduce PIH and its associated disorders.[26-29]

REFERENCES

1. Gabbe SG, Niebyl JR, Simpson JL: *Obstetrics: normal and problem pregnancies,* ed 2, New York, 1991, Churchill Livingstone.
2. Sibai BM et al: Prevention of preeclampsia with low-dose aspirin in healthy, nulliparous pregnant women, *Obstet Gynecol Surv* 49:225-227, 1994.
3. Sibai BM, Sarinoglu C, Mercer BM: Eclampsia VII: pregnancy outcome after eclampsia and long-term prognosis. I, *Am J Obstet Gynecol* 166(6): 1757-1763, 1992.
4. Krayenbrink AA et al: Endothelial vasoactive mediators in preeclampsia, *Am J Obstet Gynecol* 169(1):160-165, 1993.

5. Stone JL et al: Risk factors for severe preeclampsia, *Obstet Gynecol* 83(3):357-361, 1994.

6. Sibai BM, Ramadan MK: Acute renal failure in pregnancies complicated by hemolysis, elevated liver enzymes, and low platelets. I, *Am J Obstet Gynecol* 168(6):1682-1690, 1993.

7. Banias BB, Devoe LD, Nolan TE: Severe preeclampsia in preterm pregnancy between 26 and 32 weeks' gestation, *Am J Perinatol* 9:357, 1992.

8. Sibai BM et al: Maternal morbidity and mortality in 442 pregnancies with hemolysis, elevated liver enzymes, and low platelets (HELLP syndrome), *Am J Obstet Gynecol* 169(4):1000-1006, 1993.

9. Leduc L et al: Coagulation profile in severe preeclampsia, *Obstet Gynecol* 79(1):14-18, 1992.

10. Huddleston JF et al: A prospective comparison of two endogenous creatinine clearance testing methods in hospitalized hypertensive gravid women, *Am J Obstet Gynecol* 169(3):576-582, 1993.

11. Valcamonico A et al: Absent end-diastolic velocity in umbilical artery: risk of neonatal morbidity and brain damage, *Am J Obstet Gynecol* 170(3):796-802, 1994.

12. Leiberman JR et al: The association between increased mean arterial pressure and abnormal uterine artery resistance to blood flow during pregnancy, *Obstet Gynecol* 82(6):965-970, 1993.

13. Barton JR, Stanziano GJ, Sibai BM: Monitored outpatient management of mild gestational hypertension remote from term, *Am J Obstet Gynecol* 170(3):765-768, 1994.

14. Helewa M et al: Community-based home-care program for the management of preeclampsia: an alternative, *Obstet Gynecol Surv* 49:232-234, 1994.

15. Magann EF et al: Immediate postpartum curettage: accelerated recovery from severe preeclampsia, *Obstet Gynecol* 81(4):502-506, 1993.

16. Sibai BM: Magnesium sulfate is the ideal anticonvulsant in preeclampsia-eclampsia, *Am J Obstet Gynecol* 162(5):1141-1145, 1990.

17. Belfort MA, Moise KJ: Effect of magnesium sulfate on maternal brain blood flow in preeclampsia: a randomized, placebo-controlled study, *Am J Obstet Gynecol* 167(3):661-666, 1992.

18. Dommisse J: Phenytoin sodium and magnesium sulfate in the management of eclampsia, *Br J Obstet Gynaecol* 97:104-109, 1990.

19. Ryan G, Lange IR, Naugler MA: Clinical experience with phenytoin prophylaxis in severe preeclampsia, *Am J Obstet Gynecol* 16:1297-1304, 1989.

20. Dildy GA, Clark SL: Hypertensive crisis, *Contemp Ob/Gyn* 38(6):11-12, 1993.

21. Calhoun DA, Oparil S: Treatment of hypertensive crisis, *N Engl J Med* 323(17):1177-1183, 1990.

22. Sibai BM et al: Prevention of preeclampsia with low-dose aspirin in healthy, nulliparous pregnant women, *N Engl J Med* 329(17):1213-1266, 1993.

23. Low-dose aspirin in prevention and treatment of intrauterine growth retardation and pregnancy-induced hypertension, *Obstet Gynecol Surv* 48:523-525, 1993.

24. Belizan JM et al: Calcium supplementation to prevent hypertensive disorders of pregnancy, *N Engl J Med* 325(20):1399-1405, 1991.

25. Schiff E et al: Reduction of thromboxane A_2 synthesis in pregnancy by polyunsaturated fatty acid supplements. I, *Am J Obstet Gynecol* 168(1):122-124, 1993.

26. Spatling L, Spatling G: Magnesium supplementation in pregnancy: a double blind study, *Br J Obstet Gynaecol* 95:120-123, 1988.

27. Sibai BM, Villar MA, Bray E: Magnesium supplementation during pregnancy: a double blind randomized controlled clinical trial, *Am J Obstet Gynecol* 161(1):115-119, 1989.

28. Hunt IF et al: Zinc supplementation during pregnancy: effects on selected blood constituents and on progress and outcome of pregnancy in low-income women of Mexican descent, *Am J Nutr* 40:508-521, 1984.

29. Mahomed K et al: Zinc supplementation during pregnancy: a double blind randomized controlled trial, *Br Med J* 299:826-829, 1989.

ANTEPARTUM HEMORRHAGE

I. BACKGROUND

A. **INCIDENCE.** Antepartum bleeding occurs in 3.8% of pregnancies that progress beyond 20 weeks' gestation.[1]

B. **ETIOLOGY.** The most common causes are **abruptio placentae, placenta previa,** and **vasa previa.** Other causes of third-trimester bleeding, which most likely represent <1% of all bleeding cases, include the following:

1. Cervicitis
2. Cervical erosions
3. Endocervical polyps
4. Cancer of the cervix
5. Vaginal, vulvar, and cervical varicosities
6. Vaginal infections
7. Foreign bodies
8. Bloody show
9. Degenerating uterine fibroids

C. **PERINATAL MORBIDITY AND MORTALITY**

1. First-trimester and early second-trimester bleeding may be an indicator of total placenta previa and a decreased chance of carrying the fetus near term.
2. Modern obstetric care and neonatal intensive care units have led to a marked decrease in maternal mortality and an improvement in fetal outcome.
3. The most frequent cause for an indicated delivery is bleeding.
4. Perinatal mortality
   a. Placenta previa: <10%[1,2]
   b. Abruptio placentae: 0.4%[3]
   c. Vasa previa: >50%[4,5]

II. HEMORRHAGE ASSESSMENT

A. **CLASSIFICATION** (Table 19-1)

B. **PHYSIOLOGY**

1. Pregnant patients usually do not demonstrate the expected early signs of **volume depletion.** This is the result of the 40% blood-volume expansion achieved by 30 weeks' gestation. Thus **it is difficult for the practitioner to adequately assess the blood volume deficit** in these patients.
2. The **physiologic response** to bleeding occurs in two phases. Acutely, vasoconstriction occurs to maintain essential organ flow. Chronically (results are not manifest for at least the first 4 hours after the bleeding episode), transcapillary refill may replace up to 30% of the lost volume.

TABLE 19-1

CLASSIFICATION OF OBSTETRIC HEMORRHAGE

Clinical Signs	Bleeding		
	Mild	Moderate	Severe*
Vital signs	Within normal limits	Elevated pulse	Tachycardia
		Orthostatic blood pressure	Unrecordable blood pressure
		Tachypnea	Tachypnea
Evidence of circulation volume deficit	None	Subtle perfusion changes (delayed refilling of hypothenar area when squeezed)	Cold, clammy skin Fetal distress or death
Urine output	Within normal limits	Possibly decreased	Oliguria/anuria
Intravascular volume lost	<15%	20%-25%	>30%

*When a woman loses more than 40% of her blood volume, she will be in profound shock. Circulatory collapse and cardiac arrest occur if volume resuscitation is not begun immediately.

C. **HEMOGLOBIN (Hb) AND HEMATOCRIT (Hct).** Hb and Hct are frequently used to assess the volume loss.
1. Because effects of transcapillary refill are not manifest for at least the first 4 hours after acute bleeding, no significant change is seen in these values during this time unless the patient has bled severely.
2. The infusion of intravenous fluids may result in an earlier lowering of the measured Hb and Hct levels.
D. **URINE OUTPUT (UO).** UO usually decreases before any other signs of decreased perfusion are manifest.
1. Renal blood flow is closely correlated with urine production. If a patient is producing ≥30 ml of urine per hour, she is euvolemic.
2. If the patient produces <30 ml of urine per hour after an acute bleeding episode, she requires volume replacement and careful monitoring of her fluid status.

ABRUPTIO PLACENTAE

I. BACKGROUND
A. **DEFINITION.** *Abruptio placentae* is the premature separation of a normally implanted placenta. Different classes of abruption are defined by the size of the retroplacental blood clot at delivery or by the clinical setting. Some prefer to separately define a **marginal sinus rupture,** which is an abruption limited to the margin of the placenta.

B. INCIDENCE

1. Abruptio placentae occurs in 1% to 3% of deliveries and accounts for two thirds of antepartum hemorrhages.
2. The incidence of abruptio placentae increases as term approaches.
3. More than 90% of infants involved weigh more than 1500 g at delivery.
4. Of patients who experience an abruption, 20% manifest the condition before 28 weeks' gestation, 20% between 28 and 33 weeks' gestation, and 22% to 40% between 32 and 36 weeks' gestation.[6]

C. **ETIOLOGY.** The primary cause is unknown, but factors related to abruptio placentae include the following:

1. **Maternal hypertension and vascular disease.** Both of these are responsible for up to 50% of fatal fetal or neonatal cases.[3,7]
2. **High parity.** The incidence of abruptio placentae is 1% in primiparas and 2.5% in grand multiparas.[8]
3. **Poor nutrition,** especially folic acid deficiency. Supplementation has no apparent effect after the sixth week of pregnancy.
4. **Maternal smoking.** An increase in abruption and fetal deaths occurs in pregnant women who smoke more than 10 cigarettes per day.[3]
5. **Cocaine use**
6. Acute external trauma (rare)[9]
7. Decompression of polyhydramnios (rare)

TABLE 19-2

CONDITIONS ASSOCIATED WITH DISSEMINATED
INTRAVASCULAR COAGULATION

Obstetric	Either	Nonobstetric
Abruptio placentae	Prolonged shock of	Malignancy
Amniotic fluid	any cause	Extensive surgery
embolism	Transfusion of	Collagen vascular
Eclampsia and	incompatible	disease
severe preeclampsia	blood	Central nervous
Abortion with	Infection, especially	system trauma
hyperosmolar urea	with sepsis: bacterial,	Allergic reactions
or saline	viral, fungal, rickettsial,	Burns
Retained dead fetus	or protozoal	Vascular malformations
or missed abortion	(Most common in	Pancreatitis
Hydatidiform mole	obstetrics: septic abortion	Purpura fulminans
Retained placenta	or severe chorioam-	
(especially accreta)	nionitis/endometritis)	
Rupture of the uterus		
Significant feto-		
maternal hemorrhage		

From Main DM, Main EK: *Obstetrics and gynecology: a pocket reference,* St Louis, 1984, Mosby.

19

ANTEPARTUM HEMORRHAGE

D. RECURRENCE RATE. A 5% to 17% recurrence rate is noted after the first episode of abruption, and a 25% rate is seen after the second episode.[7] Subsequent episodes are usually more severe than the first.

E. PATHOPHYSIOLOGY. Maternal hemorrhage occurs in the decidua basalis. In most cases the source of the bleeding is small arterial vessels in the basal layer of the decidua that are pathologically prone to rupture. Infusion of thrombin-rich decidual tissue into the maternal circulation may result in disseminated intravascular coagulation (DIC). Variables affecting the extrinsic and common coagulation pathways influence the prothrombin time (PT), whereas variables affecting the intrinsic and common pathways influence the partial thromboplastin time (PTT) (Table 19-2 and Figs. 19-1 and 19-2).

F. PERINATAL MORBIDITY AND MORTALITY

1. Perinatal mortality is 4/1000, but with large retroplacental hemorrhages (>60 ml, >50%), fetal mortality may exceed 50%.[10]

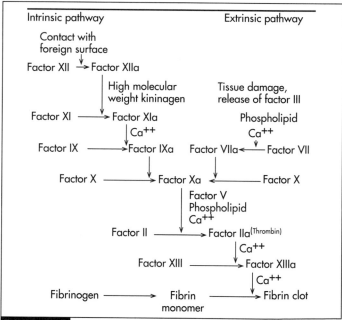

FIGURE 19-1

The intrinsic and extrinsic coagulation pathways and their convergence into a common pathway. (*Data from Lee GR et al: Clinical hematology, Philadelphia, 1993, Lea & Febiger.*)

2. Up to 40% of all fetal deaths resulting from abruptio placentae occur in gestations with fetuses alive at admission.
3. Neonatal deaths are associated with preterm birth, fetal asphyxia, and fetal exsanguination (rare).
4. Infants are often small for gestational age.
5. Congenital malformations (nonspecific) are increased two to five times more than in the general population for reasons unknown.

G. MATERNAL MORBIDITY AND MORTALITY

1. The most common complications are anemia, hemorrhage, shock, DIC, and Couvelaire uterus. As a result of hemorrhagic shock and hypotension, irreversible renal damage may occur. Although rare, uterine rupture may occur. Maternal mortality is not increased above that noted in the general pregnant population.
2. Spontaneous abortion occurs in 14% of future pregnancies.
3. Repeated abruption occurs in 9.3% of future pregnancies.

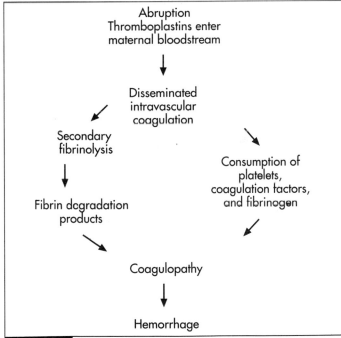

FIGURE 19-2
Pathogenesis of the coagulation disorder in abruptio placentae.

4. Rh sensitization may occur in Rh-negative mothers. Of patients with blood loss severe enough to require transfusion, 35% have evidence of fetal-maternal bleeding. Thus all Rh-negative patients should have a Kleihauer-Betke test performed and, if positive, be given 1 ampule (300 μg) of RhoGAM.

II. EVALUATION

A. **HISTORY.** Painful vaginal bleeding, usually associated with uterine contractions

B. **PHYSICAL EXAMINATION**

1. Majority of patients: external bleeding that is characteristically dark and nonclotting (occasionally serosanguineous)

2. Hypertonic frequent uterine contractions

3. Fetal distress

4. Tender uterus

5. Consideration of the diagnosis of uterine rupture if shock, diffuse abdominal pain, and tenderness are present (immediate laparotomy is indicated)

C. **DIAGNOSTIC DATA**

1. **Ultrasound** is useful to rule out placenta previa. Evidence of a retroplacental blood clot would confirm the diagnosis, especially in the minority of patients who have a concealed hemorrhage (Fig. 19-3). The presence of a clot found on ultrasound may not change management if the patient's condition is stable otherwise. Absence of a clot does not rule out abruption. An ultrasound may also be used to confirm fetal death.

2. **Complete blood cell count (CBC) with platelets and fibrinogen** and, if the possibility of DIC is present, consideration of PT, PTT, and fibrinogen degradation products testing. These six laboratory evaluations are often collectively called a **DIC panel.** Fibrinogen level and platelet count are good screening tests because other tests will not change until after the fibrinogen and platelet levels fall (Table 19-3).

3. An alum-precipitated toxoid (APT) test (Table 19-4) performed on the blood that is collected vaginally is often positive for fetal blood. A Kleihauer-Betke test of maternal venous blood also often reveals the presence of fetal blood cells. An acid elution of maternal venous blood is performed, and then a peripheral smear is made. Red blood cells (RBCs) with adult hemoglobin A are recognized as red cell ghosts (no hemoglobin within the membrane because it is soluble in acid), and the fetal RBCs remain intact, containing hemoglobin (fetal hemoglobin is less soluble). This test is usually performed by a trained technician, and, in reality, it is not routinely performed with vaginal bleeding unless a high level of clinical suspicion exists.

4. The minority of patients who have a concealed hemorrhage often present with uterine contractions nonresponsive to tocolysis.

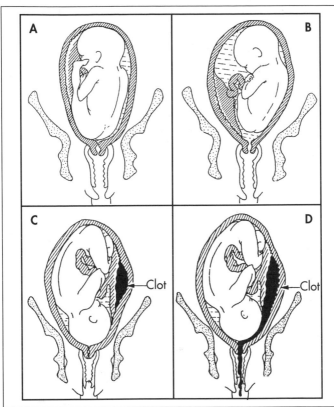

FIGURE 19-3

Placental abruption.   *(From Chamberlain G: BMJ 302[22]:1526, 1991.)*

5. A definitive diagnosis is made at the time of delivery, when gross inspection of the placenta reveals an organized or adherent clot lying within a cup-shaped depression on the maternal surface. This may not be noted if the abruption occurred recently.

D. A classification of abruptio placentae by severity is shown in Table 19-5.

E. The differential diagnosis includes **chorioamnionitis, appendicitis,** and **pyelonephritis.**

TABLE 19-3

COAGULATION STUDIES IN PLACENTAL ABRUPTION

Coagulation Study	What is Tested	Normal Value	Change Noted in Pregnancy
Fibrinogen	Fibrinogen level	400-650 mg/dl	Usually decreased
Fibrin degradation products	Fibrin and fibrinogen degradation products	$<10\ \mu g/ml$	Usually increased
Prothrombin time	Factors II, V, VII, and X (extrinsic and common pathways)	10-12 s	Normal to prolonged
Partial thromboplastin time	Factors II, V, XIII, IX, X, and XI (intrinsic and common pathways)	24-38 s	Normal to prolonged
Thrombin time	Factors I and II and circulating split-product heparin effect	16-20 s	Decreased, reflects fibrinogen change
Bleeding time	Vascular integrity and platelet function	1-5 min	Normal—no clinical value in abruption
Whole blood clotting time	Intrinsic and common pathways	Clot formation: 4-6 min	Abnormal clot formation indicates severe deficiency
	Platelet function	Retraction: <1 h	Abnormal retraction with thrombocytopenia
	Fibrinolytic activity	Lysis: none in 24 h	
Red blood cell morphology	Microangiopathic hemolysis	Absence of red blood cell distortion or fragmentation	Presence of distortion or fragmentation is uncommon but identifies a risk for renal cortical necrosis

III. THERAPEUTIC MANAGEMENT (FIG. 19-4)

A. MANAGEMENT OF PATIENT WITH A LIVING FETUS

1. Mild abruption with an immature fetus
   a. Observe on labor and delivery.
   b. When the conditions of the patient and the fetus are assessed to be stable, transfer the patient to the antepartum floor for long-term antepartum care (see section IVD).

TABLE 19-4

ALUM-PRECIPITATED TOXOID (APT) TEST FOR FETAL BLOOD

1. Mix 1 part bloody vaginal fluid with 5 to 10 parts tap water. Centrifuge for 2 min. Supernatant must be pink to proceed.
2. Take 5 parts supernatant and mix with 1 part 1% (0.25N) NaOH. Centrifuge for 2 min.
3. Interpretation: A pink color indicates fetal blood. A yellow-brown color indicates maternal blood. Adult oxyhemoglobin is less resistant to alkali than fetal oxyhemoglobin. During this reaction, adult oxyhemoglobin is converted to alkaline globin hematin.

ALTERNATIVE METHOD IF A CENTRIFUGE IS UNAVAILABLE:

1. Obtain blood from vaginal aspiration.
2. To 2 ml blood (10 drops), add 2 ml H_2O (10 drops) and 0.8 ml NaOH (5 drops).
3. Maternal blood will be brown.
4. Fetal blood remains red/pink.

From Main DM, Main EK: *Obstetrics and gynecology: a pocket reference,* St Louis, 1984, Mosby.

TABLE 19-5

CLASSIFICATION OF PLACENTAL ABRUPTION BY SEVERITY*

Clinical Signs	Classification		
	Mild	Moderate	Severe
Vaginal bleeding	Mild	Mild to moderate	Moderate to severe
Uterine tenderness	None	Slight	Marked
Uterine contractions	Irritable	Irritable vs. tetanic	Tetanic and painful
Vital signs	Stable	Tachycardia ± orthostatic blood pressure changes	Unstable
Fetal heart rate	Normal	± Distress	Distress/death
Coagulation studies	Normal	Fibrinogen: 150-250 mg/dl	Fibrinogen <150 mg/dl, platelets low, ± disseminated intravascular coagulation

*The clinical picture is often confusing, with some aspects consistent with one grade of abruption and other findings consistent with a different grade.

2. **Moderate abruption**
   a. Perform an amniotomy, and initiate an oxytocin induction if indicated (if no reason for a cesarean delivery exists).
   b. The patient with a moderate abruption has an excellent prospect for a vaginal delivery with good fetal and maternal outcomes.
   c. If the uterus becomes hypertonic during labor or if signs of fetal distress appear, assume extension of the abruption and deliver immediately, by cesarean delivery if necessary.

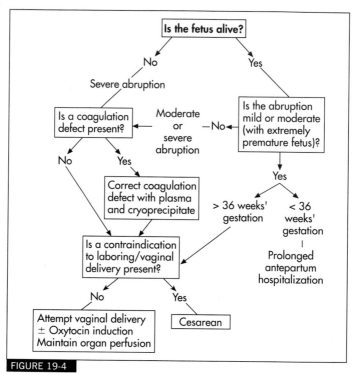

FIGURE 19-4

Management of abruptio placentae.

    d. If the baby is extremely premature, selective patients may be considered for transfusion and delayed delivery versus expectant management.

3. Severe abruption

    a. Type and cross 4 U of packed red blood cells (PRBCs).

    b. Prepare for a cesarean delivery unless special circumstances are present (maternal shock or previable fetus). A cesarean delivery should be performed only after the patient is in stable condition, with blood products infusing, even in the face of fetal distress.

    c. A severe abruption results in increased maternal mortality and morbidity.

B. MANAGEMENT OF PATIENT WITH SEVERE ABRUPTIO PLACENTAE AND FETAL DEATH

1. Initiate **blood transfusion,** preferably with fresh whole blood (or PRBCs as an alternative) (Tables 19-6 and 19-7).

TABLE 19-6

COMPARISON OF BLOOD REPLACEMENT PRODUCTS

Product	Hospital Costs ($)	Contents	Volume (ml)	Clinical Effect of Each Unit Volume Infused
Whole blood (WB)	95	Red blood cell (RBC) (2,3-DPG) White blood cell count (WBC) (not functional after 24 h) Coagulation factors (50%, V and VIII after 7 d) Plasma proteins	500	Increases intravenous volume by exact volume infused Increases hematocrit by 3%/500 ml infused
Packed red blood cells (PRBCs)	85	RBC: same as WB WBC: less than WB Plasma proteins—few	240	When compared to WB: • Same number of RBCs per unit volume (500 ml WB; 240 ml PRBCs); thus same increase in hematocrit of 3% per unit infused • Less risk of febrile reaction and WBC transfusion reaction
Platelets	51	55×10^6 platelets per unit, few WBCs, plasma	50	Increases platelet count by 5000-10,000/mm^3 per unit (of ~50 ml each) Give six packs minimum
Fresh frozen plasma	51	Clotting factors V and VIII, fibrinogen	250	Only source of factors V, XI, and XII Increases fibrinogen 10 mg/dl per unit infused
Cryoprecipitate	35	Factor VIII 25% fibrinogen, von Willebrand's factor	40	Increases fibrinogen 10 mg/dl per unit infused
Albumin 5%	70	Albumin	500	
Albumin 25%	40	Albumin	50	
Hespan (nonblood product)	45	Hespan, intravascular volume expander	500	Increases blood volume by amount corresponding to volume infused; usual volume infused: 500-1000 ml.

Modified from Gabbe SG, Niebyl JR, Simpson JL: *Obstetrics: normal and problem pregnancies*, New York, 1991, Churchill Livingstone.

ANTEPARTUM HEMORRHAGE

19

TABLE 19-7

MAJOR RISKS OF BLOOD TRANSFUSION

I. Blood products and the risk of hepatitis and human immunodeficiency virus (HIV)
   A. Each blood product unit (whole blood, packed red blood cells, platelets, fresh frozen plasma, platelets, cryoprecipitate) is from an individual donor.
   B. Each unit of blood product carries the following risks:
      1. Hepatitis B: 1/200,000
      2. Hepatitis C: 1/3300
      3. Human immunodeficiency virus (HIV): 1/225,000
      4. Human T-cell leukemia/lymphoma virus (HTLV-I/II): 1/50,000
      5. Cytomegalovirus (CMV): 1/20
      6. Immunologic reaction
         a. Fever or urticaria: 1/100
         b. Hemolytic (nonfatal): 1/25,000
         c. Hemolytic (fatal): <1/1,000,000
   C. Albumin is pooled from many donors; thus the risk of the above infections is multiplied many times for each unit administered.
II. Platelets
   A. Many hospitals are now offering plateletpheresis. This process allows a patient to receive 8 to 10 U of platelets from one donor, thus significantly decreasing the hepatitis and HIV infection risks in patients who require large infusions. The cost for 8 to 10 U of platelets obtained by plateletpheresis is $550.
   B. Each unit of platelets will raise the platelet count by about 10,000/mm³ in a normal individual. In the idiopathic thrombocytopenic purpura patient, the rise may be much less as a result of immune destruction of the transfused platelets.

---

2. Infuse adequate blood and crystalloid to **maintain Hct >30%** and **UO >30 ml/h.**
3. Send a **DIC panel;** the patient may have a consumptive coagulopathy.
   a. **Reevaluate for DIC after every 4 U of blood.**
   b. Of patients with abruptio placentae that is severe enough to kill a fetus, 38% have a plasma **fibrinogen** level <150 mg/dl, and 28% have a level <100 mg/dl.
   c. Screening for a clinically significant coagulopathy
      (1) Observe a 5-ml clot tube. If the blood fails to clot within 6 minutes or if the clot fails to retract and lyse within 2 hours, a marked coagulopathy is present. **Action, in terms of ordering appropriate replacement products, needs not await confirmatory tests.**
      (2) Strongly consider using fresh frozen plasma or cryoprecipitate (both take 60 minutes to prepare) to replace fibrinogen and clotting factors, especially if a cesarean delivery or an episiotomy is

performed. Transfuse adequate fresh frozen plasma or cryoprecipitate to achieve a fibrinogen level of 100 to 150 mg/dl. If platelets are needed, transfuse to a count of >100,000/mm^3.

(3) A vaginal delivery may be performed in the presence of very low clotting factors if unusual trauma is avoided.

d. Attempt a vaginal delivery of the fetus, regardless of fetal presentation, if the patient is in stable condition and no other obstetric indications for a cesarean delivery are present.

e. **Oxytocin induction.** If adequate spontaneous labor is not present, consider using oxytocin for induction or augmentation of labor according to hospital protocol.

f. If the maternal status is deteriorating despite blood product replacement, proceed to a cesarean delivery (the mother must be hemodynamically stable before surgery is performed). This should almost never be necessary.

g. After the fetus and placenta have been delivered, the coagulopathy will resolve within hours with appropriate blood replacement and maintenance of intravascular pressure.

h. Place a Foley catheter.

i. Start oxygen at 8 L/min via a nasal cannula.

j. If the UO is <30 ml/h or if the patient's hemodynamic status is unstable, consider placing a peripheral central venous pressure (CVP) line or central monitoring with a Swan-Ganz catheter. Normal values are CVP = 5 to 10 cm H_2O and pulmonary capillary wedge pressure = 3 to 10 mm Hg.

k. In cases of shock, place an arterial line to monitor the patient's blood pressure (BP).

PLACENTA PREVIA

I. BACKGROUND

A. DEFINITION

1. Placenta previa is classified according to the degree to which the os is covered by the placenta (Fig 19-5). This classification is based on ultrasound findings or a double setup examination.

   a. **Total (complete):** the internal os is completely covered by placental tissue. Total previas are further divided as to location of the dominant portion of the placenta (i.e., anterior, total, cervical).

   b. **Partial:** the internal os is partially covered by placental tissue.

   c. **Marginal:** the edge of the placenta is at the margin of the internal os but covers no portion of the os.

   d. **Lateral or low lying:** the edge of the placenta may be palpated by a finger introduced through the cervix.

2. The amount of **blood loss directly** correlates with the degree of previa

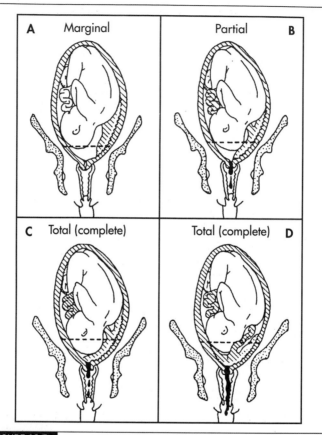

FIGURE 19-5

Placenta previa. *(From Chamberlain G: BMJ 302[22]:1527, 1991.)*

but not with the number of bleeding episodes or perinatal mortality. The origin of blood loss is presumed to be maternal.

B. ETIOLOGY

1. No specific cause has been identified.
2. Conditions associated with an increased prevalence of placenta previa
   a. Increased parity (It is thought that previous gestations permanently damage the endometrium, making every area of placental attachment unsuitable for placental attachment in subsequent pregnancies.)

   b. Closely spaced pregnancies
   c. Previous abortion
   d. Previous cesarean delivery[11]
   e. Multiple gestations
   f. Advanced maternal age
   g. Anemia
   h. Abnormal fetal presentation
   i. Congenital malformations
   j. Tumors that distort the contour of the uterus
   k. Endometritis
   l. Male fetus
   m. Smoking[12]

C. INCIDENCE
1. Incidence of placenta previa
   a. 1/250 pregnancies beyond 24 weeks' gestation[13]
   b. 1/1500 nulliparas
   c. 1/20 grand multiparas
2. Frequency of the different classes of placenta previa
   a. Total previa: 23% to 31%
   b. Partial previa: 21% to 33%
   c. Marginal previa: 37% to 55%
3. The incidence is affected by the **gestational age** at the time of diagnosis.
   a. The ultrasound diagnosis of placenta previa in the second trimester is 5%.[13]
   b. The ultrasound diagnosis of placenta previa at term is 0.5%. (The 90% conversion rate is thought to result from differential growth of the uterus.)[14]
   c. If an ultrasound at 26 to 28 weeks' gestation demonstrates placenta previa, the condition will most likely persist until the delivery, and thus the patient should be managed expectantly (i.e., pelvic rest, no heavy work).
4. The **recurrence rate** for placenta previa is 12 times the expected incidence.

D. PERINATAL MORBIDITY AND MORTALITY
1. Perinatal mortality is <10%.
2. Prematurity is the primary cause of perinatal morbidity and mortality. Increased perinatal mortality is associated with early bleeding, larger blood losses, and larger placenta previas (i.e., complete vs. marginal).
3. **Congenital malformations** (nonspecific) are two to four times more frequent in patients with placenta previa.

E. MATERNAL MORBIDITY AND MORTALITY
1. Maternal mortality is <1%.
2. Placenta accreta (placenta has grown into the myometrium) occurs in 5% of patients with placenta previa and in 24% of those with placenta previa and a prior cesarean delivery.[15] Treatment is a hysterectomy un-

19

ANTEPARTUM HEMORRHAGE

less the attachment is limited and the bleeding is controlled with local sutures.

3. Abruptio placentae recurs more frequently than in the general population (5% to 17% recurrence rate).

4. Rh sensitization may occur in Rh-negative mothers. Of patients with blood loss that is severe enough to require transfusion, 35% have evidence of fetal-to-maternal bleeding. Thus all Rh-negative patients should have a Kleihauer-Betke test performed and, if positive, should be given 1 ampule (300 μg) of RhoGAM.

5. DIC rarely occurs, and, when it does, it usually results from hemorrhagic shock or abruptio placentae.

6. Irreversible renal damage is rare but is the most common long-term complication of hemorrhagic shock and hypotension.

II. EVALUATION

A. CLINICAL PRESENTATION

1. **Vaginal bleeding** is usually painless and of sudden onset in the second or third trimester.
   a. The peak incidence is at 34 weeks' gestation; 65% of patients have their first bleeding after 30 weeks' gestation. No maternal fatality has been associated with the first bleeding episode (barring an inappropriate vaginal examination, which may result in a massive maternal hemorrhage).
      (1) Bleeding may begin without an obvious inciting cause (i.e., vaginal examination, intercourse, onset of labor). In these cases, it may be precipitated by formation of the lower uterine segment with consequent detachment of a portion of the placenta.
      (2) In 10% of cases, bleeding begins only with the onset of labor.

2. **Abnormal fetal presentations** are increased in the presence of placenta previa at the following rates:
   a. Breech, shoulder, and compound presentations occur in up to 35% of placenta previa cases.
   b. Of all transverse lies, 60% are associated with placenta previa.
   c. Of all breech and compound lies, 24% are associated with placenta previa.

B. DIAGNOSTIC EVALUATION

1. **Ultrasound** provides a 98% accuracy rate in localizing the placenta. In a small percentage of patients, ultrasound cannot unequivocally diagnose placenta previa. (In these patients, a double setup examination may be indicated.) This usually occurs beyond 32 weeks' gestation, when elevation of the presenting part is essential for obtaining adequate resolution.
   a. Areas of ultrasound confusion include a blood clot at the level of the internal os, the presence of a succenturiate lobe, or a thick "decidual reaction."

b. The diagnosis is confirmed by finding the placenta covering at least a portion of the cervix at the time of a double setup examination or cesarean delivery.

2. A **gentle speculum examination** should be performed for evaluation of the vagina and cervix on admission and intermittently as indicated.

III. MANAGEMENT OF PLACENTA PREVIA

A. MILD BLEEDING

1. If mature (>36 weeks' gestation), the fetus should be delivered.
2. In the patient whose fetus is <36 weeks' gestation with a mature lung profile, whose bleeding ceases, and who has no need for transfusion, delaying delivery should be considered.
3. If the fetal lungs are immature, the patient may receive long-term antepartum care.

B. MODERATE HEMORRHAGE. When the acute bleeding episode has subsided and the maternal condition has stabilized, evaluate fetal lung maturity for all gestations between 32 and 36 weeks. Assume pulmonary immaturity if the gestation is <32 weeks, and assume maturity if the gestation is >36 weeks.

1. **Mature.** Deliver immediately.
2. **Immature**
   a. Provide intensive care on labor and delivery for the first 24 to 48 hours. Maintain Hb ≥10 g/dl (Hct ≥30). Consider using steroids to accelerate fetal lung maturation.
   b. Give $MgSO_4$ for tocolysis if the uterus is irritable or if preterm labor develops.[13]
   c. If the patient's condition remains unstable with steady moderate blood loss, or if the patient requires more than 2 U of blood in 24 hours, deliver.
   d. If the patient's condition becomes stable and remains so for 24 to 48 hours, she is a candidate for long-term antepartum care. Most patients fit into this category.

C. SEVERE HEMORRHAGE

1. Place **two large-bore IV lines,** one for lactated Ringer's solution and the second for blood.
2. Blood samples to be drawn on admission include the following:
   a. DIC panel (CBC, PT, PTT, platelets, fibrinogen, fibrinogen degradation products).
   b. Type and crossmatch for 4 U of PRBCs.
   c. If necessary, start infusing **O-negative blood** immediately. Keep the blood bank informed of the patient's status. Infuse **type-specific** blood as soon as it is available.
   d. Type-specific blood takes 15 to 30 minutes to prepare.
   e. A complete crossmatch requires 45 to 60 minutes to prepare if no major antibodies are found.
   f. Keep **4 U of PRBCs** available at all times.

g. Fresh whole blood, platelets, and cryoprecipitate (rarely) may be necessary.

3. Place a Foley catheter and treat a decreased UO aggressively, maintaining UO $\geq$30 ml/h. Hydrate the patient adequately. Later, if indicated, give a 20- to 60-mg bolus of furosemide (Lasix). Hypovolemic shock may result in acute tubular and cortical necrosis.

4. Consider placing a peripheral **CVP** or a central **Swan-Ganz** catheter for accurate assessment of fluid status.

5. Perform an ultrasound for gestational dating.

6. Perform a cesarean delivery.

IV. LONG-TERM ANTEPARTUM CARE

A. PATIENT SELECTION. Patients with proved fetal pulmonary immaturity and those with gestations $\leq$36 weeks, stable vital signs, and resolution of bleeding are eligible.

B. CONTINUOUS HOSPITALIZATION. Hospitalization for a minimum of 72 hours is advised because nearly one third of all patients with placenta previa who are initially selected for expectant management require delivery within this time.

C. ORDERS FOR THE FLOOR

1. Bed rest with bathroom privileges

2. Stool softeners

3. Prenatal vitamins, $FeSO_4$

4. Laboratory tests
   a. Hb obtained weekly; keep Hb $\geq$10 g/dl
   b. For patients with placenta previa, type and hold 2 U of PRBCs. Have this available at all times. Blood specimens for type and hold will probably need to be drawn every 2 to 3 days.

5. Antepartum testing if indicated

6. Daily uterine monitoring if indicated

D. Perform an amniocentesis for fetal pulmonary studies at 36 weeks' gestation, and, if fetal lungs are immature, repeat every 7 to 10 days. When fetal lungs are mature, the patient with placenta previa should be scheduled for a cesarean delivery.

E. If the patient has had no further bleeding and the following are true, she may go home at strict bed and pelvic rest[16] after being observed for 72 hours on the antepartum floor:

1. She lives within 15 minutes of the hospital.

2. She has a responsible adult who will be at home with her.

3. The companion has access to an automobile at all times.

VASA PREVIA

A. DEFINITION. Umbilical vessels insert velamentously in a low-lying placenta and traverse the membranes in front of the fetal presenting part (Fig. 19-6).

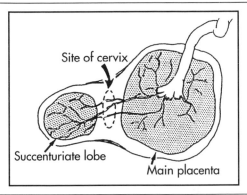

FIGURE 19-6

Vasa previa. *(From Chamberlain G: BMJ 302[22]:1530, 1991.)*

B. PATHOLOGY. The vessels are not protected by Wharton's jelly.
C. INCIDENCE
1. Vasa previa occurs in 0.1% to 1.8% of all pregnancies, with the trend toward the lower end of this range.[16]
2. Singletons: 0.25% to 1.25%
3. Twins: 6% to 10%
4. Triplets: 95%
D. PERINATAL MORTALITY. It is >50%, resulting from a vasa previa tear or rupture with resultant fetal exsanguination. Compression of the fetal vessels by the presenting part may cause hypoxia and eventual death.
E. DIAGNOSIS
1. Painless vaginal bleeding is common but not mandatory for the diagnosis.
2. Diagnosis of fetal bleeding
   a. Examination of blood for nucleated RBCs, normoblasts
   b. Hemoglobin electrophoresis (takes 60 minutes)
   c. APT test (Table 19-4)
3. Fetal distress is a common presentation. Frequently seen fetal heart rate patterns include sinusoidal changes, tachycardia, late decelerations, or prolonged decelerations.
F. TREATMENT. Treatment is an emergent cesarean delivery.

SUMMARY

Relationship of signs and treatment modalities to differential diagnosis is shown in Table 19-8.

TABLE 19-8

RELATIONSHIP OF SIGNS AND TREATMENT MODALITIES TO
DIFFERENTIAL DIAGNOSIS

Signs and Treatment Modalities	Differential Diagnosis		
	Placenta Previa	Abruptio Placentae	Vasa Previa
Pain with uterine contractions	No	Yes	No
Tender uterus	No	Yes	No
Primary danger	Mother	Fetus/mother	Fetus
Blood	Maternal	Maternal	Fetal
Ultrasound helpful	Yes	Maybe	Yes
Cesarean mandatory	Yes	No	Yes

REFERENCES

1. Creasy RK, Resnik R: *Maternal-fetal medicine: principles and practice,* ed 3, Philadelphia, 1994, Saunders.
2. Gorodeski IG, Bahari CM: The effect of placenta previa localization upon maternal and fetalneonatal outcome, *J Perinat Med* 16:169-177, 1987.
3. Naeye R, Harkness WL, Utts J: Abruptio placentae and perinatal death: a prospective study, *Am J Obstet Gynecol* 28:740, 1977.
4. Torrey EW: Vasa previa, *Am J Obstet Gynecol* 63:146, 1952.
5. Sirivongs B: Vasa previa report of 3 cases, *J Med Assoc Thai* 57:261, 1974.
6. Blair RG: Abruption of placenta: a review of 189 cases occurring between 1965 and 1969, *Br J Obstet Gynaecol* 80:242, 1973.
7. Pritchard J: The genesis of severe placental abruption, *Am J Obstet Gynecol* 208:22, 1970.
8. Hibbard BM, Jeffcoate TNA: Abruptio placentae, *Obstet Gynecol* 27:155, 1966.
9. Kettel ML, Branch W, Scott JR: Occult placental abruption after maternal trauma. II, *Obstet Gynecol* 71(3):449-453, 1988.
10. Gabbe SG, Niebyl JR, Simpson JL: *Obstetrics: normal and problem pregnancies,* ed 2, New York, 1991, Churchill Livingstone.
11. Taylor VM et al: Placenta previa and prior cesarean delivery: how strong is the association? *Obstet Gynecol* 84(1):55-58, 1994.
12. Handler AS et al: The relationship between exposure during pregnancy to cigarette smoking and cocaine use and placenta previa, *Am J Obstet Gynecol* 170(3):884-890, 1994.
13. Cotton DB et al: The conservative aggressive management of placenta previa, *Am J Obstet Gynecol* 137(6):687, 1980.
14. Rizos N, Doran T, Miskin M: Natural history of placenta previa ascertained by diagnostic ultrasound, *Am J Obstet Gynecol* 133:287, 1979.
15. Clark SL, Koonings PP, Phelan JP: Placenta previa/accreta and prior cesarean section, *Obstet Gynecol* 66(1):89-92, 1985.
16. Droste S, Keil K: Expectant management of placenta previa: cost-benefit analysis of outpatient treatment. I, *Am J Obstet Gynecol* 170(5):1254-1257, 1994.

VENOUS THROMBOEMBOLISM IN PREGNANCY

I. BACKGROUND

A. DEFINITION. Thromboembolism is the obstruction of a blood vessel by material carried within the bloodstream from a different site of origin. Thromboembolism in pregnancy is subdivided into two categories:

1. Venous thromboembolism (VTE)

2. Pulmonary embolism (PE)

VTE and PE have similar diagnostic work-ups and treatments. This chapter addresses both these problems in pregnancy when the etiology is of hematologic product origin.

20

B. ETIOLOGY. The increased incidence of VTE and PE during gestation is due to biochemical and physical changes during pregnancy that promote coagulation. These changes, which are related to prevention of hemorrhage during delivery, include the following:

1. Biochemical factors
   a. Increased plasma concentration of coagulation
   b. Increased plasma concentration of fibrinolysis inhibitors (protein S, protein C, antithrombin III)
   c. Increased plasma concentration of procoagulants

2. Physiologic factors
   a. Venous dilation
   b. Obstruction of venous system by gravid uterus

3. Activated protein C resistance (APC-R; factor V [Leiden]) has been implicated in up to 60% of thromboembolic complications of pregnancy. APC-R is an autosomal dominantly inherited mutation of factor V present in up to 5.2% of Northern European descendants (much less common in the Asian American and African American populations: 0.4% and 1.2%, respectively). The specific mutation substitutes a glutamine for arginine at position 506. In those individuals with this mutation, factor V still functions as a procoagulant protein but is rendered resistant to degradation by activated protein C. APC-R has also been associated with an increase of preeclampsia, fetal loss, intrauterine growth restriction (IUGR), and placental infarction.[1,2]

C. INCIDENCE. Thromboembolic complications occur in only approximately 1/1000 to 2/10,000 pregnancies but are the most common cause of maternal death.[3] This incidence is increased twofold to threefold further in the puerperium. The overall risk is six times greater in pregnancy than in the nonpregnant state. The following factors predispose patients to VTE in pregnancy and the puerperium:

1. Increased maternal age

2. Operative delivery

3. Bed rest

4. Obesity
5. Immobilization in general
6. Malignancy
7. Dehydration
8. Previous VTE
9. Blood group other than O
10. Caucasian race
11. Sickle cell disease
12. Thrombophilia syndrome (Table 20-1)

D. **PERINATAL MORBIDITY AND MORTALITY.** The majority of fetal morbidity and mortality is related to maternal treatment. Warfarin has been associated with a number of congenital defects. With fetal exposure occurring in the first 6 to 9 weeks of gestation, warfarin embryopathy may result. Characteristic features of this syndrome include nasal hypoplasia, depression of the bridge of the nose, and epiphyseal stippling. Thirty percent of these babies will be mentally retarded. Exposure to warfarin during the second and third trimesters results in an increased incidence of central nervous system (CNS) abnormalities (including agenesis of the corpus callosum), ophthalmologic abnormalities (including optic atrophy), and microcephaly. Many of the CNS abnormalities are thought to be a result of recurrent intracranial hemorrhage. A safer alternative is heparin, which does not cross the placenta and has been shown to be free of any adverse effects on the fetus.

E. **MATERNAL MORBIDITY AND MORTALITY**
1. Mortality secondary to PE occurs in 1/100,000 pregnancies. Thirteen percent of untreated patients will die, making it the leading cause of maternal mortality. Patients who recover from the PE usually have no residual effects.

TABLE 20-1

THROMBOPHILIA SYNDROME

One or more of the following may be present:
1. A deficiency (inherited or acquired) in one of the following:
   a. Antithrombin III
   b. Protein S
   c. Protein C
2. Activated protein C resistance (Leiden factor V)
3. Hemoglobinuria
4. Paroxysmal homocystinuria
5. Antiphospholipid antibodies
   a. Anticardiolipin
   b. Lupus anticoagulant

2. VTE damages the valves of the vein, resulting in venous insufficiency that can range from mild edema to skin ulceration.
3. Heparin side effects are greatest in those receiving unfractionated heparin but still may occur in those treated with low–molecular-weight (LMW) heparin. The following side effects are seen primarily:
   (a) Thrombocytopenia (occurs in 2% treated with unfractionated heparin)
   (b) Osteopenia (may occur in those who receive >20,000 U/d for >3 months)

F. DIFFERENTIAL DIAGNOSIS
1. PE
   a. Pneumonia
   b. Asthma
   c. Pleurodynia
   d. Pleuritis
   e. Musculoskeletal
   f. Hyperventilation syndrome
   g. Myocardiopathy

2. VTE
   a. Muscle strain or injury
   b. Lymphatic obstruction
   c. Venous reflux
   d. Baker's cyst
   e. Cellulitis
   f. Internal abnormality

II. EVALUATION

A. HISTORY. Identify the patient's risk factors other than pregnancy for VTE. Inquire specifically about family history, as well as whether the patient has been traveling (and thus has been immobile for a prolonged period) or experienced any recent trauma. Patients with a PE often appear anxious and complain of a cough, palpitations, or lightheadedness.

B. PHYSICAL EXAMINATION
1. **PE:** Tachypnea is present in 90% of patients with PE. Other significant findings include dystonia, tachycardia, diaphoresis, wheezing or rales, and hypotension (see Table 20-2 for additional signs and symptoms).
2. **VTE:** The patient may present with pain and swelling without a recent history of travel or trauma. Occasionally hard veins may be palpated. Patients may also be asymptomatic and progress to symptomatic PE if untreated.

C. DIAGNOSTIC DATA. An initial laboratory work-up should include an **antithrombin III, PT** (prothrombin time), and **PTT** (partial thromplastin time). In addition:
1. **PE:** Tests may include **ABG** (arterial blood gas), **CXR** (chest x-ray), **ECG** (electrocardiogram) and **ventilation-perfusion (V̇/Q̇) scan.** How-

TABLE 20-2

SYMPTOMS AND SIGNS IN 117 PATIENTS WITH ACUTE PULMONARY
EMBOLISM WITHOUT PREEXISTING CARDIAC OR PULMONARY DISEASE

Symptoms	Patients (%)	Signs	Patients (%)
Dyspnea	73	Tachypnea (≥20 respirations per minute)	70
Pleuritic pain	66	Rales (crackles)	51
Cough	37	Tachycardia (>100/bpm)	30
Leg swelling	28	Fourth heart sound	24
Leg pain	26	Increased pulmonary component of second sound	23
Hemoptysis	13		
Palpitations	10	Deep venous thrombosis	11
Wheezing	9	Diaphoresis	11
Angina-like pain	4	Temperature >38.5°C	7
		Wheezes	5
		Homans' sign	4
		Right ventricular lift	4
		Pleural friction rub	3
		Third heart sound	3
		Cyanosis	1

Modified from Stein PD et al: *Chest* 100:598, 1991.

ever, **pulmonary arteriography** (0.05 rad of fetal exposure) should be considered the gold standard. An ABG less than 85 mm Hg is suspicious yet nonspecific. An S1Q3T3 pattern on ECG is specific but present in less than 10% of patients with a PE. The patient's CXR may show nonspecific findings, including atelectasis, pleural effusion, parenchymal densities, or an elevated hemidiaphragm. Use of pulmonary arteriography may show a filling defect representing the clot. In addition, a ventilation/perfusion scan (0.01 and 0.015 rads, respectively of exposure to the fetus) is useful to determine if a V̇/Q̇ mismatch is present (Table 20-3). A mismatch, however, may represent any disease process that alters perfusion, including pneumonia, atelectasis, or a tumor.

2. **VTE**

   a. **Ultrasound with Doppler flow** is the first diagnostic procedure that should be performed when this diagnosis is strongly suspected. With this imaging modality, the clot may be visualized or decreased flow appreciated. Ultrasound does not work well above the inguinal region or in the calf. If an ultrasound appears to be inadequate, consider a **venogram** (which may show a filling defect). **Impedance plethysmography's** sensitivity and specificity are also poor for calf deep venous thromboses (DVTs) but high for proximal DVTs. This objective test is used infrequently because of Doppler sonography's superiority in noninvasive diagnostic accuracy.

TABLE 20-3

COMPARISON OF SCAN CATEGORY WITH ANGIOGRAPHIC FINDINGS

Scan Category	Pulmonary Embolism Present	Pulmonary Embolism Absent	Pulmonary Embolism Uncertain	No Angiogram	Total No.
High probability	102	14	1	7	124
Intermediate probability	105	217	9	33	364
Low probability	39	199	12	62	312
Near-normal/normal	5	50	2	74	131
TOTAL	251	480	24	176	931

From PIOPED Investigators: *JAMA* 263:2753-2759, 1990.

20

VENOUS THROMBOEMBOLISM IN PREGNANCY

b. **Venography** remains the gold standard for diagnosis of DVT. To perform this test, a vein on the dorsum of the foot is cannulated, and then dye is injected through this port. This process is moderately painful. An intraluminal filling defect seen in many projections diagnoses DVT.

c. **D-dimer,** measured by running a blood sample through an enzyme-linked immunosorbent assay (ELISA) assay or a latex agglutination assay, has a significant negative predictive value. A normal ultrasound and D-dimer virtually exclude DVT from the diagnosis.

III. THERAPEUTIC MANAGEMENT

If the clinical picture is highly suggestive of a thromboembolic complication, *therapy may be initiated without definitive test results.*

A. Acute treatment options for PE include **heparin** therapy as detailed in C below, thrombolytic therapy, and inferior vena cava (IVC) interruption.[4] **Thrombolytic therapy** is used to speed the reduction of the thromboembolic burden. Agents used include streptokinase, urokinase, and recombinant tissue plasminogen activator (tPA). In patients who cannot receive anticoagulants, consultation with a vascular surgeon is needed. Surgical **IVC filter** placement may be necessary in these patients.

B. Hemodynamic management[5] will be necessary when hypotension and severe hypoxemia result from massive PE. See Figure 20-1 for care.

C. HEPARIN THERAPY[6-8]

1. Acute therapy

a. This is often initiated with continuous IV administration of heparin followed by a maintenance dose (totaling 40,000 U of heparin over 24 hours). Dosing in this range is continued for 7 days.

b. Therapeutic levels are considered a doubled PTT (INR >2.0) or a heparin level of 0.8 to 1 U/ml as measured by protamine-sulfate neutralization test.

c. Check platelet levels approximately twice weekly in the first 2 weeks of treatment. After this, they may be checked one or two times per month or more frequently if indicated.

d. Heparins, including the LMW forms, are large uncharged molecules that *do not cross* the placenta or cause any known fetal problems.

2. Chronic prophylactic therapy in high-risk women should follow acute therapy.

a. Standard heparin doses are 10,000 U SC bid. The goal is to maintain heparin's effect without altering the PTT.

b. LMW heparin can be given SC once daily and is considered an acceptable alternative to standard heparin.

c. Osteoporosis may occur in those individuals receiving more than 20,000 U/d SC for more than 3 months. Preliminary studies suggest that LMW heparin might carry a lower risk of osteoporosis than preparations used before this time. It is currently seen in 1 of 100 patients treated (up to 2% more may have a vertebral fracture). Ter-

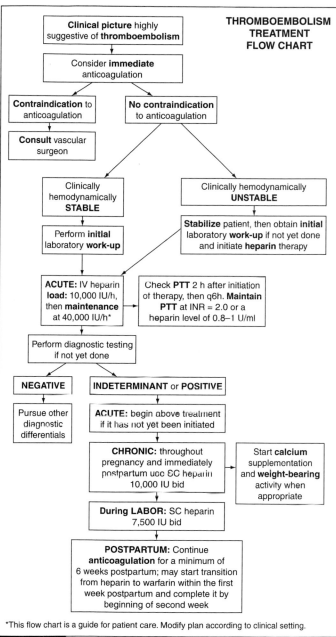

THROMBOEMBOLISM TREATMENT FLOW CHART

Clinical picture highly suggestive of **thromboembolism**

Consider **immediate** anticoagulation

Contraindication to anticoagulation

Consult vascular surgeon

No contraindication to anticoagulation

Clinically hemodynamically **STABLE**

Clinically hemodynamically **UNSTABLE**

Stabilize patient, then obtain **initial** laboratory **work-up** if not yet done and initiate **heparin** therapy

Perform **initial** laboratory **work-up**

ACUTE: IV heparin **load:** 10,000 IU/h, then **maintenance** at 40,000 IU/h*

Check **PTT** 2 h after initiation of therapy, then q6h. **Maintain PTT** at INR = 2.0 or a heparin level of 0.8–1 U/ml

Perform diagnostic testing if not yet done

NEGATIVE

Pursue other diagnostic differentials

INDETERMINANT or **POSITIVE**

ACUTE: begin above treatment if it has not yet been initiated

CHRONIC: throughout pregnancy and immediately postpartum use SC heparin 10,000 IU bid

Start **calcium** supplementation and **weight-bearing** activity when appropriate

During LABOR: SC heparin 7,500 IU bid

POSTPARTUM: Continue **anticoagulation** for a minimum of 6 weeks postpartum; may start transition from heparin to warfarin within the first week postpartum and complete it by beginning of second week

*This flow chart is a guide for patient care. Modify plan according to clinical setting.

FIGURE 20-1

Thromboembolism treatment flow chart.

mination of therapy usually causes these reversible changes to spontaneously regress.

    d. Precaution to avoid bleeding is to be taken during anticoagulation. Specifically advise patients as to the following:

        (1) Brush teeth gently.

        (2) Avoid use of nonsteroidal antiinflammatory drugs (NSAIDs), which will decrease platelet activity and further increase risk for hemorrhage.

        (3) If emergency surgery is needed, rapid reversal of heparin's effects can be achieved using protamine sulfate.

3. During **labor** SC heparin should be decreased to approximately 7500 U bid. Anticoagulation treatment should continue for at least 6 weeks postpartum. At 1 week postpartum the patient may be switched to warfarin. Neither warfarin nor heparin is found in breast milk. In addition, it has been found that individual responses to heparin are highly variable during pregnancy, and prophylactic doses may need to be increased. Therefore it is important to monitor heparin levels closely until a therapeutic dose is found.

IV. AFTER RECOVERY AND TREATMENT FOR VTE

Discuss these points with your patients:

A. Increased risk for future thromboembolic event

B. APC-R gene testing for certain high-risk populations

C. Lifestyle modification to avoid high-risk activities: encourage women to get out and stretch for 15 minutes intermittently during long car trips, and encourage mild physical activity

I would like to acknowledge the assistance of Nicole Nilson, a third-year medical student at the Universary of Colorado School of Medicine, for her assistance in preparing this chapter.

REFERENCES

1. Hooper CW, Evatt BL: The role of activated protein C resistance in the pathogenesis of venous thrombosis, *Am J Med Sci* 316(2):120-128, 1998.
2. Hellgren M, Svensson PJ, Dahlback B: Resistance to activated protein C as a basis for venous thromboembolism associated with pregnancy and oral contraceptives, *Am J Obstet Gynecol* 173(1):210-213, 1995.
3. Tegborn L et al: Recurrent thromboembolism in pregnancy and puerperium, *Am J Obstet Gynecol* 160(1):90-94, 1989.
4. Clark SL et al: *Critical care obstetrics,* Malden, Mass, 1997, Braun-Brumfield.
5. James DK et al: *High risk pregnancy: management options,* ed 2, Philadelphia, 1999, Saunders.
6. Barbour LA, Smith JM, Marlar RA: Heparin levels to guide thromoembolism prophylaxis during pregnancy, *Am J Obstet Gynecol* 173(6):1869-1873, 1995.
7. Bennett JC, Plum F: *Cecil textbook of medicine,* ed 20, Philadelphia, 1996, Saunders.
8. Goldman L, Bennett JC: *Cecil textbook of medicine,* ed 21, Philadelphia, 2000, Saunders.

PREGNANCY LOSS: SPONTANEOUS ABORTION AND STILLBIRTHS

Pregnancy loss is an unfortunate occurrence. Many losses occur preclinically (before a missed menstrual cycle), whereas the majority of clinically recognized pregnancies are lost in the first trimester. Spontaneous abortion rates increase with advancing maternal age (women over 40 years old have twice the likelihood of experiencing fetal loss as women in their 20s). Even in couples with recurrent losses, the overall prognosis for a live-born infant is 60% to 70%.[1]

21

I. PRECLINICAL LOSSES

A. **DEFINITION.** Spontaneous abortion is a pregnancy loss before 5 to 6 weeks after the last menstrual period (LMP), as detected by β-human chorionic gonadotropin (hCG) assays performed 28 to 35 days after the previous menses.

B. **INCIDENCE.** When 40% to 60% of all pregnancies are lost, 30% to 40% are a result of preclinical losses and 10% to 20% are a result of clinical losses.[2]

C. **ETIOLOGY**

1. Morphologic abnormalities of embryos

2. Chromosomal abnormalities are noted in 25% of in-vitro fertilized embryos.[3] This is thought to result in morphologically normal and abnormal embryos and to be the primary cause of all preclinical losses. Autosomal monosomy is unviable, and most monosomies are noted to abort around implantation. Trisomies generally survive only until just after implantation.[4,5]

II. FIRST-TRIMESTER LOSSES

A. **DEFINITION.** Clinical loss through 13 completed weeks of pregnancy.

B. **INCIDENCE.** Of clinically recognized pregnancies, 12% are lost in the first trimester. Studies with ultrasound demonstrate that fetal viability ceases weeks before maternal symptoms occur; thus fetuses aborting clinically at 10 to 12 weeks' gestation usually died weeks before.[6] A recent study of 232 pregnancies observed with ultrasound demonstrated that embryonic losses occured by 8.5 weeks' gestation, no losses occurred between 8.5 and 14 weeks' gestation, and 2% were lost after 14 weeks' gestation. This suggests that early pregnancy loss is complete by the end of the embryonic period (70 days after the woman's LMP).[7]

C. ETIOLOGY

1. Chromosomal abnormalities
   a. **Autosomal trisomy** is responsible for 53% of all chromosomal abnormalities (in this group, chromosome 1 is the only chromosome not to demonstrate a trisomy; trisomy 16 is the most frequent). Maternal age increases the rate of most trisomies. Double trisomy is lethal.
   b. **Polyploidy** (the presence of more than two haploid chromosomal complements) usually is seen as triploidy (69,XXY or 69,XXX). Polyploidy pregnancies are rare and usually only progress to 2 to 3 weeks embryologically.
   c. **Monosomy X** is responsible for 15% to 20% of chromosomal abnormalities and is the single most common chromosomal abnormality. It is usually caused by the loss of the paternal sex chromosome.
   d. **Structural rearrangements** are found in 1.5% of all aborted fetuses. These may arise de novo, or they may be inherited. They are not a common cause of sporadic losses but are important in recurrent abortions.
   e. **Sex chromosomal polysomy:** 47,XXY or 47,XYY occurs in 1/800 male births; 47,XXX occurs in 1/800 female births. These polysomies are only slightly more common in abortuses (noted in 0.6% of abortus specimens and 1.3% of chromosomally abnormal abortuses).

2. Neural tube defects and other polygenic or multifactorial traits are responsible for a large number of the other abortuses.

3. Luteal phase defects (LPDs), or a hypothesized progesterone deficiency that might fail to prepare the estrogen-primed uterine lining for implantation, may potentially be caused by decreased gonadotropin-releasing hormone, decreased follicle-stimulating hormone, inadequate luteinizing hormone, inadequate ovarian steroidogenesis, and endometrial receptor defects.[8] It is thought that LPDs may occur in up to 35% of women with recurrent pregnancy loss.

4. Infections: *Variola vaccinia, Salmonella typhi, Vibrio fetus, Listeria,*[9] malaria, cytomegalovirus, *Brucella, Toxoplasma, Mycoplasma hominis, Chlamydia trachomatis,* and *Ureaplasma urealyticum* are all associated with fetal wastage,[10,11] but definitive data proving cause and effect are lacking for almost all. Transplacental infection occurs with many of these organisms, and thus losses may occur. *U. urealyticum* is the most commonly implicated organism in recurrent abortions.

5. Irradiation: diagnostic radiographs (<10 rads [see Appendix E]) place a patient at no increased risk.

6. Chemotherapy administered for medical indications can cause embryonic loss. Medical personnel should avoid exposure to chemotherapeutic agents, even though exposure doses are much lower than therapeutic ones. Some of these agents are known abortifacients.

7. Cigarette smoking during pregnancy is associated with increased abortion rates of normal karyotype fetuses.

8. Caffeine intake >150 mg/d is inconsistently associated with increased fetal loss rates.[12]

9. Consumption of alcoholic drinks twice weekly has been associated with an increased miscarriage rate in some studies but not in others.[13-15]

10. Environmental chemicals associated with fetal loss are anesthetic gases, arsenic, aniline, benzene, ethylene oxide, formaldehyde, and lead.[16,17] Video display terminals do *not* appear to cause fetal wastage.

11. Maternal illness caused by a debilitating disease rarely causes abortion.

D. EVALUATION

1. History: the patient has a history of uterine contractions, bleeding, and passage of tissue. Inquire as to any history of pregnancy loss as well as pelvic surgery, chemical exposure (i.e., smoking, alcohol use), or presence of any known medical illnesses.

2. Examination: a full examination should be performed. On pelvic examination, check for opening of the cervical os, lesions of the cervix and vagina, size of the uterus, and size and tenderness of the adnexa.

3. Diagnostic data: if bleeding has been heavy, a blood count is indicated. All patients must have their Rh status documented. Ultrasound, if available, may be used to assess fetal viability.

4. Differential diagnosis includes ectopic pregnancy, threatened abortion, inevitable abortion, complete abortion, red degeneration of fibroid uterus, or lesion of the cervix (e.g., polyp) or the vagina.

E. THERAPEUTIC MANAGEMENT

1. **Threatened abortion** (i.e., os closed or bleeding and cramping present). Studies do not demonstrate that conservative management (i.e., bed rest and pelvic rest) affects outcome, although many physicians recommend these measures because of empiric common sense.

   a. Consider evaluation of serial quantitative β-hCG.

   b. Administer 1 ampule (300 μg; this covers up to 30 ml of Rh-positive blood or 15 ml of red blood cells)[18] RhoGAM if the patient is Rh negative. If gestation is <13 weeks, the physician may administer only 50 μg (minidose) of RhoGAM (the total blood volume of a first-trimester gestation is less than 2.5 ml).[19]

2. An **inevitable abortion** is present when a patient presents with bleeding and cramping and examination demonstrates an open cervical os and a viable fetus within the uterine cavity. Discuss the option of elective dilation and curettage (D&C) versus expectant management. The decision is primarily based on the degree of bleeding and cramping and the patient's emotional status. Tissue should be sent to the pathology department for documentation of products of conception (see section IIE3 for additional management considerations).

3. **Incomplete abortion.** Part of the fetus or placenta is retained within the uterus.
   a. Perform suction and sharp D&C.
   b. Check blood count if bleeding is heavy.
   c. Administer RhoGAM (300 μg for gestations >13 weeks, 50 μg for gestations <13 weeks) if the patient is Rh negative.
   d. Consider methylergonovine (Methergine; 200 μg orally every 6 hours for six doses) if bleeding is heavy.
   e. Consider providing a narcotic or nonsteroidal antiinflammatory prescription for pain relief.
   f. If this is the patient's second or third spontaneous abortion (SAB), consider sending tissue for karyotyping (place specimen in normal saline).
   g. Provide resources for emotional support.
   h. Counsel patient as to frequency of fetal wastage (10% to 20% of clinically recognized pregnancies) and its etiologies.
4. **Complete abortion.** The entire contents of the uterus have been spontaneously expelled (see section IIE3b-f).
5. A **missed abortion** (an embryonic gestation) should be suspected when the uterus fails to enlarge on subsequent examinations and symptoms of pregnancy may regress. A collapsed gestational sac and lack of fetal heart motion may be seen on ultrasound. Treat as detected in section IIE3.
6. **Recurrent abortion**
   a. Evaluation is usually indicated after three SABs and considered after two, based on the patient's age and desires.
   b. Obtain **karyotyping of patient and partner** (antenatal chromosomal studies should be offered if a balanced chromosomal rearrangement is detected in either parent).
   c. **Karyotype** abortus. Trisomic tissue suggests that recurrent aneuploidy may be occurring.
   d. Perform **a late luteal phase biopsy** to exclude an LPD. The diagnosis is made by histologic dating demonstrating an endometrium 2 or more days less than expected. Progesterone therapy (25-mg suppository intravaginally, twice daily, starting from midcycle for 6 to 8 weeks) may be indicated (inform the patient of unproven efficacy), or consider using clomiphene citrate.
   e. Check **a thyroid panel and fasting blood sugar.** Endocrine causes other than poorly controlled diabetes are unlikely etiologies of recurrent abortion.
   f. **Culture** the endometrium for *U. urealyticum,* or consider empiric treatment for the couple with doxycycline (250 mg twice daily for 10 days).
   g. If the abortion occurred after ultrasound documentation of fetal viability (7 to 10 weeks' gestation), obtain a **hysterosalpingogram** or perform hysteroscopy to rule out a uterine anomaly or submucosal leiomyoma.

h. Consider obtaining a **lupus anticoagulant** (LAC) and **anticardiolipin antibody** (ACA) to exclude autoimmune disease. The role of **autoimmune diseases** in first-trimester SABs is not well documented; however it is currently being investigated. No consensus has occurred on evaluation and treatment for antisperm antibodies and other antibodies.

i. Encourage cessation of smoking and of alcohol and caffeine consumption.

III. EARLY SECOND-TRIMESTER LOSSES

A. DEFINITION. Fetal loss between 14 and 20 weeks' gestation.

B. INCIDENCE. Of clinical pregnancies, 5% result in early second-trimester losses.

C. ETIOLOGY

1. Chromosomal abnormalities are less frequent than in the first trimester. Abnormalities present are more similar to those seen in live-born infants (trisomies 13, 18, 21; monosomy X; sex chromosomal polysomies).

2. Anatomic defects resulting from polygenic or multifactorial factors are found in a greater number of second- and third-trimester losses. Concomitant cytogenetic data are necessary to delineate the precise role of anatomic defects in second-trimester losses.

3. Endocrine abnormalities
    a. Overt thyroidism, hypothyroidism, or hyperthyroidism is associated with decreased conception rates and fetal loss.[20]
    b. Diabetes mellitus: patients with poorly controlled disease are at increased risk for early pregnancy loss.[21-23]

4. Muellerian fusion defects are a known cause of second-trimester abortion. Abortions occur in up to 20% to 35% of women with fusion defects,[24] with higher loss rates in those with septate and bicornate uteri than in those with unicornate or uterus didelphys. Fetal loss is thought to be caused by uterine inability to accommodate an enlarging fetus as well as implantation of the fetus on a poorly vascularized septum.

5. Leiomyomas are infrequently a cause of pregnancy wastage. Submucous leiomyomas are the type most likely to cause abortion as a result of thinning of the endometrium over the leiomyoma (implantation would occur in a poorly decidualized site). In addition, leiomyomas may undergo rapid growth with a resultant compromise in blood supply to the leiomyoma and subsequent necrosis, which could in turn cause uterine contractions and result in an abortion. Leiomyomas may also encroach on the space required by the fetus, resulting in a less optimal vascular supply to the growing fetus.

6. Incompetent cervix (painless dilation and effacement of the cervix) may be caused by cervical conization, cervical dilation (forceful), or cervical lacerations. An inherent weakness may also be present (see Chapter 12).

7. Infections play a prominent role in second-trimester loss (see section IIC4). Placental infection is thought to be the culprit in many second-

21

PREGNANCY LOSS

trimester abruptions (45% of patients with placental hematomas have documented chorioamnionitis).

8. Antifetal antibodies (i.e., Rh-negative women and anti-P antibodies)[25]
9. Autoimmune disease
    a. Patients with LAC and ACA have an increased risk of fetal wastage. LAC has been associated with subplacental clotting and fetal losses in all trimesters (thought to be a decidual abortifacient mechanism). The frequency of midtrimester fetal death in women with LAC or ACA is markedly increased[26]; in addition, growth retardation and preeclampsia occur in surviving fetuses.
    b. The association of antisperm antibodies and antinuclear antibodies with early losses is less well established.

IV. STILLBIRTH/FETAL DEATH

A. **DEFINITION.** Fetal death after 20 weeks of pregnancy (Table 21-1).
B. **INCIDENCE.** 7.5/1000 live births
C. **ETIOLOGY.** See Table 21-2 for a list of all possible causes of fetal death. A few of these conditions are discussed below.
1. Chromosomal abnormalities are present in 5% of stillborn infants (vs. a live-born rate of 0.6%).
2. Infants with anatomic defects caused by polygenic or multifactorial etiologies, as detailed in section III, need cytogenetic testing to delineate the role of the anatomic defect in a fetal loss. Neural tube defects are generally not considered cytogenetic in origin and are noted in 1% of stillbirths.
3. Autoimmune diseases (see section IIIC). The presence of antiphospholipid antibodies (APAs) in association with an unexplained second-trimester elevation of maternal serum α-fetoprotein (present in 22% with APA [only 1.6% of general population])[28] is significantly associated with fetal loss, often as a result of placental pathology (i.e., decreased placental weight, placental infarction, intraplacental hematoma).
D. **EVALUATION** (Table 21-3)
1. Mother
    a. Review prenatal records for blood pressure, serologic tests, glucose tolerance, and isoimmunization.
    b. Consider endocrine evaluation if not already performed during pregnancy, including a thyroid panel (rule out hypothyroidism and hyperthyroidism) as well as a fasting blood sugar (to screen for diabetes).
    c. Consider autoimmune disease evaluation with LAC and ACA.
    d. Obtain a Kleihauer-Betke stain of maternal blood to look for evidence of a fetal-maternal hemorrhage.
2. Fetus and products of conception (See Table 21-1 for current reporting requirements.)
    a. Evaluate for a cord accident (i.e., true knot or a tight cord around the infant's neck), placental pathologic findings (abruption), and gross fetal anomalies.

TABLE 21-1

CURRENT REPORTING REQUIREMENTS

The following general fetal death reporting requirements are as of March 1991.

20 WK OR MORE OF GESTATION	20 WK OR MORE OF GESTATION OR BIRTH WEIGHT OF 500 g OR MORE	BIRTH WEIGHT OF 500 g OR MORE
Alabama	District of Columbia	New Mexico
Alaska		South Dakota
Arizona*	**20 WK OR MORE OF GESTATION OR BIRTH WEIGHT OF 350 g OR MORE**	Tennessee*
California		
Connecticut		**16 WK OR MORE OF GESTATION**
Florida		Pennsylvania
Guam	Idaho	**ALL PRODUCTS OF HUMAN CONCEPTION**
Illinois	Kentucky	
Indiana	Louisiana	American Samoa
Iowa	Massachusetts	Arkansas
Maryland*	Mississippi	Colorado
Minnesota	Missouri	Georgia
Montana	New Hampshire	Hawaii
Nebraska	South Carolina	Maine
Nevada	Wisconsin	New York
New Jersey		Northern Mariana Islands
North Carolina	**BIRTH WEIGHT IN EXCESS OF 350 g**	Rhode Island
North Dakota		Virginia
Ohio	Kansas	Virgin Islands
Oklahoma		
Oregon*	**20 WK OR MORE OF GESTATION OR BIRTH WEIGHT OF 400 g OR MORE**	
Puerto Rico		
Texas		
Utah	Michigan	
Vermont*		
Washington		
West Virginia		
Wyoming		

From American College of Obstetricians and Gynecologists: *Diagnosis and management of fetal death.* Tech Bull No. 176, Washington, DC, 1993. The College.
*Specific modifiers apply.

b. If fetal weight is <500 g, all products of conception are to be sent to the pathology department for evaluation.

c. For fetal weights >500 g, obtain consent from the family for autopsy (this may be the most important factor for diagnosing the cause of death) and x-ray scans.

d. Obtain tissue for culture and karyotype.

(1) Cultures should be obtained in a sterile fashion for aerobic and anaerobic bacteria and viruses or fungi, as clinically indicated (obtain from fetal surface of placenta).

TABLE 21-2

CAUSES OF STILLBIRTH AND FETAL DEATH

Maternal Conditions	Fetal Conditions	Obstetric Conditions
Severe anemia (i.e., sickle cell disease)	Chromosomal abnormalities	Multiple gestation
Collagen vascular diseases	Postdate pregnancy	Intrauterine growth retardation
Systemic lupus erythematosus	Structural malformations	Oligohydramnios
Antiphospholipid syndrome		Premature rupture of membranes
Drugs of abuse (e.g., cocaine, amphetamines)		Preeclampsia
Endocrine abnormalities		Placental abruption
Diabetes		Cord accidents (e.g., knot or prolapse)
Hyperthyroidism or hypothyroidism		Fetal-to-maternal hemorrhage
Infections		
Cytomegalovirus		
Toxoplasmosis		
Parvovirus B-19		
Listeriosis		
Syphilis		

TABLE 21-3

EVALUATION OF FETAL DEATH

Maternal Testing	Tissue Testing
Random glucose	Fetal/placental gross examination
Complete blood cell count with platelet count	Autopsy/pathology evaluation
Venereal Disease Research Laboratory (test for syphilis)	Bacterial and viral cultures
Antibody screen	Photographs
Kleihauer-Betke	X-ray scans
Urine toxicology	Karyotyping of fetal tissues
Consider obtaining the following:	
Lupus anticoagulant/anticardiolipin antibody	
CMV (IgM and IgG), TORCH, or parvovirus titers	
Thyroid function testings	

CMV, Cytomegalovirus; *Ig,* immunoglobulin; *TORCH,* toxoplasmosis, rubella, cytomegalovirus, herpes simplex.

   (2) Karyotyping may be performed on placental tissue or intracardiac blood. Chromosomal abnormalities are more likely to be identified with fetal anomalies, growth retardation, stigmata of aneuploidy, or recurrent pregnancy losses.
   e. Notify the appropriate hospital personnel (e.g., fetal loss support services) of the patient's status so they may provide the family with emotional support and burial options.
3. Further work-up should be guided by the gross and histopathologic findings of the fetus and stillbirth.
   a. Nonrecurrent causes (e.g., cord accidents, large fetal-maternal hemorrhage) may negate the need for further work-up.
   b. Inflammatory findings may guide the need for cultures or immunologic tests of recent infection (i.e., TORCH [toxoplasmosis, rubella, cytomegalovirus, herpes simplex] titers).
   c. Vascular findings may suggest careful scrutiny of the mother for occult microvascular disease (e.g., renal disease, systemic lupus erythematosus, LAC).
E. THERAPEUTIC MANAGEMENT. The cause of the stillbirth dictates subsequent pregnancy management.
1. A **cytogenetic** abnormality indicates consideration of antenatal testing in subsequent pregnancies.
2. The presence of placental **abruption** indicates prevention of another stillbirth could potentially be achieved by antepartum surveillance beginning 2 to 4 weeks before the time of the current death.
3. **Morphologic abnormalities** indicate the need for imaging studies in a subsequent pregnancy.
4. **Endocrine** diseases require appropriate treatment.
5. Studies show that women with **LAC** or **ACA** and a second- or third-trimester pregnancy loss may benefit from treatment with one baby aspirin taken daily and prednisone (10 mg/d orally).
6. Antepartum testing for unknown causes or those with recurrent causes.

21

PREGNANCY LOSS

REFERENCES

1. Vlaanderen W, Treffers PE: Prognosis of subsequent pregnancies after recurrent spontaneous abortion in first trimester, *BMJ* 295:92, 1987.
2. Sciarra JJ, editor: *Early abortion,* Philadelphia, 1994, Lippincott.
3. Papadopoulos G et al: The frequency of chromosome anomalies in human preimplantation embryos after in-vitro fertilization, *Hum Reprod* 4:91, 1989.
4. Berry L, Poswillo DE, editors: Chromosomal animal model of human disease: fetal trisomy and development failure. In *Teratology,* Berlin, 1975, Springer-Verlag.
5. Boué A, Thibault C, editors: Fetal mortality due to euploidy and irregular meiotic segregation in the mouse. In *Les accidents chromosomiques de la reproduction,* Paris, 1973, INSERM.
6. Gabbe SG, Niebyl JR, Simpson JL: *Obstetrics: normal and problem pregnancies,* ed 2, New York, 1991, Churchill Livingstone.

7. Goldstein SR: Embryonic death in early pregnancy: a new look at the first trimester, *Obstet Gynecol* 84(2):294-297, 1994.
8. Jones GS:The luteal phase defect, *Fertil Steril* 27:351, 1976.
9. Linnan MJ et al: Epidemic listeriosis associated with Mexican-style cheese, *N Engl J Med* 319:823-828, 1988.
10. Gellin BG, Broome CV: Listeriosis, *JAMA* 261(9):1313-1320, 1989.
11. Gaillard DA et al: Spontaneous abortions during the second trimester of gestation, *Arch Pathol Lab Med* 117:1022-1026, 1993.
12. Mills JL et al: Moderate caffeine use and the risk of spontaneous abortion and intrauterine growth retardation, *JAMA* 269(5):593-597, 1993.
13. Kline J et al: Drinking during pregnancy and spontaneous abortion, *Lancet* 2:176, 1980.
14. Harlap S, Shino PH: Alcohol, smoking and incidence of spontaneous abortions in the first and second trimester, *Lancet* 2:173, 1980.
15. Halmesmaki E et al: Maternal and paternal alcohol consumption and miscarriage, *Br J Obstet Gynaecol* 96:188, 1989.
16. Fija-Talamanaca I, Settimi L: Occupational factors and reproductive outcome. In Hafez ESE, editor: *Spontaneous abortion,* Lancaster, United Kingdom, 1984, MTP Press.
17. Barlow S, Sullivan FM: *Reproductive hazards of industrial chemicals: an evaluation of animal and human data,* San Diego, 1982, Academic Press.
18. Pollock W, Ascari WQ, Kochesky RJ: Studies on Rh prophylaxis: relationship between doses of anti Rh and size of antigen stimulus, *Transfusion* 11:333, 1971.
19. Bowman JM, Pollock JM: Transplacental fetal hemorrhage after amniocentesis, *Obstet Gynecol* 66:749-754, 1985.
20. Montero M et al: Successful outcome of pregnancy in women with hypothyroidism, *Ann Intern Med* 94:31, 1981.
21. Miodnovik M et al: Spontaneous abortion among insulin dependent diabetic women, *Am J Obstet Gynecol* 150:372, 1984.
22. Miodovnik M et al: Glycemic control and spontaneous abortion in insulin dependent diabetic women, *Obstet Gynecol* 68:366, 1986.
23. Miodovnik M et al: Elevated maternal glycohemoglobin in early pregnancy and spontaneous abortion among insulin dependent diabetic women, *Am J Obstet Gynecol* 153:439, 1985.
24. Heinonen P, Saarikoski S, Pystynen P: Reproductive performance of women with uterine anomalies: an evaluation of 182 cases, *Acta Obstet Gynecol Scand* 61:157, 1982.
25. American College of Obstetricians and Gynecologists: *Diagnosis and management of fetal death.* Tech Bull No. 176, Washington, DC, 1993, The College.
26. Scott JR, Rote NS, Branch DW: Immunologic aspects of recurrent abortions and fetal death, *Obstet Gynecol* 70:645, 1987.
27. Grubb DK, Rabello YA, Paul RH: Post-term pregnancy: fetal death rate with antepartum surveillance, *Obstet Gynecol* 79:1024-1026, 1992.
28. Silver RM et al: Unexplained elevations of maternal serum alpha-fetoprotein in women with antiphospholipid antibodies: a harbinger of fetal death, *Obstet Gynecol* 83(1):150-156, 1994.

PART IV

Appendices

MATERNAL PHYSIOLOGY
Temperature Conversion Chart

TABLE A-1

TEMPERATURE EQUIVALENTS

Centigrade	Fahrenheit	Centigrade	Fahrenheit
35.0	95.0	38.2	100.7
35.2	95.4	38.4	101.1
35.4	95.7	38.6	101.4
35.6	96.1	38.8	101.8
35.8	96.4	39.0	102.2
36.0	96.8	39.2	102.5
36.2	97.1	39.4	102.9
36.4	97.5	39.6	103.2
36.6	97.8	39.8	103.6
36.8	98.2	40.0	104.0
37.0	98.6	40.2	104.3
37.2	98.9	40.4	104.7
37.4	99.3	40.6	105.1
37.6	99.6	40.8	105.4
37.8	100.0	41.0	105.8
38.0	100.4	41.2	106.1

To convert Centigrade to Fahrenheit: $(9/5 \times \text{Temperature}) + 32$
To convert Fahrenheit to Centigrade: $(\text{Temperature} - 32) \times 5/9$

Common Laboratory Values in Pregnancy

TABLE B-1			
Test	Normal Range (Nonpregnant)	Change in Pregnancy	Timing
SERUM CHEMISTRIES			
Albumin	3.5-4.8 g/dl	↓ 1 g/dl	Most by 20 wk, then gradual
Bilirubin			
Total	0.25-1.5 mg/dl	No sig. change	
Direct	0-0.2 mg/dl	No sig. change	
Blood gases (arterial, whole blood)			
pH	7.35-7.45	No sig. change	
P_{O_2}	80-105 mm Hg	↑ 7 mm Hg	By end of first trimester
P_{CO_2}	35-45 mm Hg	↓ 7 mm Hg	By end of first trimester
Calcium			
Total	9.0-10.3 mg/dl	↓ 10%	Gradual fall
Free	4.5-5.0 mg/dl	↓ slight	
Carbon dioxide content	24-32 mmol/L	↓ 4-5 mmol/L	By 12 wk, then stable
Ceruloplasmin	15-16 mg/dl	↑ 75%	Gradual rise
Chloride	95-105 mmol/L	No sig. change	
Copper	70-155 g/dl	↑ 75%	Gradual rise
Complement (total)	150-250 CH50	↑ 25%	Gradual rise
C3	690-1470 mg/L	↑ 40%-50%	Gradual rise
C4	105-305 mg/L	No data—probably behaves like C3	
Creatinine (female)	0.6-1.1 mg/dl	↓ 0.3 mg/dl	Most by 20 wk
Fibrinogen	1.5-3.6 g/L	↑ 0.1-2 g/L	Progressive
Folate			
Serum	3 ng/ml	↓ 50%	Gradual fall
Red cell	117-541 ng/ml	↓ 12%	Gradual fall
Glucose, fasting (plasma)	65-105 mg/dl	↓ 10%	Gradual fall
Ferritin	15-300 μg/L	↓ 40-50 μg/L	Second trimester, less in supplemented women

Continued

TABLE B-1 —cont'd

Test	Normal Range (Nonpregnant)	Change in Pregnancy	Timing
SERUM CHEMISTRIES—cont'd			
Immunoglobulin			
IgA	39-358 mg/dl	No sig. change	
IgM	33-229 mg/dl	No sig. change	
IgG	679-1537 mg/dl	↓ 100 mg/dl	Gradual
Iron (female)	60-135 g/dl	↓ 35%	Gradual, less with supplements
Iron binding capacity	250-350 g/dl	↑ 40%-50%	Second trimester
Lactate (plasma)	0.3-1.3 mmol/L	No change	
Lipids			
Cholesterol	120-330 mg/dl	↑ 60-80 mg/dl	Progressive after 13 wk
Triglyceride	10-190 mg/dl	↑ 100 mg/dl	Progressive
Magnesium	1.5-2.4 mEq/L (1.8-2.9 mg/dl)	↓ 10%-20%	By 20 wk, then stable
Osmolality	270-290 mOsm/kg	↓ 10 mOsm/kg	By 8 wk, then stable
Phosphorus, inorganic	2.5-6 mg/dl	No sig. change	
Potassium (plasma)	3.5-4.5 mmol/L	↓ 0.2-0.3 mmol/L	By 20 wk
Protein electrophoresis			
Albumin	3.5-4.8 g/dl	↓ 1 g/dl	Most by 20 wk, then gradual
α_1-Globulin	0.1-0.5 g/dl	↑ 0.1 g/dl	Gradual
α_2-Globulin	0.3-1.2 g/dl	↑ 0.1 g/dl	Gradual
β-Globulin	0.7-1.7 g/dl	↑ 0.3 g/dl	Gradual
Gamma globulin	0.7-1.7 g/dl	↓ 0.1 g/dl	Gradual
Protein (total)	6.5-8.5 g/dl	↓1 g/dl	By 20 wk, then stable
Sodium	135-145 mmol/L	↓ 2-4 mmol/L	By 20 wk, then stable
Urea nitrogen	12-30 mg/dl	↓ 50%	First trimester
Uric acid	3.5-8 mg/dl	↓ 33%	First trimester, rise at term
URINARY CHEMISTRIES			
Creatinine	15-25 mg/kg/d (1-1.4 g/d)	No sig. change	
Protein	Up to 150 mg/d	Up to 250-300 mg/d	By 20 wk
Creatinine clearance	90-130 ml/min/ 1.73 m^2	↑ 40%-50%	By 16 wk

TABLE B-1 —cont'd

Test	Normal Range (Nonpregnant)	Change in Pregnancy	Timing
SERUM ENZYMATIC ACTIVITIES			
Amylase	23-84 IU/L	↑ 50%-100%	←Controversial
Creatinine phosphokinase	25-145 mU/ml	↓ 25%-30%	8-20 wk, then returns to normal
Lactic dehydrogenase (LDH)	90-250 mU/ml	Slight ↑, not sig.	
Lipase	4-24 IU/dl	↓ 50%	Gradual
Phosphatase, alkaline	30-95 mU/ml	↑ by 100%-200%	Mostly in third trimester
Transaminase			
Alanine amino (SGPT)	5-35 mU/ml	No sig. change	
Aspartate amino (SGOT)	5-40 mU/ml	No sig. change	
Gamma-glutamyl transpeptidase	1-45 IU/L	No sig. change	
HEMATOLOGIC STUDIES			
Coagulation studies			
Bleeding time (template)	2.5-9.5 min	No sig. change	
Partial thromboplastin time	24-36 s	No sig. change	
Prothrombin time	70%-100%	No sig. change	
Thrombin time	11.3-18.5 s	No sig. change	
Factors			
VIII, VIII antigen	60%-160%	↑ 100%-150%	Beginning second trimester
X, IX	60%-160%	↑ 30%	Gradual
VII, XII	60%-160%	No change	Controversial
II, V, XI	60%-160%	No sig. change	
V	60%-160%	↓ 30%	Gradual
Hematocrit (female)	37%-47%	↓ 4%-6%	Bottoms at 30-34 wk
Hemoglobin (female)	12.0-16.0 g/dl	↓ 1.5-2.0 g/dl	Bottoms at 30-34 wk
Erythrocyte count (female)	$4.2\text{-}10.9 \times 10^6/\text{mm}^3$	$\downarrow 0.8 \times 10^6/\text{mm}^3$	Bottoms at 30-34 wk

Continued

B

COMMON LABORATORY VALUES IN PREGNANCY

TABLE B-1 —cont'd

Test	Normal Range (Nonpregnant)	Change in Pregnancy	Timing
HEMATOLOGIC STUDIES—cont'd			
Leukocyte count	4.8-10.8 × 10³/ mm³	↑ 3.5 × 10³/ mm³	Gradual
Polymorphs	48%-82%	↑ 3 × 10³/ mm³	Gradual
Lymphocytes	8%-44%	↑ 0.3 × 10³/ mm³	Gradual
Monocytes	2%-8%	No sig. change	
Eosinophils	0%-6%	No sig. change	
Platelet count	150-400 × 10³/ mm³	Slight ↓	
Erythrocyte indexes			
Mean corpuscular hemoglobin (MCH)	27-31 pg/cell	No sig. change	
Mean corpuscular hemoglobin concentration (MCHC)	32-36 g/dl	No sig. change	
Mean corpuscular volume (MCV)	81-99 μm³	No sig. change	
Sedimentation rate (whole blood ESR by the Westergren method in women <50 years of age)	Up to 30 mm/h	↑ 2-6 X	Most by 20 wk, then gradual
SERUM HORMONE VALUES			
Adrenocorticotropic hormone (ACTH)	20-100 pg/ml	No sig. change	Early, gradual after 24 wk
Aldosterone	20-90 ng/L	↑ 300%-800%	Gradual
Cortisol (plasma)	8-21 μg/dl	↑ 20 μg/dl	
Growth hormone, fasting	5 ng/ml	No sig. change	
Insulin, fasting	10 mU/L	No sig. change Slight ↑ (?)	First half of pregnancy Second half of pregnancy

TABLE B-1 —cont'd

Test	Normal Range (Nonpregnant)	Change in Pregnancy	Timing
Parathyroid hormone	2-10 U/ml	↑ 200%-300%	Progressive after 24 wk
Prolactin (female)	25 ng/ml	↑ 50-400 ng/ml	Gradual, peaks at term
Renin activity (plasma)	0.9-3.3 ng/ml/h	↑ 100%	Early, stable
Thyroxine, total (T_4)	5-11 g/dl	↑ 5 mg/dl	Early sustained
T_3 resin uptake	35%-45%	↓ to 25%-35%	Early sustained
Free thyroxine index (T_7)	1.75-4.95	No sig. change	
Triiodothyronine (T_3)	125-245 ng/dl	↑ 50%	Early sustained
TSH	Up to 8 U/ml	No sig. change	
Free T_4	1-2.3 ng/dl	No sig. change	

From Main DM, Main EK: *Obstetrics and gynecology: a pocket reference,* St Louis, 1984, Mosby.

B

COMMON LABORATORY VALUES IN PREGNANCY

Analgesia and Anesthesia in Labor and Delivery

I. PAIN PATHWAYS AND THE STAGES OF LABOR

The first stage of labor begins with the onset of regular contractions and ends with the cervix being completely dilated. The pain from the first stage of labor is conducted via the T10 to L1 nerve roots. The second stage of labor begins at full cervical dilation and ends with the delivery of the infant. Second-stage pain, caused by distention of the vulva and perineum, is conducted by the pudendal nerve via the S2 to S4 nerve roots.

II. PAIN RELIEF DURING LABOR AND DELIVERY

A. PARENTERAL MEDICATIONS

1. **Sedative tranquilizers** are generally used during the first stage of labor, often in conjunction with a narcotic. The use of barbiturates (i.e., Seconal, Nembutal, Amytal) is generally restricted to the early, latent phase of labor when delivery is not anticipated for at least 12 hours because they have depressant effects on the neonate. The phenothiazines, promethazine (Phenergan), and hydroxyzine (Vistaril) are effective in reducing anxiety without causing neonatal depression. Diazepam (Valium), a benzodiazepine, has been safely used in small doses (2.5 to 10 mg intravenously [IV] as needed) to relieve extreme maternal anxiety without producing significant adverse neonatal effects. Midazolam (Versed), also a benzodiazepine, can cause an anterograde amnesia that is undesirable at the time of birth.

2. **Narcotics** are used to provide pain relief during labor and to supplement regional and general anesthesia during a cesarean delivery. All currently used narcotics produce some degree of respiratory depression and can cause orthostatic hypotension as well as nausea and vomiting. Narcotics are transferred rapidly across the placenta and can cause neonatal respiratory depression. Meperidine (Demerol) is currently the most commonly used narcotic in obstetrics. It has replaced morphine as an obstetric analgesic because of the latter's prolonged duration of action and greater neonatal respiratory depression. Fentanyl (Sublimaze) may be used as an adjuvant for both regional and general anesthesia for cesarean delivery. The use of IV fentanyl for analgesia during labor is currently under investigation. The synthetic narcotic agonist-antagonists, butorphanol (Stadol) and nalbuphine (Nubain), cause only limited respiratory depression, making them useful for labor analgesia. However, both drugs may cause dizziness or drowsiness, making them unsuitable for ambulating patients.

The author would like to acknowledge the valuable assistance of George Mattione, M.D., in the preparation of this appendix.

3. **Dissociative drugs and neuroleptanalgesia.** The dissociative drugs, such as ketamine and scopolamine, are rarely used as sedatives during labor. Neuroleptanalgesia, using a combination of a narcotic and a major tranquilizer (i.e., fentanyl and droperidol [Innovar]), is not a popular technique because of its potential for profound neonatal depression.

B. **REGIONAL ANALGESIA FOR LABOR AND DELIVERY**

1. **Classification of blocks**

   a. The **lumbar epidural block** is one of the most popular forms of analgesia during labor and can be performed as a single injection (when the cervix, if fully dilated, and the fetal head are in position for delivery) or as a continuous technique consisting of intermittent boluses of local anesthetic through an epidural catheter (usually initiated when cervical dilation reaches 4 to 6 cm). An epidural block is capable of providing uninterrupted analgesia throughout labor and delivery. However, maternal blood pressure and fetal heart rate must be monitored after each injection so that maternal hypotension can be treated before fetal bradycardia occurs. It has become common practice to administer a low concentration of combined local anesthetic and narcotic via continuous infusion. This technique has the advantage of providing a continuous and stable level of anesthesia with fewer occurrences of hypotensive episodes while better maintaining pelvic muscle tone (Figs. C-1 and C-2). Recent studies suggest an increase in cesarean delivery rates when epidurals are administered before 5 cm of dilation (see Thorp et al. in Suggested Readings).

   b. The **caudal block** is a form of epidural analgesia in which the epidural space is entered through the sacral hiatus. It is less frequently used for vaginal delivery than lumbar epidural analgesia because it is less effective in providing analgesia during the first stage of labor and is more painful to administer. Caudal block also requires more local anesthetic agent than a lumbar epidural does, thus increasing the risk of total spinal anesthesia should dural puncture occur during needle placement for the caudal block. Puncture of the fetal head and injection of local anesthetic into the fetus have been reported during caudal placement. Before injection of the local anesthetic, a rectal examination should be performed to rule out this possibility. Perineal anesthesia and muscle relaxation are more rapid than with lumbar epidural analgesia (Fig. C-1).

   c. The **subarachnoid (spinal) block** is not commonly used for vaginal delivery because the urge to bear down is abolished and the mother is unable to cooperate in the delivery. However, this block provides excellent anesthesia for cesarean delivery (Fig. C-1).

   d. The **paracervical block** is used for pain relief during the first stage of labor. A paracervical block is generally performed when the cervix is dilated 4 to 6 cm in the multiparous patient and 5 to 6 cm in the primiparous patient. Fetal bradycardia is the most common and se-

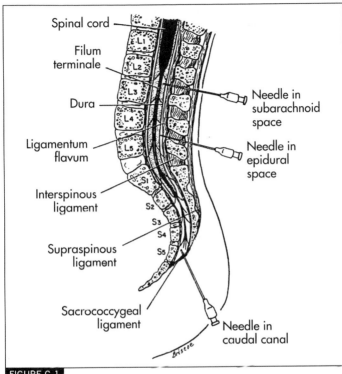

FIGURE C-1

Schematic diagram of lumbosacral anatomy. *(From Shnider SM, Levinson G: Anesthesia for obstetrics, ed 3, Baltimore, 1993, Williams & Wilkins.)*

rious complication of this block, and the incidence may be as high as 50%. Although the mechanism of this effect is controversial, this block should not be done in the presence of impaired uteroplacental circulation or if the fetus is at risk.

e. The **pudendal block** is administered for pain relief during the second stage of labor and produces adequate perineal analgesia for outlet forceps delivery as well as episiotomy and repair. For optimal effect, this block can be administered at the start of the second stage of labor in the primiparous patient and at 6 to 8 cm dilation in the multiparous patient.

f. The **local block** is generally used before an episiotomy is done during vaginal delivery.

2. **Effect of regional anesthesia on labor and delivery.** Because of the number of variables present in any given delivery, the effect of regional analgesia on the progress and outcome of labor and delivery is difficult

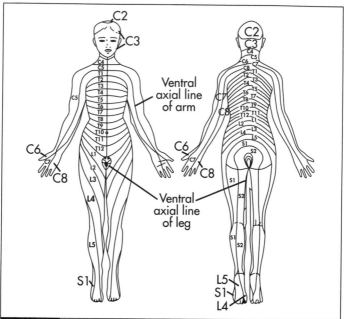

FIGURE C-2

Dermatomes. Knowledge of spinal dermatomes is helpful in determining levels of epidural or spinal anesthesia. Two dermatomal charts that are commonly used are in general agreement as to levels on the trunk (a good guidepost is that the umbilicus = T10) but disagree markedly on distribution on the limbs. This perhaps more widely used chart shows dermatomes extending as strips that are nearly the length of the limb. The alternative chart (Forester) indicates a more patchy distribution. Relative clinical correctness is not resolved. There is a clear mistake on the above chart, however, in that C5 and T1 do not extend significantly onto the thorax; rather, C3 and C4 supply this area. *(From Keegan JJ, Garrett FD: Anat Rec 102:409, 1948.)*

to ascertain. Contrary to earlier studies, it has been shown that the initiation of epidural analgesia had minimal effect on the duration or quality of the first phase of labor if hypotension is avoided and uterine displacement is maintained. Epidural analgesia has also been reported to increase the duration of the second phase of labor as well as increasing the frequency of instrumental delivery. This effect can be minimized through the use of more dilute concentrations of local anesthetics in combination with a low dose of narcotic (fentanyl or sufentanil) using a continuous infusion technique. In addition, if arbitrary time limits on the length of the second stage of labor are avoided, there is no significant increase in the incidence of instrumental delivery. Finally, it has not been shown that the administration of a "perineal dose" of local anesthetic just before delivery results in an increased incidence of instrumental delivery.

C. **INHALATION ANESTHETICS FOR LABOR AND DELIVERY.** Although nitrous oxide (N_2O) has been found to have little effect on the uterus, the halogenated agents (halothane, flurane, isoflurane) can produce profound, dose-dependent uterine relaxation. Therefore general anesthesia can be used to relax the uterus during tetanic contractions or to facilitate intrauterine manipulation. Although such relaxation can lead to increased blood loss after vaginal delivery (or during cesarean delivery), this effect can be reversed by the administration of oxytocin.

D. **ANESTHESIA FOR CESAREAN DELIVERY**

1. **Regional.** Both spinal and epidural anesthesia can be used for cesarean delivery. The use of regional techniques allows for a decreased risk of pulmonary aspiration (compared with general anesthesia) and decreases the risk of neonatal respiratory depression by lessening the need for systemic narcotics. Also, the fact that the mother is awake and able to participate may enhance the birth experience. The disadvantages of using a regional technique include the possibilities of a prolonged onset time (especially compared with general anesthesia), spinal headache, and maternal hypotension with resulting fetal hypoxia. Contraindications to the use of regional anesthetic techniques include patient refusal, hypovolemic shock, uteroplacental insufficiency, septicemia or infection at the site of injection, coagulation disorders (including hemolysis, elevated liver enzymes, and low platelet count [HELLP] syndrome), and certain neurologic disorders, such as multiple sclerosis. In addition, spinal anesthesia is contraindicated in the patient who is preeclamptic because its use may result in profound maternal hypotension with a subsequent decrease in uteroplacental perfusion and fetal asphyxia.

2. **General.** The major advantage of general anesthesia for cesarean delivery is the speed in which it can be administered and in which a distressed fetus can be delivered. General anesthesia tends to cause less maternal hypotension than regional anesthesia, has greater cardiac stability, and allows for control of the airway and ventilation. General anesthesia may also be preferable in patients with coagulopathies, preexisting neurologic diseases (including lumbar disk disease), local infections, or generalized sepsis. Important considerations, if general anesthesia is anticipated, include the increased possibility of aspiration pneumonitis in the pregnant patient, maintenance of maternal ventilation and oxygenation, and the prevention of maternal hypotension. It is important to note that the incidence of difficult or failed intubation is much higher in the obstetric surgical patient. Inability to control the airway, with the resulting lack of oxygenation, or the aspiration of gastric contents resulting in pneumonitis remains the leading cause of anesthetic-related maternal morbidity and mortality.

III. ANESTHETIC CONSIDERATIONS IN THE PREGNANT PATIENT

Although no anesthetic drug has yet been demonstrated to be teratogenic in humans, fetal exposure to any drug should be minimized, especially during the first trimester. It is preferable that elective surgery be postponed until 6 weeks postpartum so that the physiologic changes associated with pregnancy and the increased risk of aspiration of gastric contents have abated. If possible, surgery should be postponed until the second or third trimester and a regional anesthetic technique selected to minimize fetal exposure to drugs. If general anesthesia with N_2O is to be employed, consider pretreating patients with folinic acid because N_2O inactivates vitamin B_{12}, which is essential in folate metabolism and thymidine synthesis. After the sixteenth week of gestation, continuous fetal heart rate monitoring and uterine tocodynamometry should be employed to detect preterm labor, especially in the postoperative period. Regardless of the anesthetic technique selected, the pregnant or postpartum patient has an increased risk of aspiration of gastric contents and must be treated as having a full stomach, regardless of nothing-by-mouth (NPO) status. Appropriate measures to decrease this risk include the preoperative administration of nonparticulate oral antacids (Bicitra, 30 ml orally, 15 to 30 minutes before the procedure) to neutralize existing gastric acid, dopamine agonists (metoclopramide [Reglan], 10 mg orally or intramuscularly, 1 hour before the procedure) to increase gastric emptying, or H_2-receptor antagonists (famotidine [Pepcid]), 20 mg orally, 2 hours before the procedure) to decrease gastric acid production. The administration of preoperative anticholinergics (atropine, scopolamine, glycopyrrolate) has not been shown to effectively decrease the risk of gastric aspiration in humans. When general anesthesia is required for the pregnant patient, the airway must be protected via the placement of a cuffed endotracheal tube. The use of cricoid pressure (pressing the cricoid cartilage dorsally against the body of the sixth cervical vertebra) during intubation has been shown to be effective in preventing the passive regurgitation of stomach contents but not active vomiting (Fig. C-3). The tube is generally placed immediately after consciousness is lost. If difficulty in placement is anticipated, intubation should be performed while the patient is awake.

IV. LOCAL ANESTHETIC AGENTS

A. **MECHANISM OF ACTION.** Local anesthetic agents block the sodium channels in the nerve membrane, thus impairing propagation of the action potential in axons. In general, myelinated fibers are more readily blocked than nonmyelinated fibers, and thinner fibers are more easily blocked than thick ones.

B. **TYPES OF LOCAL ANESTHETICS.** Local anesthetics are classified as esters (procaine, chloroprocaine, tetracaine) or amides (bupivacaine, etidocaine, lidocaine, mepivacaine). The esters are metabolized by

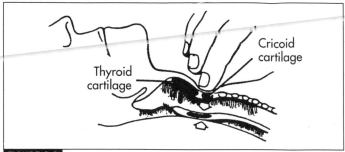

FIGURE C-3

Technique of posterior pressure on cricoid cartilage. *(From Shnider SM, Levinson G: Anesthesia for obstetrics, ed 2, Baltimore, 1993, Williams & Wilkins.)*

plasma cholinesterase and thus have short half-lives in the circulation. Paraamino benzoic acid, a degradation product of ester metabolism, can cause a hypersensitivity reaction in susceptible individuals. Amide local anesthetics are metabolized primarily in the liver (Table C-1).

C. **ESTER LOCAL ANESTHETIC AGENTS.** Procaine (Novocain) is a short-acting agent used for local infiltration and spinal anesthesia. Chloroprocaine (Nesacaine) is a short-acting agent used for local infiltration and epidural anesthesia. Rapid hydrolysis of this agent by plasma cholinesterase makes this the least cardiotoxic of the local anesthetics. Previous reports of arachnoiditis and neurotoxicity with this agent are now attributed to the preservative metabisulfite, which has been replaced with ethylenediamine tetraacetic acid (EDTA). However, this new formulation has been reported to cause severe backache when dosage exceeds 25 ml of solution. In addition, chloroprocaine or one of its metabolites can impair the actions of other epidural agents, such as bupivacaine or fentanyl. Tetracaine (Pontocaine) is a long-acting agent used primarily for spinal anesthesia.

D. **AMIDE LOCAL ANESTHETIC AGENTS.** Bupivacaine (Marcaine, Sensorcaine) can be used for all forms of local and regional anesthesia. It provides a sensory block of high quality (in relation to the degree of motor blockade) and long duration. However, its slow onset of action (up to 30 minutes) can make it impractical for urgent procedures. In addition, intravascular injection of bupivacaine can result in cardiac arrest that is resistant to treatment. It has been shown that pregnant patients in labor are more susceptible to this effect, and 0.75% bupivacaine is contraindicated for epidural anesthesia or obstetric practice. Lidocaine (Xylocaine) is the most frequently used local anesthetic for all forms of local and regional anesthesia. Although lidocaine does have a high rate of placental transfer, Apgar scores are statistically unaffected. Mepivacaine (Carbocaine) is used for local

TABLE C-1

LOCAL ANESTHETIC AGENTS AND THEIR USES

Agent	Concentration	Duration (h) Without Epidural	Duration (h) With Epidural	Dosage*
INFILTRATION ANESTHESIA				
Procaine	0.5%-1%	0.25-0.5	0.5-1.5	Up to 40 ml of 1% (60 ml with epidural)
Chloroprocaine	0.5%-1%	0.25-0.5	0.5-1.5	Up to 80 ml of 1% (100 ml with epidural)
Lidocaine	0.5%-1%	0.5-2	1-3	Up to 30 ml of 1% (50 ml with epidural)
Mepivacaine	0.5%-1%	0.5-2	1-3	Up to 30 ml of 1% (50 ml with epidural)
Bupivacaine	0.25%-0.5%	2-4	4-8	Up to 35 ml of 0.5% (45 ml with epidural)
PERIPHERAL NERVE BLOCK				
Chloroprocaine	2%-3%	0.5-1.5		Up to 40 ml of 2%
Lidocaine	1%-1.5%	1-2	2-4	Up to 50 ml of 1%
Mepivacaine	1%-2%	1-2	3-5	Up to 50 ml of 1%
Bupivacaine	0.25%-0.5%	1.5-6	6-12	Up to 45 ml of 0.5%
SPINAL ANESTHESIA				
Procaine	5% in 5% glucose	0.5-1		120 mg†
Lidocaine	5% in 7.5% glucose	0.75-1.5	1.5-2	60 mg†
Tetracaine	0.5% in 5% glucose	2-3	3-5	12 mg†
Bupivacaine	0.75% in 8.25% glucose	2-4	4-8	9.0 mg†
EPIDURAL AND CAUDAL ANESTHESIA				
Chloroprocaine	2%-3%	0.5-1	0.5-1.5	25 ml of 3% solution (see text)
Lidocaine	1%-2%	0.75-1.5	1-2	Up to 400 mg (600 mg with epidural)
Mepivacaine	1%-2%		1-2	Up to 300 mg (500 mg with epidural)
Bupivacaine	0.25%-0.5%		2-4	Up to 175 mg (225 mg with epidural)

*Spinal and epidural dosage requirements vary with height. A dosage reduction of 25% to 50% may be required in the pregnant or elderly patient.

†Local anesthetic agents for spinal anesthesia must be diluted with 10% dextrose to appropriate volume.

infiltration, nerve blocks, and epidural anesthesia with a duration of action slightly longer than lidocaine. However, it has an increased half-life in the neonate, which has lead to a decline in its use in obstetrics. Etidocaine (Duranest) is not frequently used in anesthetic practice.

V. COMPLICATIONS OF REGIONAL ANESTHESIA

A. **HYPOTENSION.** The most common complication of spinal or epidural anesthesia is hypotension. Blood pressure must be monitored frequently after administration of regional anesthesia because even mild reductions in maternal blood pressure may adversely affect uterine blood flow. The degree and duration of maternal hypotension necessary to cause fetal distress are variable. Fortunately, it has been shown that if hypotension from regional anesthesia is promptly corrected, it has little adverse effect on neonatal outcome. The most effective means to prevent maternal hypotension include hydration before administration of regional anesthesia and continuous left uterine displacement to minimize aortocaval compression. Prophylactic administration of a vasopressor (ephedrine, 10 to 15 mg IV) is effective in decreasing the incidence of hypotension associated with spinal anesthesia. Treatment of hypotension after spinal or epidural anesthesia includes rapid infusion of fluids, increasing left uterine displacement, administration of IV ephedrine, and use of the Trendelenburg position to increase venous return. The administration of supplemental oxygen to the mother will not necessarily raise fetal PaO_2 if maternal hypotension is not corrected.

B. **TOTAL SPINAL ANESTHESIA.** Total spinal anesthesia can result from extensive spread of local anesthetic administered subdurally. However, it is more commonly the result of injecting the epidural dose of local anesthetic into an epidural needle or catheter that has been improperly placed or that has migrated into the subarachnoid space. Nausea and profound hypotension may be followed by loss of consciousness and cardiac or respiratory arrest. Treatment is supportive, with an airway established, the patient ventilated with oxygen, and the trachea intubated (using succinylcholine, 1 to 1.5 mg/kg) to prevent aspiration of gastric contents. The patient should be placed in the Trendelenburg position with left uterine displacement and fluids and ephedrine administered to maintain blood pressure. Maternal bradycardia must be treated promptly by administering atropine and ephedrine. If these are ineffective, IV epinephrine should be administered. In cases of cardiac arrest secondary to high spinal anesthesia, a full resuscitation dose of epinephrine should be administered immediately.

C. **LOCAL ANESTHETIC CONVULSIONS.** High blood levels of a local anesthetic may be a result of accumulation during repeated injections over a period of time or rapid systemic absorption from a highly vascular area. However, they are generally caused by the inadvertent intravascular injection of local anesthetic during epidural anesthesia. Seizures are generally preceded by loss of consciousness. Early recognition of this reaction is important because small doses of barbiturates (diazepam [Valium], 5 mg, or thiopental [Pentothal], 50 mg, IV, repeated as necessary) may prevent convulsions. Treatment is generally supportive with ventilation and circulation supported as previously described. The incidence of intravascular injection can be decreased by judiciously aspirating needles and catheters before dosing and by routinely injecting test doses of local anesthetics with epinephrine.

D. NEUROLOGIC COMPLICATIONS. The most common complication of spinal and epidural anesthesia is the postdural puncture (spinal) headache. For a spinal anesthetic, the incidence of headache can be minimized by using the smallest needle possible, inserting the needle with the bevel parallel to the longitudinal dural fibers, and using a "pencil-point" type of needle (Sprotte or Whitacre). Prophylactic bed rest and increased hydration have little or no effect on the incidence of postpuncture headache. The incidence of dural puncture with epidural anesthesia is usually between 1% and 2% with headache occurring almost 80% of the time. Treatment is generally supportive and consists mainly of bed rest, hydration, and use of oral analgesics. IV caffeine sodium benzoate and oral caffeine have been shown to relieve these headaches, but such treatment is associated with a high rate of recurrence. In severe headaches lasting longer than 24 hours, 20 ml of aseptically obtained autologous blood may be injected into the epidural space at the site of dural puncture. This epidural "blood patch" has a success rate greater than 90% but may need to be repeated should the headache recur. A prophylactic blood patch within 24 hours of the dural puncture has not been shown to be effective.

SUGGESTED READINGS

Barash PG, Cullen BF, Stoelting RK: *Clinical anesthesia,* ed 2, Philadelphia, 1992, Lippincott.

Danforth DN et al: *Obstetrics and gynecology,* Philadelphia, 1982, Harper & Row.

Firestone LL, Lebowitz PW, Cook CE: *Clinical anesthesia procedures of the Massachusetts General Hospital,* ed 3, Boston, 1998, Little, Brown.

Katz J: *Atlas of regional anesthesia,* Norwalk, Conn, 1985, Appleton-Century-Crofts.

Miller RD: *Anesthesia,* ed 3, San Franciso, 1990, Churchill Livingstone.

Shnider SM, Levinson G: *Anesthesia for obstetrics,* ed 3, Baltimore, 1993, Williams & Wilkins.

Thorp JA et al: The effect of intrapartum epidural analgesia on nulliparous labor: a randomized controlled prospective trial, *Am J Obstet Gynecol* 169:851-858, 1993.

Tunstall ME, Sheick A: Failed intubation protocol: oxygenation without aspiration, *Clin Anesthesiol* 4:171-188, 1986.

FETAL PHYSIOLOGY
Chromosomal Abnormalities

TABLE D-1

ESTIMATES OF RATES PER THOUSAND OF CHROMOSOME ABNORMALITIES IN LIVE BIRTHS BY SINGLE-YEAR INTERVAL

Maternal Age (y)	Down's Syndrome	Edwards' Syndrome (Trisomy 18)	Patau's Syndrome (Trisomy 13)	XXY	XYY	Turner's Syndrome Genotype	Other Clinically Significant Abnormality*	Total†
<15	1.0‡	<0.1‡	<0.1-0.1	0.4	0.5	<0.1	0.2	2.2
15	1.0‡	<0.1‡	<0.1-0.1	0.4	0.5	<0.1	0.2	2.2
16	0.9‡	<0.1‡	<0.1-0.1	0.4	0.5	<0.1	0.2	2.1
17	0.8‡	<0.1‡	<0.1-0.1	0.4	0.5	<0.1	0.2	2.0
18	0.7‡	<0.1‡	<0.1-0.1	0.4	0.5	<0.1	0.2	1.9
19	0.6‡	<0.1‡	<0.1-0.1	0.4	0.5	<0.1	0.2	1.8
20	0.5-0.7	<0.1-0.1	<0.1-0.1	0.4	0.5	<0.1	0.2	1.9
21	0.5-0.7	<0.1-0.1	<0.1-0.1	0.4	0.5	<0.1	0.2	1.9
22	0.6-0.8	<0.1-0.1	<0.1-0.1	0.4	0.5	<0.1	0.2	2.0
23	0.6-0.8	<0.1-0.1	<0.1-0.1	0.4	0.5	<0.1	0.2	2.0
24	0.7-0.9	0.1-0.1	<0.1-0.1	0.4	0.5	<0.1	0.2	2.1
25	0.7-0.9	0.1-0.1	<0.1-0.1	0.4	0.5	<0.1	0.2	2.1
26	0.7-1.0	0.1-0.1	<0.1-0.1	0.4	0.5	<0.1	0.2	2.1
27	0.8-1.0	0.1-0.2	<0.1-0.1	0.4	0.5	<0.1	0.2	2.2
28	0.8-1.1	0.1-0.2	<0.1-0.2	0.4	0.5	<0.1	0.2	2.3
29	0.8-1.2	0.1-0.2	<0.1-0.2	0.5	0.5	<0.1	0.2	2.4
30	0.9-1.2	0.1-0.2	<0.1-0.2	0.5	0.5	<0.1	0.2	2.6
31	0.9-1.3	0.1-0.2	<0.1-0.2	0.5	0.5	<0.1	0.2	2.6
32	1.1-1.5	0.1-0.2	0.1-0.2	0.6	0.5	<0.1	0.2	3.1
33	1.4-1.9	0.1-0.3	0.1-0.2	0.7	0.5	<0.1	0.2	3.5

Age							
34	1.9-2.4	0.2-0.4	0.1-0.3	0.7	0.5	<0.1	0.2	4.1
35	2.5-3.9	0.3-0.5	0.2-0.3	0.9	0.5	<0.1	0.3	5.6
36	3.2-5.0	0.3-0.6	0.2-0.4	1.0	0.5	<0.1	0.3	6.7
37	4.1-6.4	0.4-0.7	0.2-0.5	1.1	0.5	<0.1	0.3	8.1
38	5.2-8.1	0.5-0.9	0.3-0.7	1.3	0.5	<0.1	0.3	9.5
39	6.6-10.5	0.7-1.2	0.4-0.8	1.5	0.5	<0.1	0.3	12.4
40	8.5-13.7	0.9-1.6	0.5-1.1	1.8	0.5	<0.1	0.3	15.8
41	10.8-17.9	1.2-2.1	0.6-1.4	2.2	0.5	<0.1	0.3	20.5
42	13.8-23.4	1.4-2.7	0.7-1.8	2.7	0.5	<0.1	0.3	25.5
43	17.6-30.6	1.8-3.5	0.9-2.4	3.3	0.5	<0.1	0.3	32.6
44	22.5-40.0	2.3-4.6	1.2-3.1	4.1	0.5	<0.1	0.3	41.8
45	28.7-52.3	2.9-6.0	1.5-4.1	5.1	0.5	<0.1	0.3	53.7
46	36.6-68.3	3.7-7.9	1.9-5.3	6.4	0.5	<0.1	0.3	68.9
47	46.6-89.3	4.7-10.3	2.4-6.9	8.2	0.5	<0.1	0.3	89.1
48	59.5-116.8	6.0-13.5	3.0-9.0	10.6	0.5	<0.1	0.3	115.0
49	75.8-152.7	7.6-17.6	3.8-11.8	13.8	0.5	<0.1	0.3	149.3

From Hook EB: *Obstet Gynecol* 58:282, 1981.

*XXX is excluded.

†Calculation of the total at each age assumes rate for autosomal aneuploidies is at the midpoint of the ranges given.

‡No range can be constructed for those under 20 y by the same methods as for those 20 y and over. These age-related risk estimates are for women who present with no other risk factor except age. They are derived from multiple regression studies of *live births* of chromosomally abnormal infants.

FETAL PHYSIOLOGY D

Diagnostic Radiology and the Fetus

I. DIAGNOSTIC RADIOLOGIC PROCEDURES AND LEVEL OF FETAL RADIATION EXPOSURE

A. RADIOGRAPHS

1. **X-ray scans** (Table E-1)
2. **Computed tomography.** The fetal exposure with this radiologic modality has been difficult to determine. Table E-2 is a rough guide to estimated fetal dosage.

B. MAGNETIC RESONANCE IMAGING. No radiation is used with this form of scanning.

C. OCCUPATIONAL EXPOSURE. The National Council of Radiation Protection and Measurement recommends that mothers facing occupational radiation exposure not be exposed to more than 0.5 radiation absorbed dose (rad) throughout their pregnancy.

II. EFFECTS OF RADIATION ON THE FETUS

A. TIME OF EXPOSURE

1. Fetal radiation exposure soon after conception results either in abortion or an unaffected fetus.
2. Fetal radiation exposure between 8 and 15 weeks' gestation demonstrates a linear relationship between the absorbed fetal dose and severe mental retardation. The risk has been estimated at 0.4% per rad.*
Columbia Presbyterian Medical Center cites this estimate as a follow-up study of children born to mothers who received pelvic irradiation in Hiroshima and Nagasaki. According to Harrison (see Suggested Readings), microcephaly showed a statistic increase at doses at or above 10 to 19 rads, small stature at 25 rads, and mental retardation at 50 rads. This is far above current radiographic dosages (Table E 3).

B. EXPOSURE DOSE

1. At a level of >50 rads of fetal exposure, a significant chance of an embryopathic event is present.
2. At a level of >15 rads of fetal exposure, the number of malformations is significantly higher than control levels. Only exposures above this level warrant consideration of pregnancy termination.
3. Many authors claim never to have seen congenital defects at a dose level of ≤10 rads. However, Harrison found that low levels of intrauterine radiation (1 to 3 rads) may be associated with a small increase in the risk (1.5 to 2×) of leukemia and of chromosomal abnormalities in

---

*Quoted in Columbia Presbyterian draft policy concerning occupationally exposed women who are or could be pregnant, *Br J Radiol* 57:409-414, 1984.

ESTIMATED DOSE TO UTERUS FROM EXTRAABDOMINAL EXAMINATIONS (FLUOROSCOPIC DOSE EXCLUDED)

Examination	Estimated Mean Dose (mrad/Examination)			Reported Range§
	BRH*	ICRP†	UNSCEAR‡	
Dental		<10	0.06	0.03-0.1
Head-cervical spine	<0.5	<10	<10	<0.5-3.0
Extremities	<0.5	<10	<10	<0.5-18.0
Shoulder	<0.5	<10		<0.5-3.0
Thoracic spine	11	<10		<10-55
Chest (radiographic)	1		2	0.2-43
Chest (photofluorographic)	3	<10	3	0.9-40
Mammography			<10	
Femur (distal)		50	1	1-50
Upper gastrointestinal series	171	150		5-1230
Cholecystography	78	150	120	14-1600
Cholangiography				
Lumbar spine	990		560	27-3970
Lumbosacral spine		550	470	100-2440
Pelvis	290	340	320	55-2190
Hips and femur (proximal)	170	690	330	73-1370
Urography, intravenous, or retrograde pyelogram	810	960 1100	810 715	70-5480 120-5480
Urethrocystography		2060		275-4110
Lower gastrointestinal tract (barium enema)	1240	1100	1200	28-12,600
Abdomen	300	690	290	25-1920
Abdomen (obstetric)		1370 (fetal)	410	150-2200
Pelvimetry		5480	850	220-5480
Hysterosalpingography		1650	1740	270-9180

Modified from National Council on Radiation Protection and Measurements (NCRP), 1977; Wagner LK, Lester RG, Saldana LR: *Exposure of the pregnant patient to diagnostic radiations: a guide to medical management,* Philadelphia, 1985, Lippincott. All values are for radiography only (no fluoroscopy). Doses listed for lower abdominal studies are 37% higher than those in NCRP (1977).
*Bureau of Radiological Health (BRH) (1976).
†International Commission of Radiological Protection (CRP) (1970).
‡United Nations Scientific Committee on the Effects of Atomic Radiation (UNSCEAR) (1972).
§Includes BRH (1976), ICRP (1970), UNSCEAR (1972), and Lindell and Dobson (1961).

ESTIMATED AVERAGE FETAL DOSE PER DIAGNOSTIC RADIOLOGIC EXAMINATION: COMPUTED TOMOGRAPHY

Examination	Typical Dose to Fetus
Head scan	Insignificant
Extremity	Insignificant
Chest	Insignificant to low
Abdominal with or without contrast	Below 10 rads*

*Varies with fetal proximity to the area being studied.

SUMMARY OF EFFECTS OF DIAGNOSTIC LEVELS OF RADIATION (0-25 RADS) ON THE UNBORN*

Weeks After Conception	Gestation Stage	Effect				
		Prenatal Death	Small Head Size	Severe Mental Retardation (SMR)	Other Malformation	Childhood Cancer
0–	Preimplantation	Possible radiation-induced resorption	None established for humans at diagnostic levels	None established for humans at diagnostic levels	None established for humans at diagnostic levels	Higher risk period
2–	Major organogenesis	None established for humans at diagnostic levels	Incidence of 1%/rad at Hiroshima, but causal nature of radiation is uncertain		Animal data suggest this is most sensitive stage, but none established for humans at diagnostic levels	
6–						

(First trimester)

Continued

E

DIAGNOSTIC RADIOLOGY AND THE FETUS

231

TABLE E-3

SUMMARY OF EFFECTS OF DIAGNOSTIC LEVELS OF RADIATION (0-25 RADS) ON THE UNBORN*—cont'd

Weeks After Conception	Gestation Stage	Effect					
		Prenatal Death	Small Head Size	Severe Mental Retardation (SMR)	Other Malformation	Childhood Cancer
8-	Synaptogenesis Rapid neuron development and migration			SMR at 0.4%/rad from A-bomb, but radiation may not have been sole cause of this effect	None established for humans at diagnostic levels	Lesser risk period
15-						
16-			None established for humans at diagnostic levels	None established or humans at diagnostic levels		
38-						

(Second and third trimesters)

Modified from Wagner LK, Lester RG, Saldana LR: *Exposure of the pregnant patient to diagnostic radiations: a guide to medical management*, Philadelphia, 1985, Lippincott.
*Effects from placental transfer of radionuclides are not included.

germ cells, although this is controversial. (For example, in one large study the control risk of leukemia was 1/2880, and the risk of those exposed to pelvimetry was 1/2000 [Harrison, 1977].)

4. Intrauterine growth retardation and central nervous system (CNS) abnormalities (microcephaly, cerebral and cerebellar hypoplasia) may be seen throughout gestation with *therapeutic* doses of radiation. It is unlikely that a major anomaly in an infant is caused by radiation if fetal growth or the CNS has not been affected.

5. All pregnant women exposed to radiation must be made aware of the possible long-term effects of this exposure.

III. CONVERSION OF RADIOLOGIC UNITS

A. A **roentgen (R)** is a measure of the quantity of X or gamma ionizing radiation in the air.

B. The **rad** is a measure of the energy absorbed by tissue from ionizing radiation equivalent to 100 ergs of energy per gram. For practical purposes, the R and the rad are equivalent.

C. A **rem** is the dose in rads multiplied by the quality factor (the quality factor equals 1 for the radiations encountered with x-rays and gamma rays and electrons and photons). This unit allows radiologists to describe the observation that some forms of radiation, such as neutrons, may produce a greater biologic effect per dose of absorbed energy.

D. *Rad* and *rem* are commonly used terminology in the United States. Internationally, they are comparable to the gray and the sievert in the following manner:

$$100 \text{ rads} - 1 \text{ gray (Gy)}$$

$$100 \text{ rems} = 1 \text{ sievert (Sv)}$$

SUGGESTED READINGS

Harrison JA: Radiation in pregnancy. In Goldstein AI, editor: *Advances in perinatal medicine,* New York, 1977, Symposia Specialists Medical Books.

Main DM, Main EK: *Obstetrics and gynecology: a pocket reference,* St Louis, 1984, Mosby.

Howland WJ, editor: *Radiation biology syllabus and questions for diagnostic radiology residents,* Oak Brook, Ill, 1982, Radiological Society of North America.

National Council on Radiation Protection and Measurements: *Medical radiation exposure of pregnant and potentially pregnant women.* NCRP Report No. 54, Bethesda, Md, May 1, 1985.

Mossman KL, Hill LT: Radiation risks in pregnancy, *Obstet Gynecol* 60:237-242, 1982.

Policy Concerning Occupationally Exposed Women Who Are or Could Be Pregnant, New York, 1990, Columbia Presbyterian Medical Center (draft).

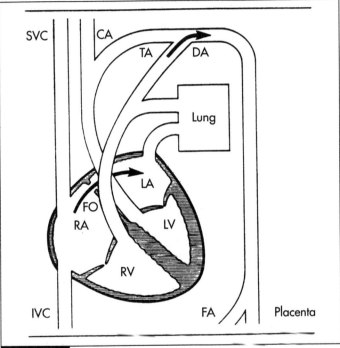

FIGURE F-1

Anatomy of fetal heart and central shunts. *SVC,* Superior vena cava; *CA,* carotid artery; *TA,* thoracic aorta; *DA,* ductus arteriosus; *RA,* right atrium; *FO,* foramen ovale; *LA,* left atrium; *RV,* right ventricle; *LV,* left ventricle; *IVC,* inferior vena cava; *FA,* femoral artery. *(From Anderson DF et al: Am J Physiol 241:H60, 1981.)*

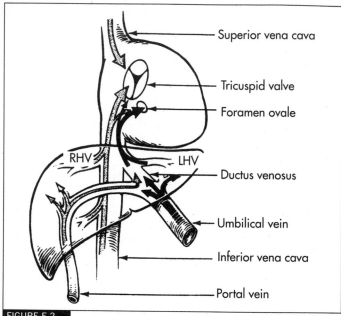

FIGURE F-2

Anatomy of umbilical and hepatic circulation. *RHV*, Right hepatic vein; *LHV*, left hepatic vein. *(From Rudolph AM: Hepatology 3:254, 1983.)*

TABLE F-1

Fetal Structure	From/To	Adult Remnant
Umbilical vein	Umbilicus/ductus venosus	Ligamentum teres hepatitis
Ductus venosus	Umbilical vein/inferior vena cava (bypasses liver)	Ligamentum venosum
Foramen ovale	Right atrium/left atrium	Closed atrial wall
Ductus arteriosus	Pulmonary artery/descending aorta	Ligamentum arteriosum
Umbilical artery	Common iliac artery/umbilicus	Superior vesicle arteries Lateral vesicoumbilical ligaments

From Gabbe SG, Niebyl JR, Simpson JL: *Obstetrics: normal and problem pregnancies,* ed 2, New York, 1991, Churchill Livingstone.

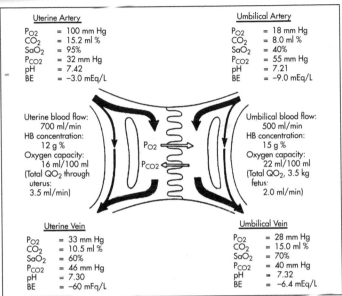

Uterine Artery		Umbilical Artery	
P_{O2}	= 100 mm Hg	P_{O2}	= 18 mm Hg
CO_2	= 15.2 ml %	CO_2	= 8.0 ml %
SaO_2	= 95%	SaO_2	= 40%
P_{CO2}	= 32 mm Hg	P_{CO2}	= 55 mm Hg
pH	= 7.42	pH	= 7.21
BE	= −3.0 mEq/L	BE	= −9.0 mEq/L

Uterine blood flow:
700 ml/min
HB concentration:
12 g %
Oxygen capacity:
16 ml/100 ml
(Total QO_2 through
uterus:
3.5 ml/min)

P_{O2}

P_{CO2}

Umbilical blood flow:
500 ml/min
HB concentration:
15 g %
Oxygen capacity:
22 ml/100 ml
(Total QO_2, 3.5 kg
fetus:
2.0 ml/min)

Uterine Vein		Umbilical Vein	
P_{O2}	= 33 mm Hg	P_{O2}	= 28 mm Hg
CO_2	= 10.5 ml %	CO_2	= 15.0 ml %
SaO_2	= 60%	SaO_2	= 70%
P_{CO2}	= 46 mm Hg	P_{CO2}	= 40 mm Hg
pH	= 7.30	pH	= 7.32
BE	= −60 mFq/L	BE	= −6.4 mEq/L

FIGURE G-1

Placental transfer of oxygen and carbon dioxide. These data represent a synthesis of estimations from clinical material and extrapolations from sheep models. *(From Bonica JJ: Obstetric analgesia and anesthesia, ed 2, Amsterdam, 1980, World Federation of Societies of Anesthesiologists.)*

TABLE G-1

DEFINITIONS

Term	Definition
Acidemia	Increased concentration of hydrogen ions in the blood
Acidosis	A pathologic condition marked by an increased concentration of hydrogen ions in tissue
Hypoxemia	Decreased oxygen content in blood
Hypoxia	A pathologic condition marked by a decreased level of oxygen in tissue
Asphyxia	Hypoxia and metabolic acidosis

TABLE G-2

CLASSIFICATION OF FETAL OR NEWBORN ACIDEMIA*

Acidemia Type	P_{CO_2} (mm Hg)	HCO_3^- (mEq/L)	Base Deficit (mEq/L)†
Respiratory	High (>65)	Normal (≥22)	Normal (−6.4 ± 1.9)
Metabolic	Normal (<65)	Low (≤17)	High (−15.9 ± 2.8)
Mixed	High (≥65)	Low (≤17)	High (−9.6 ± 2.5)

From *Assessment of Fetal and Newborn Acid-Base Status.* ACOG Tech Bull No. 127, Washington, DC, April 1989, American College of Obstetricians and Gynecologists.
*Umbilical artery pH less than 7.2.
†Means ± standard deviations are given in parentheses.

TABLE G-3

NORMAL UMBILICAL CORD BLOOD pH AND BLOOD GAS VALUES IN TERM NEWBORNS (MEAN ± ONE STANDARD DEVIATION)

Value	Yeomans* ($n = 146$)	Ramin* ($n = 1,292$)	Riley† ($n = 3,522$)
Arterial blood			
pH	7.28 (0.05)	7.28 (0.07)	7.27 (0.069)
P_{CO_2} (mm Hg)	49.2 (8.4)	49.9 (14.2)	50.3 (11.1)
HCO_3^- (mEq/L)	22.3 (2.5)	23.1 (2.8)	22.0 (3.6)
Base excess (mEq/L)	—‡	−3.6 (2.8)	−2.7 (2.8)
Venous blood			
pH	7.35 (0.05)	—	7.34 (0.063)
P_{CO_2} (mm Hg)	38.2 (5.6)	—	40.7 (7.9)
HCO_3^- (mEq/L)	20.4 (4.1)	—	21.4 (2.5)
Base excess (mEq/L)	—	—	−2.4 (2)

Ramin SM et al: Umbilical artery acid–base status in the preterm infant. *Obstet Gynecol* 74: 256-258, 1989.
Riley RJ, Johnson JWC: Collecting and analyzing cord blood gases. *Clin Obstet Gynecol* 36:13-23, 1993.
Yeomans ER et al: Umbilical cord pH, P_{CO_2} and bicarbonate following uncomplicated term vaginal deliveries. *Am J Obstet Gynecol* 151:798-800, 1985.
*Data are from infants of selected patients with uncomplicated vaginal deliveries.
†Data are from infants of unselected patients with vaginal deliveries.
‡Data were not obtained.

TABLE G-4

NORMAL UMBILICAL ARTERY BLOOD pH AND BLOOD GAS VALUES IN PREMATURE INFANTS (MEAN ± ONE STANDARD DEVIATION)

Value for Arterial Blood	Ramin* (n = 77)	Dickinson† (n = 949)	Riley† (n = 1,015)
pH	7.29 (0.07)	7.27 (0.07)	7.28 (0.089)
Pco₂ (mm Hg)	49.2 (9.0)	51.6 (9.4)	50.2 (12.3)
HCO₃⁻ (mEq/L)	23.0 (3.5)	23.9 (2.1)	22.4 (3.5)
Base excess (mEq/L)	−3.3 (2.4)	−3.0 (2.5)	−2.5 (3)

Dickinson JE et al: The effect of preterm birth on umbilical cord blood gases. *Obstet Gynecol* 79:575-578, 1992.

Ramin SM et al: Umbilical artery acid–base status in the preterm infant. *Obstet Gynecol* 74: 256-258, 1989.

Riley RJ, Johnson JWC: Collecting and analyzing cord blood gases. *Clin Obstet Gynecol* 36:13-23, 1993.

*Data are from infants of selected patients with uncomplicated vaginal deliveries.

†Data are from infants of unselected patients with vaginal deliveries.

Ultrasound Evaluation: Fetal Growth

H

Weeks of gestation	4	5	6	7	8	9	10	11	12
Gestational sac only	100	→							
Yolk sac	0	90	100	→					
Fetal pole with heart motion	0	0	86	100	→				
Single ventricle	0	0	6	82	100	25	0	0	0
Falrx	0	0	0	0	30	75	100	100	100
Midgut herniation	0	0	0	0	100	100	100	50	0
Total cases	6	11	15	17	10	13	15	11	6

FIGURE H-1

Transvaginal sonography. Percentage of six embryonic structures present *(white areas)* or absent *(gray areas)* during first trimester of pregnancy in patients evaluated with transvaginal sonography. Solid lines separate weeks of gestation at which a majority of embryos demonstrated a change in sonographic appearance. NOTE: The yolk sac is usually not seen after 12 weeks' gestation. *(From Timor-Tritsch IE, Monteagudo A: Obstet Gynecol Rep 2:210, 1990.)*

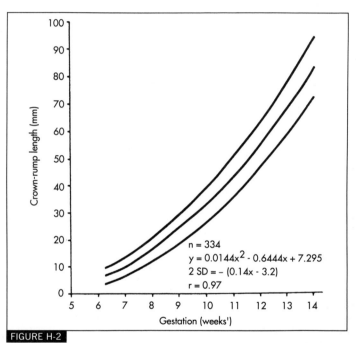

FIGURE H-2

Nomogram showing the correlation between the crown-rump length measurement and gestational age. *(From Robinson H, Fleming J: Br J Obstet Gynaecol 82:703, 1975.)*

H

ULTRASOUND EVALUATION: FETAL GROWTH

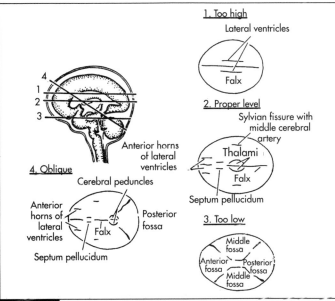

1. Too high
Lateral ventricles
Falx

2. Proper level
Sylvian fissure with middle cerebral artery
Thalami
Falx
Septum pellucidum

3. Too low
Middle fossa
Anterior fossa
Posterior fossa
Middle fossa

4. Oblique
Cerebral peduncles
Anterior horns of lateral ventricles
Anterior horns of lateral ventricles
Posterior fossa
Falx
Septum pellucidum

FIGURE H-3

Landmarks for obtaining a proper biparietal diameter. These drawings demonstrate the landmarks seen when placing the ultrasound transducer in too high, correct, too low, or oblique positions. *(Modified from materials developed by JP Crane at Washington University, St Louis. In Main DM, Main EK, editors: Obstetrics and gynecology: a pocket reference, St Louis, 1984, Mosby.)*

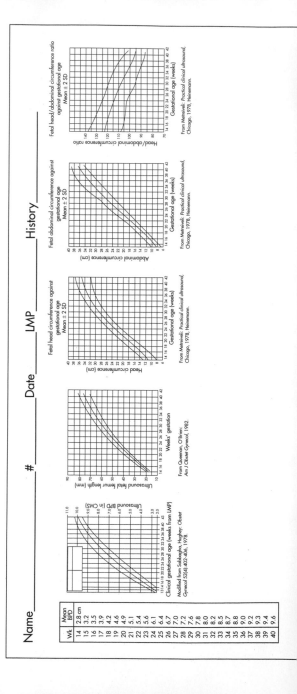

Name_____ #_____ Date_____ LMP_____ History_____

Wk	Mean BPD
14	2.8 cm
15	3.2
16	3.5
17	3.9
18	4.2
19	4.6
20	4.9
21	5.1
22	5.4
23	5.6
24	6.1
25	6.4
26	6.7
27	7.0
28	7.2
29	7.6
30	7.8
31	8.0
32	8.2
33	8.5
34	8.7
35	8.8
36	9.0
37	9.2
38	9.3
39	9.4
40	9.6

Ultrasound BPD (in CMS)

Modified from Sabbagha, Hughey, Obster Gynecol 52(4):402-406, 1978.

Fetal head circumference against gestational age
Mean ± 2 SD

From Metreveli: Practical clinical ultrasound, Chicago, 1978, Heinemann.

Fetal abdominal circumference against gestational age
Mean ± 2 SD

From Metreveli: Practical clinical ultrasound, Chicago, 1978, Heinemann.

Fetal head/abdominal circumference ratio against gestational age
Mean ± 2 SD

From Metreveli: Practical clinical ultrasound, Chicago, 1978, Heinemann.

Ultrasound fetal femur length (mm)

From Queenan, O'Brien: Am J Obstet Gynecol, 1982.

Weeks' gestation

ULTRASOUND EVALUATION: FETAL GROWTH

FIGURE H-4
Sequential analysis of ultrasonic fetal growth parameters. *(From Gabbe SG, Niebyl JR, Simpson JL: Obstetrics: normal and problem pregnancies, ed 2, New York, 1991, Churchill Livingstone.)*

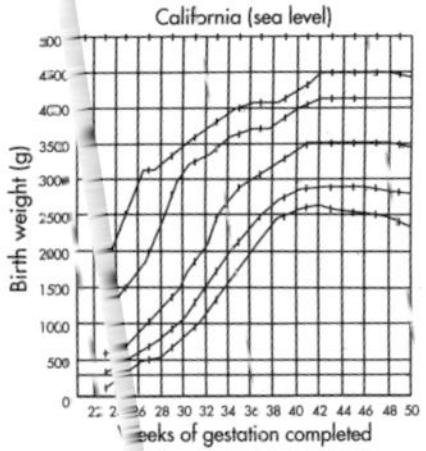

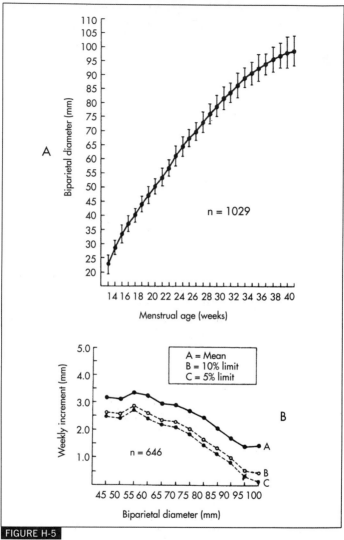

FIGURE H-5

A, Mean fetal biparietal diameter (mm) ±2 standard deviations for each week of pregnancy from 13 weeks' gestation to term. **B,** Mean growth rate of the fetal biparietal diameter. The mean weekly increase in the biparietal diameter is rapid and almost linear from 14 until 30 weeks' menstrual age (3.3 mm/wk). The growth slows significantly between 30 and 36 weeks (2 mm/wk) and then falls rapidly until term, with a mean rate of increase of 1.2 mm/wk. *(From Campbell S. In Beard RS, Nathaniels PW, editors: Fetal physiology in medicine: the basis of perinatology, Philadelphia, 1976, Saunders.)*

Ultrasound Evaluation:
Amniotic Fluid Volume

TABLE I-1

AMNIOTIC FLUID INDEX PERCENTILE VALUES (mm)

Week	Percentile					n
	2.5th	5th	50th	95th	97.5th	
16	73	79	121	185	201	32
17	77	83	127	194	211	26
18	80	87	133	202	220	17
19	83	90	137	207	225	14
20	86	93	141	212	230	25
21	88	95	143	214	233	14
22	89	97	145	216	235	14
23	90	98	146	218	237	14
24	90	98	147	219	238	23
25	89	97	147	221	240	12
26	89	97	147	223	242	11
27	85	95	146	226	245	17
28	86	94	146	228	249	25
29	84	92	145	231	254	12
30	82	90	145	234	258	17
31	79	88	144	238	263	26
32	77	86	144	242	269	25
33	74	83	143	245	274	30
34	72	81	142	248	278	31
35	70	79	140	249	279	27
36	68	77	138	249	279	39
37	66	75	135	244	275	36
38	65	73	132	239	269	27
39	64	72	127	226	255	12
40	63	71	123	214	240	64
41	63	70	116	194	216	162
42	63	69	110	175	192	30

From Moore TR, Cayle JE: *Am J Obstet Gynecol* 162:1168, 1990.

TABLE I-2

OLIGOHYDRAMNIOS

DEFINITION

<200 ml amniotic fluid at term

Ultrasound definition: Amniotic fluid index (AFI) less than 5 cm

DIAGNOSIS

1. Antenatal diagnosis is clinically difficult. It has been suggested that oligohydramnios can be diagnosed by ultrasound when the largest pocket of amniotic fluid measures less than 1 cm in its broadest diameter.
2. Presence of amnion nodosum on placenta at delivery is highly correlated with oligohydramnios.

CLINICAL ASSOCIATIONS

1. Fetal malformations, particularly renal agenesis, polycystic kidneys, ureteral and urethral obstruction, and agenesis of the penis
2. Extramembranous pregnancies
3. Prolonged leakage of amniotic fluid
4. Intrauterine growth retardation, particularly secondary to pregnancy-induced hypertension and other conditions that induce placental insufficiency
5. Postmaturity syndrome

FETAL ANOMALIES ASSOCIATED WITH PROLONGED OLIGOHYDRAMNIOS (USUALLY AFTER A MINIMUM OF 3 WK OF OLIGOHYDRAMNIOS)

1. Potter's facies: Increased space between eyes, prominent fold that arises from inner canthus and sweeps downward and laterally below the eyes, nasal flattening, excessive recession of the chin, enlarged and low-set ears
2. Pulmonary hypoplasia and insufficiency
3. Limb malpositions, such as clubbed feet
4. Fetal growth retardation

Modified from Main DM, Main EK: *Obstetrics and gynecology: a pocket reference,* St Louis, 1984, Mosby.

TABLE I-3

INCIDENCE OF POLYHYDRAMNIOS AND ASSOCIATED CONDITIONS

	Incidence*	
	No.	%
Total deliveries	86,301	100.00
Polyhydramnios†	358	0.41
Associated conditions		
Diabetes	88	24.6
Erythroblastosis fetalis	41	11.5
Multiple gestation	33	9.2
Congenital malformations‡	72	20.1
Idiopathic	124	34.6
TOTAL	358	100.0

From Main DM, Main EK: *Obstetrics and gynecology: a pocket reference*, St Louis, 1984, Mosby.
*Data from Queenan JT, Gadow EC: *Am J Obstet Gynecol* 108:349, 1970. Based on a 20-year retrospective study in one institution (1948-1967). Polyhydramnios defined as ≥2000 ml amniotic fluid; 1.7% acute, 98.3% chronic.
†Polyhydramnios, clinical definition: ≥2000 ml amniotic fluid. Polyhydramnios, ultrasound definition: amniotic fluid Index >25 cm or a single pocket >8 cm.
‡Approximately 50% of the congenital anomalies will involve the central nervous system, 20% the gastrointestinal tract, and 20% the heart. (From Murray SR: *Am J Obstet Gynecol* 88:65, 1964; Jocaby HE, Charles D: *Am J Obstet Gynecol* 94:110, 1966.)

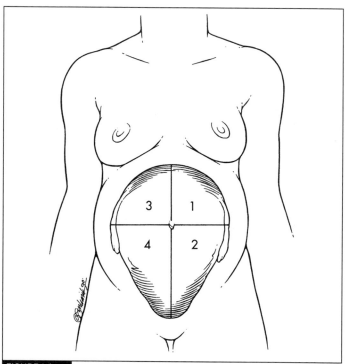

FIGURE I-1

The amniotic fluid index measurement uses ultrasound to assess depth of fluid pockets in each quadrant of uterus. Note that umbilicus divides uterus into upper and lower halves, and linea nigra divides uterus into right and left halves. *(From Gabbe SG, Niebyl JR, Simpson JL: Obstetrics: normal and problem pregnancies, ed 2, New York, 1991, Churchill Livingstone.)*

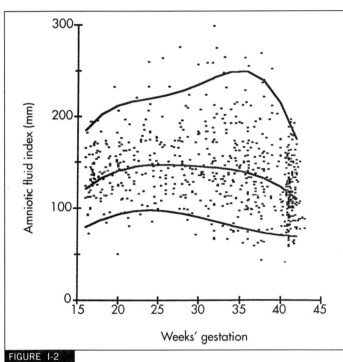

FIGURE I-2

Graph demonstrating the **amniotic fluid index** in millimeters plotted against **gestational week** in a population of normal patients. Upper, middle, and lower lines represent 95th, 50th, and 5th percentiles, respectively. *(From Moore TR: Am J Obstet Gynecol 163:762, 1990.)*

Ultrasound Evaluation: Placental Grading

The placenta may be assessed by ultrasound evaluation. As the placenta matures, its ultrasonic appearance changes. Table J-1 and Figure J-1 illustrate the commonly used placental grading system.

J

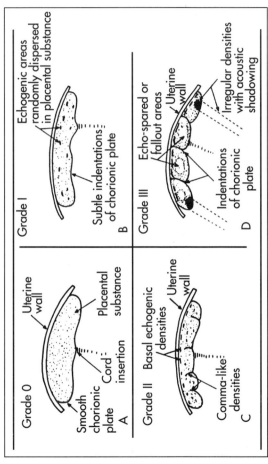

FIGURE J-1

Four stages of placental maturation based on appearance of basal and chorionic plate of placenta and placental substance. *(From Grannum PAT, Berkowitz RL, Hobbins JC: Am J Obstet Gynecol 133:915, 1979.)*

TABLE J-1
SUMMARY OF PLACENTAL GRADING

Section of Placenta	Placental Grade			
	0	1	2	3
Chorionic plate	Straight and well defined	Subtle undulations	Indentations extending into placenta but not to basal layer	Indentations communicating with basal layer
Placental substance	Homogeneous	Few scattered EGAs	Linear echogenic densities (comma-like densities)	Circular densities with echo-spared areas in center; large, irregular densities casting acoustic shadows
Basal layer	No densities	No densities	Linear arrangement of small EGAs (basal stippling)	Large and somewhat confluent basal EGAs; can create acoustic shadows

From Grannum P, Berkowitz R, Hobbins J: *Am J Obstet Gynecol* 133:915, 1979.
EGAs, Echogenic areas.

J

ULTRASOUND EVALUATION: PLACENTAL GRADING

255

Intrapartum Fetal Heart Rate Monitoring

Fetal heart rate (FHR) analysis allows antepartum and intrapartum assessment of the unborn child. Intrapartum monitoring may be done externally (through the abdomen and anterior uterine wall) or internally (by placement of an electrode on the infant's presenting part). When external FHR analysis does not confirm fetal well-being, internal monitoring should be considered. If internal monitoring does not indicate adequate oxygenation of the infant, traditionally a physician facilitates delivery in the most expeditious way. If a vaginal delivery is predicted shortly a physician may elect to perform "scalp sampling," i.e., making a small incision on the infant's scalp and obtaining an aliquot of capillary blood to be tested for pH. The pH value helps the physician determine whether the fetus is maintaining adequate oxygenation so that a vaginal delivery may be attempted.

In early 2000 the FDA approved an additional method for evaluating fetal health. Oxygen saturation of the fetal red blood cells can now be assessed in real time. After rupture of membranes a sensor is placed into the uterine cavity and rests against the fetal cheek or temple. Real-time measurement of fetal oxygenation by pulse oximetry ($FSpo_2$) may be tracked continuously. Mallinckrodt (St. Louis, MO) makes this monitor, which is called Oxifirst. If available at your institution, consider its use in the presence of a nonreassuring fetal heart rate tracing.

K

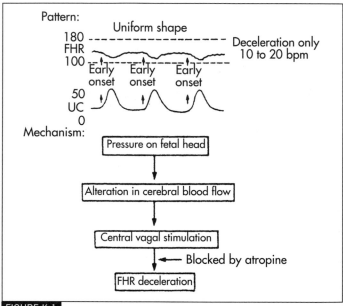

FIGURE K-1

Pattern and mechanism of early decelerations. Early decelerations generally occur at 4 to 7 cm of cervical dilation. They can be reproduced by pressing a doughnut pessary with an internal diameter of 4 to 6 cm over neonatal head, thus causing compression of anterior fontanelle. This pattern is not associated with fetal hypoxia, acidosis, or low Apgar scores. *FHR,* Fetal heart rate; *UC,* uterine contraction. *(From Main DM, Main EK: Obstetrics and gynecology: a pocket reference, St Louis, 1984, Mosby.)*

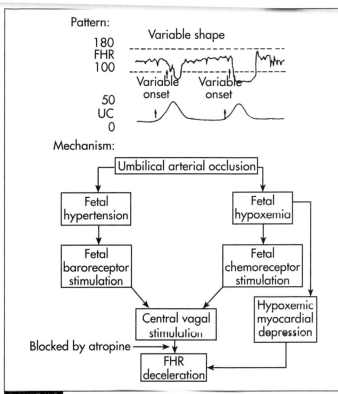

FIGURE K-2

Pattern and mechanism of variable decelerations. Variable decelerations are changeable in duration, intensity, and timing relative to contractions. Characteristically, they are abrupt in onset and return to baseline. Degree of fetal compromise varies directly with duration and degree of cord compression. If compression is prolonged and repetitive, fetal hypoxia and acidosis may occur. Associated loss of variability and tachycardia suggest fetal compromise. *FHR,* Fetal heart rate; *UC,* uterine contraction. *(From Main DM, Main EK: Obstetrics and gynecology: a pocket reference, St Louis, 1984, Mosby.)*

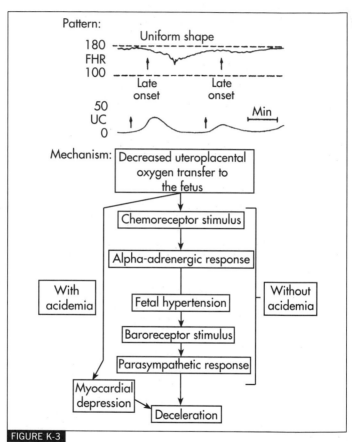

FIGURE K-3

Pattern and mechanism of late decelerations. *FHR,* Fetal heart rate; *UC,* uterine contraction. *(From Main DM, Main EK: Obstetrics and gynecology: a pocket reference, St Louis, 1984, Mosby.)*

TABLE K-1

CAUSES OF FETAL TACHYCARDIA

Fetal hypoxia
Maternal fever
Parasympatholytic drugs
    Atropine
    Hydroxyzine (Vistaril, Atarax)
    Phenothiazines
Maternal hypothyroidism
Fetal anemia
Fetal heart failure
Amnionitis
Fetal cardiac tachyarrhythmia
β-Sympathomimetic drugs

From Freeman RK, Garite TJ, Nageotte MP: *Fetal heart rate monitoring,* ed 2, Baltimore, 1991, Williams & Wilkins.

TABLE K-2

CAUSES OF DECREASED FETAL HEART RATE VARIABILITY

Hypoxia/acidosis
Drugs
    Central nervous system depressants
    Parasympatholytics
Fetal sleep cycles
Congenital anomalies
Extreme prematurity
Fetal tachycardia
Preexisting neurologic abnormality

From Freeman RK, Garite TJ, Nageotte MP: *Fetal heart rate monitoring,* ed 2, Baltimore, 1991, Williams & Wilkins.

TABLE K-3

EXAMPLES OF DRUGS CAUSING DECREASED FETAL HEART RATE VARIABILITY

Central nervous system depressants
   Analgesics/narcotics
      Meperidine (Demerol)
      Heroin
      Alphaprodine (Nisentil)
      Morphine
   Barbiturates
      Phenobarbital
      Secobarbital
   Tranquilizers
      Diazepam
   Phenothiazines
      Propiomazine hydrochloride (Largon)
      Promethazine (Phenergan)
Parasympatholytics
   Phenothiazines
   Atropine
General anesthetics

Modified from Freeman RK, Garite TJ, Nageotte MP: *Fetal heart rate monitoring,* ed 2, Baltimore, 1991, Williams & Wilkins.

TABLE K-4

CAUSES OF FETAL BRADYCARDIA

1. Physiologic (not associated with fetal acidosis)
   a. 100-120 bpm with good variability during the first stage of labor
   b. 85-120 bpm with good variability during the second stage of labor
2. Congenital complete heart block
   a. Associated with high incidence of structural heart lesions
   b. Associated with maternal connective tissue disease (e.g., systemic lupus erythematosus)
   c. Maternal viral infection
   d. Maternal hypothermia
3. Maternal medications depressing atrioventricular nodal conduction
   a. Antegrade (slow) limb
      (1) Digitalis
      (2) β-Blockers
      (3) Calcium channel blockers
   b. Retrograde (fast) limb
      (1) Quinidine
      (2) Procainamide
4. Central nervous system
5. Prolonged deceleration
6. Fetal death (with transmitted maternal signal)

Modified from Freeman RK, Garite TJ, Nageotte MP: *Fetal heart rate monitoring,* ed 2, Baltimore, 1991, Williams & Wilkins.

TABLE K-5

CAUSES OF PROLONGED FETAL HEART RATE DECELERATIONS

Fetal-placental etiologies
  Tetanic contraction (spontaneous)
  Prolapsed umbilical cord
  Central nervous system anomalies
  Prolonged umbilical cord compression (as seen with rapid descent of fetus during
    expulsion)
Maternal etiologies
  Maternal convulsion
  Supine hypotension
  Maternal respiratory arrest (high spinal or intravenous narcotic) or cardiac
    decompensation
Iatrogenic etiologies
  Tetanic contraction (oxytocin-induced)
  Vaginal examination
  Application of internal fetal scalp electrode
  Fetal scalp blood sampling
  Paracervical block
  Epidural block

Data from Freeman RK, Garite TJ, Nageotte MP: *Fetal heart rate monitoring,* ed 2, Baltimore, 1991,
Williams & Wilkins.

TABLE K-6

GRADING OF VARIABLE DECELERATIONS

Definition: The onset of the deceleration is usually at the onset of the contraction, with
the nadir of the deceleration at the peak of the contraction.

	Grades of Deceleration		
	Mild	Moderate	Severe
Amplitude in drop of fetal heart tones	Not below 70-80 bpm	<80 bpm	<70 bpm
Duration	<30 s	Any	>60 s

Other parameters of the fetal heart rate tracing must be evaluated to determine the fetal
response and toleration of variable decelerations.

Data from Freeman RK, Garite TJ, Nageotte MP: *Fetal heart rate monitoring,* ed 2, Baltimore, 1991,
Williams & Wilkins.

TABLE K-7

GRADING OF LATE DECELERATIONS

Definition: The onset of the deceleration is usually more than 30 seconds after the onset of the contraction with the nadir of the deceleration following the peak of the contraction. The descent from and return to baseline are smooth and gradual.

	Grades		
	Mild	Moderate	Severe
Amplitude of drop in fetal heart tones	<15 bpm	15-45 bpm	>45 bpm

All late decelerations must be considered significant and potentially ominous *regardless of* severity grade. Associated lack of variability and tachycardia are further predictors of fetal acidosis.

From Main DM, Main EK: *Obstetrics and gynecology: a pocket reference,* St Louis, 1984, Mosby.

TABLE K-8

FETAL SCALP pH IN RELATION TO FETAL HEART RATE PATTERNS

Fetal Heart Tone Pattern	Scalp pH	Number of Samples
No deceleration	7.30 ± 0.042	71
Early deceleration	7.30 ± 0.041	16
Variable deceleration (mild)	7.29 ± 0.046	42
Variable deceleration (moderate)	7.26 ± 0.044	35
Late deceleration (mild)	7.22 ± 0.060	27
Late deceleration (moderate)	7.21 ± 0.054	7
Variable deceleration (severe)	7.15 ± 0.069	10
Late deceleration (severe)	7.12 ± 0.066	10

From Main DM, Main EK: *Obstetrics and gynecology: a pocket reference,* St Louis, 1984, Mosby.

Antepartum Fetal Surveillance

I. BACKGROUND

A. At least 70% of fetal deaths occur before the onset of labor. Antepartum surveillance is designed to identify those fetuses at risk of intrauterine compromise and death at a time when intervention could improve fetal outcome.

1. Causes of **stillbirth**

   a. Chronic uteroplacental insufficiency (UPI)—60% to 70%

   b. Congenital anomalies—20% to 25%

   c. Acute UPI (abruptio placentae, placenta previa)—5% to 10%

   d. Infection—5% to 10%

   e. Unexplained—5% to 10%

2. **Acute events** that occur randomly or suddenly and may result in fetal death (may not be identifiable by antepartum testing)

   a. Cord accidents

   b. Abruptio placentae

   c. Hydrops fetalis

   d. Intrauterine infection

B. CANDIDATES FOR TESTING

1. It is not practical to monitor all patients. Patients at high risk for UPI are appropriate candidates for antepartum testing. Those with the most serious and unpredictable conditions require testing soon after fetal viability. When a disorder that predisposes to UPI is diagnosed during pregnancy (i.e., preeclampsia), begin testing at the time of diagnosis. Patients at risk for UPI are also at risk for intrauterine growth retardation (IUGR). It is important to perform an ultrasound at 24 to 28 weeks' gestation to rule out IUGR because earlier testing is indicated if IUGR is suspected.

   a. **Conditions** that indicate the need for **testing at a specific time**

     (1) Diabetes, classes A2 to R—32 to 33 weeks' gestation

     (2) Diabetes class A, complicated by hypertension—32 to 34 weeks' gestation

     (3) Chronic hypertension—32 to 34 weeks' gestation

     (4) Autoimmune disease—32 to 34 weeks' gestation

     (5) Maternal cyanotic cardiac disease—32 to 34 weeks' gestation

     (6) Hemoglobinopathy—32 to 34 weeks' gestation

     (7) Maternal renal disease—32 to 34 weeks' gestation

     (8) Diabetes class A, uncomplicated—40 weeks' gestation

     (9) Postdate pregnancy—42 weeks' gestation

     (10) Maternal hyperthyroidism

   b. The following conditions indicate the **need for testing on diagnosis.** Testing should not be started before intervention would be considered (i.e., <24 to 26 weeks' gestation).

     (1) Preeclampsia

     (2) Suspected IUGR

(3) Discordant twins
  c. Conditions that **may indicate a need for testing,** depending on the clinical setting
    (1) Decreased fetal movement
    (2) Maternal age $\geq$35 years
    (3) Rh isoimmunization
    (4) Maternal hyperthyroidism

II. SURVEILLANCE TECHNIQUES

A. FETAL MOVEMENT COUNTS (may be considered for all patients, including those at low risk for UPI)

1. Women with term gestations, who are trained in detecting fetal movement, are able to detect 85% of gross fetal movements. This mode of testing is a particularly useful surveillance tool for all patients, including those at low risk.

2. A common method of determining fetal movement is to instruct the patient to do the following:
  a. Lie down on her left side after a meal.
  b. Count the number of fetal movements that occur.
  c. If less than three movements are felt per hour for 2 consecutive hours, inform the physician.

B. NONSTRESS TEST (NST)

1. The NST monitors the fetal heart rate (FHR) in the absence of regular uterine activity. The presence of FHR accelerations is considered reassuring. The FHR is interpreted according to the level of FHR reactivity.
  a. **Reactive** (Fig. L-1) identifies the fetus with both of the following:
    (1) Two FHR accelerations of 15 seconds' duration occur in a 20-minute period.
    (2) The peak amplitude of accelerations is 15 bpm above the baseline.
  b. **Nonreactive** (Fig. L-2) is the lack of either (1) or (2) above.

2. Reactivity is decreased in the presence of fetal sleep or inactivity and in gestations less than 30 weeks. Sound stimulation with an artificial larynx may arouse an inactive fetus.

3. The testing interval is every 3 or 4 days.

4. The false-negative rate is 1.9 to 8.6/1000 (fetal deaths within 3 or 4 days after a reactive test).

5. Acoustic stimulation may be used if the FHR tracing does not meet criteria for reactivity. Recommendations for performing acoustic stimulation include the following:
  a. Applying an artificial larynx over the fetal head and stimulating for 1 second, *or*
  b. Placing a metal pot or pie tin over the fetal head and tapping it loudly with a metal spoon
  c. Either a or b may be repeated within 10 seconds if no acceleration has occurred within that time (may repeat up to four times).
  d. Monitor for at least 15 minutes following accelerations.

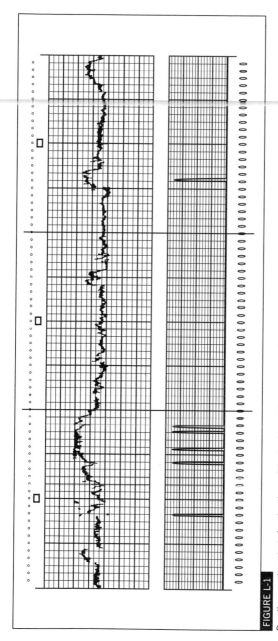

FIGURE L-1

Reactive nonstress test. Accelerations of the fetal heart that are greater than 15 bpm and last longer than 15 seconds can be identified. When the patient appreciates a fetal movement, she presses an event marker on the monitor, creating the arrows on the lower portion of the tracing. (*From Gabbe SG. In Gabbe SH, Niebyl JR, Simpson JL, editors: Obstetrics: normal and problem pregnancies, ed 2, New York, 1991, Churchill Livingstone.*)

ANTEPARTUM FETAL SURVEILLANCE **L**

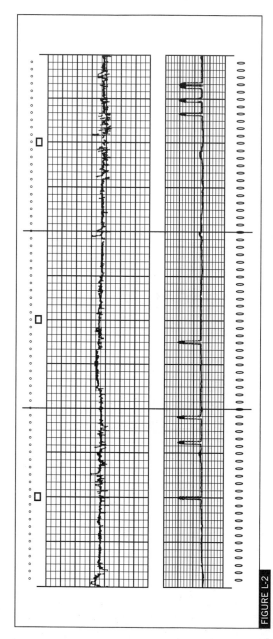

FIGURE L-2

Nonreactive nonstress test. No accelerations of the fetal heart rate are observed. Patient has perceived fetal activity, as indicated by arrows in lower portion of tracing. *(From Gabbe SG. In Gabbe SH, Niebyl JR, Simpson JL, editors: Obstetrics: normal and problem pregnancies, ed 2, New York, 1991, Churchill Livingstone.)*

C. CONTRACTION STRESS TEST (CST) (Tables L-1 and L-2)

1. The CST evaluates fetal oxygen reserves. In the presence of a uterine contraction >25 mm Hg, blood flow is restricted through the uterus. Fetuses with adequate oxygen reserves tolerate the stress of a uterine contraction, but those with diminished reserves demonstrate a fall in heart rate.

TABLE L-1

INTERPRETATION OF THE CONTRACTION STRESS TEST

Interpretation	Description	Incidence (%)
Negative	No late decelerations appearing anywhere on the tracing with adequate uterine contractions (three in 10 min)	80
Positive	Late decelerations that are consistent and persistent, present with the majority (greater than 50%) of contractions without excessive uterine activity; if persistent late decelerations are seen before the frequency of contractions is adequate, the test is interpreted as positive	3-5
Suspicious	Inconsistent late decelerations	5
Hyperstimulation	Uterine contractions closer than every 2 min or lasting longer than 90 s or five uterine contractions in 10 min; if no late decelerations seen, test interpreted as negative	5
Unsatisfactory	Quality of the tracing inadequate for interpretation, or adequate uterine activity cannot be achieved	5

From Gabbe SG, Niebyl JR, Simpson JL: *Obstetrics: normal and problem pregnancies*, ed 2, New York, 1991, Churchill Livingstone.

TABLE L-2

TESTING SCHEME: CONTRACTION STRESS TEST (CST)

Negative	Equivocal	Positive Reactive	Nonreactive
Repeat in 1 wk	Repeat in 1 d	If term or amniocentesis demonstrates pulmonary maturity, deliver. If fetus is immature, repeat the CST	Consider delivery

2. A CST may be performed weekly if the results are reactive and negative, **except for diabetic patients** in whom a **midweek NST** is recommended.

3. An **absolute contraindication** to a CST is a **previous classic cesarean** delivery or other **uterine surgery** where the **endometrial cavity was entered.** The exception is a low transverse cesarean delivery.

D. BIOPHYSICAL PROFILE (BPP)

1. In a BPP, fetal biophysical parameters are studied ultrasonically and five independent variables that correlate with fetal well-being are investigated (Table L-3).

2. The technique of BPP scoring is detailed in Table L-3, and suggested management based on results of the BPP is given in Table L-4.

3. Studies have demonstrated the following:
   a. Fetuses with **low scores** are frequently **acidotic.**
   b. **Higher scores** (8 and 10) usually indicate that the fetus is **healthy.** The false-negative rate is 1 to 2/1000. (This number represents fetuses who die within 7 days of a reassuring test.)
   c. In patients with premature rupture of membranes, absent fetal breathing may be predictive of fetal infection.
   d. Equivocal tests are uncommon.
   e. No contraindications exist to the test.

4. The BPP testing interval is 7 days, except in patients with diabetes, significant IUGR, or a postdates fetus where testing is recommended every 3 to 4 days.

E. MODIFIED BPP

1. The modified BPP includes both an NST and calculation of the amniotic fluid volume (AFV) (Fig. L-3). Clinical results and failure rates are similar to those obtained with a full BPP. Estimations of the AFV correlate well with the actual fluid volume and fetal outcome. Perinatal mortality has been demonstrated to correlate well with the amniotic fluid index (AFI) (Table L-5).

2. All modalities for calculating the AFV include measuring the largest pocket of fluid while the ultrasound transducer is held perpendicular to the floor. The AFI is the sum of the depths (in centimeters) of the amniotic fluid in the four abdominal quadrants, divided at the umbilicus (from 30 weeks' gestation onward). A rough guide for fluid volume determination is as follows:
   a. AFI <5 cm = oligohydramnios
   b. AFI 5 to 8 cm = borderline oligohydramnios
   c. AFI 8 to 25 cm = normal
   d. AFI >25 cm = polyhydramnios

F. A summary of antepartum fetal surveillance modalities is shown in Table L-6, and a branched scheme for using the NST, CST, and modified BPP is shown in Figure L-4.

TABLE L-3

TECHNIQUE OF BIOPHYSICAL PROFILE SCORING

Biophysical Variable	Normal (Score = 2)	Abnormal (Score = 0)
Fetal breathing movements	At least one episode of at least 30-s duration in 30-min observation	Absent or no episode of ≥30-s duration in 30 min
Gross body movement	At least three discrete body or limb movements in 30 min (episodes of active continuous movement considered a single movement)	Up to two episodes of body or limb movements in 30 min
Fetal tone	At least one episode of active extension with return to flexion of fetal limb(s) or trunk; opening and closing of hand considered normal tone	Either slow extension with return to partial flexion or movement of limb in full extension or absent fetal movement
Reactive fetal heart rate	At least two episodes of acceleration of ≥15 bpm and at least 15-s duration associated with fetal movement in 30 min	Fewer than two accelerations or acceleration <15 bpm in 30 min
Qualitative amniotic fluid volume	At least one pocket of amniotic fluid measuring at least 1 cm in two perpendicular planes	Either no amniotic fluid pockets or a pocket <1 cm in two perpendicular planes

From Gabbe SG, Niebyl JR, Simpson JL: *Obstetrics: normal and problem pregnancies,* ed 2, New York, 1991, Churchill Livingstone.

L

ANTEPARTUM FETAL SURVEILLANCE

TABLE L-4

MANAGEMENT BASED ON THE BIOPHYSICAL PROFILE

Score	Interpretation	Management
10	Normal infant; low risk of chronic asphyxia	Repeat testing at weekly intervals; repeat twice weekly in diabetics and patients at ≥42 weeks' gestation.
8	Normal infant; low risk of chronic asphyxia	Repeat testing at weekly intervals; repeat testing twice weekly in diabetics and patients at ≥42 weeks' gestation; oligohydramnios is an indication for delivery.
6	Suspect chronic asphyxia	Repeat testing within 24 h; deliver if oligohydramnios is present.
4	Suspect chronic asphyxia	If ≥36 weeks' gestation and conditions are favorable, deliver; if at <36 weeks and L/S <2.0, repeat test same day; if repeat score ≤4, deliver.
0-2	Strongly suspect chronic asphyxia	Extend testing time to 120 min; if persistent score ≤4, deliver, regardless of gestational age.

From Gabbe SG, Niebyl JR, Simpson JL: *Obstetrics: normal and problem pregnancies,* ed 2, New York, 1991, Churchill Livingstone.
L/S, Lecithin/sphingomyelin ratio.

MODIFIED BIOPHYSICAL PROFILE

Nonstress test (NST) twice per week
and
Amniotic fluid index (AFI) once per week

↓

If nonreactive NST or AFI < 5 cm

↓

Backup test
Contraction stress test (CST)
or
biophysical profile (BPP)

↓

Manage as with BPP or CST

FIGURE L-3

Modified biophysical profile decision tree.

TABLE L-5

RELATIONSHIP OF AMNIOTIC FLUID LEVELS TO PERINATAL MORTALITY

Amniotic Fluid Index*	Perinatal Mortality
Normal (8-24 cm)	1.97/1000
Marginal (5-8 cm)	37.74/1000
Decreased (<5 cm)	109.4/1000

*The amniotic fluid index (AFI) is the measurement, in centimeters, of the deepest fluid pockets found in all four quadrants of the uterus, as demonstrated on ultrasound with the transducer perpendicular to the floor.

TABLE L-6

SUMMARY OF ANTEPARTUM FETAL SURVEILLANCE MODALITIES

Test	Patient Indications	Testing Interval	Equipment Required	Expertise Required	Equivocal Results	False-Negative Rate	Cost
FMC	Low risk	Daily	None	Minimal	—	—	None
NST	High risk	3-4 d	1. FHR monitor	Intermediate	Frequent	1.9-8.6/1000	Modest
CST	High risk	Weekly	1. FHR monitor 2. Possible IV infusion	Intermediate	Frequent	0-2.2/1000	Modest
BPP	High risk	Weekly	1. FHR monitor 2. Ultrasound	Advanced	Uncommon	1-2/1000	Expensive
Mod BPP	High risk	3-4 d	1. FHR monitor 2. Ultrasound	Advanced	Uncommon	1-2/1000	Expensive

FMC, Fetal movement count; *NST,* nonstress test; *CST,* contraction stress test; *BPP,* biophysical profile; *Mod BPP,* modified biophysical profile; *IV,* intravenous; *FHR,* fetal heart rate.

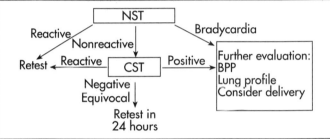

FIGURE L-4

Branched testing scheme with use of nonstress test (NST), contraction stress test (CST), and biophysical profile (BPP). Delivery is considered when NST result is nonreactive and CST results are positive. Delivery is also considered when a bradycardia is observed during NST. Fetal BPP may be used to decrease incidence of unnecessary premature intervention. *(From Gabbe SG. In Gabbe SH, Niebyl JR, Simpson JL, editors: Obstetrics: normal and problem pregnancies, ed 2, New York, 1991, Churchill Livingstone.)*

Fetal Lung Maturity: Glucocorticoids for Accelerated Fetal Lung Maturation

I. FETAL LUNG MATURITY

A. Fetal lung maturity may be determined by analyzing a specimen of amniotic fluid (usually obtained by amniocentesis).

B. The methods of assessing fetal lung maturity are detailed in Tables M-1 and M-2.

M

C. Modifiers of pulmonary maturity tests are detailed in Table M-3.

D. The relationship of phospholipid production, phosphatidylinositol, and phosphatidylglycerol in amniotic fluid and the lecithin/sphingomyelin (L/S) ratio are detailed in Figures M-1, M-2, and M-3. When determining the lung maturity in infants of diabetic mothers, an L/S ratio higher than that of nondiabetic patients is required. The absolute value depends on the institution in which the study is performed.

E. The **foam stability,** or **"shake,"** test is detailed in Figures M-4 and M-5.

F. Microviscosimetry is the evaluation of relative lipid content in fluids. When amniotic fluid is assessed (cannot be contaminated with blood) it is incubated for 30 minutes with the lipid-soluble dye 1,6-diphenyl-1,3,5-hexatriene. The amount of absorbed dye is then measured by passing polarized light through the specimen and evaluating the amount of polarization seen by fluorescence (the P value). As the L/S ratio increases, the P value decreases. This test is very sensitive and has a low false-maturity rate.

G. Surfactant/albumin ratio (TDX test). A ratio of greater than or equal to 70 mg of surfactant to 1 g of albumin is considered mature. As in F above, few false-mature results occur, and 50% of newborns with immature TDX results will develop respiratory distress syndrome (RDS).

H. Foam stability index (FSI). This assay is a modification of the shake test. The FSI value is the highest value tube in which a stable ring of foam persists. A value greater than or equal to 47 is considered mature.

I. Tap test. In this test, amniotic fluid is placed in a test tube with hydrochloric acid and diethylether. This mixture is then tapped until 200 to 300 bubbles occur in the top ether layer. Mature amniotic fluid reveals bubbles that rise to the surface and burst, whereas the bubbles of immature fluid are stable. Blood, mucus, and meconium will affect the results and may be separated out before processing by centrifuging the specimen. As with the other studies detailed above, this test has few false-mature results.

TABLE M-1

ASSESSMENT OF FETAL LUNG MATURITY (FLM): PRINCIPLE AND LEVELS OF MATURITY

Test	Principle	Maturity Level
L/S ratio	Quantity of surfactant lecithin compared with sphingomyelin	≥2.0 (method dependent)
Lung profile	Includes determination of L/S ratio, percentage precipitable lecithin, PG, and PI	L/S ratio ≥2.0; >50% acetone precipitable lecithin, 15%-20% PI, 2%-10% PG
Amniostat-FLM*	Immunologic test with agglutination in presence of PG	Test positive with PG ≥2 μg/ml of amniotic fluid
Disaturated phosphatidylcholine (DSPC)	Direct measure of primary phospholipid in surfactant	≥500 μg/dl
Microviscosimeter*	Fluorescence depolarization used to determine phospholipid membrane content	P <0.310-0.336
Shake test*	Generation of stable foam by pulmonary surfactant in presence of ethanol	Complete ring of bubbles 15 min after shaking at 1:2 dilution
Lumadex-FSI*	Modification of manual FSI; stable foam in presence of increasing concentration of ethanol	≥47
Optical density	Evaluates turbidity changes dependent on total phospholipid concentration	At 650 nm, ≥0.15

From Gabbe SG, Niebyl JR, Simpson JL: *Obstetrics: normal and problem pregnancies*, ed 2, New York, 1991, Churchill Livingstone.
L/S, Lecithin/sphingomyelin; *PG*, phosphatidylglycerol; *PI*, phosphatidylinositol; *FSI*, foam stability index.
*Denotes screening test.

ASSESSMENT OF FETAL LUNG MATURITY (FLM): TESTING MODALITY ADVANTAGES AND DISADVANTAGES

Test	Advantages	Disadvantages
L/S ratio	Few falsely mature values; not altered by changes in amniotic fluid volume	Many falsely immature values, long turnaround time, special laboratory equipment required
Lung profile	Reduces falsely immature L/S ratios; PG not altered by blood, meconium	Requires more time and equipment than L/S ratio
Amniostat-FLM*	Rapid, few falsely mature tests; can be used with contaminated specimens	Many falsely immature results
Disaturated phosphatidylcholine (DSPC)	Few falsely mature tests; may reduce falsely immature tests	May be altered by changes in amniotic fluid volume
Microviscosimeter*	Few falsely mature tests; fast, easily performed	Requires expensive equipment
Shake test*	Few falsely mature tests; fast, easily performed	Concentration of reagents critical; many falsely immature results
Lumadex-FSI*	Few falsely mature tests; fast, easily performed	Concentration of reagents critical; some falsely immature results
Optical density at 650 nm*	Few falsely mature tests; fast, easily performed	Many falsely immature results; need clear amniotic fluid

From Gabbe SG, Niebyl JR, Simpson JL: *Obstetrics: normal and problem pregnancies,* New York, 1991, Churchill Livingstone.
L/S, Lecithin/sphingomyelin; *PG,* phosphatidyl glycerol; *FSI,* foam stability index.
*Denotes screening test.

M

FETAL LUNG MATURITY

TABLE M-3
MODIFIERS OF PULMONARY MATURITY TESTS

Test	Blood	Meconium	Temperature	Collection Location
L/S	Inconsistent effect appears to raise immature L/S and lower mature L/S. L/S ratio of serum is 1.31-1.46.	Inconsistent effect reported to increase L/S by 0.1-0.5, which is an effect more pronounced in term infants	Room temperature storage × 24 h may decrease L/S. However, another study suggests that L/S is stable at 22°C (room temperature) for 72 h, 4°C for 72 h, and −40°C for 1 y.	Vaginal collection of free-flowing amniotic fluid is reliable. Amniocentesis near fetal mouth may increase L/S relative to collection far from fetal mouth.
PG	Reliable even in face of bloody fluid		Tendency to decrease PG at room temperature, but decrease not significant. Stable at 4°C for 48 h and at −20°C for 1 y.	Vaginal samples are clinically reliable.
Shake	May produce false-mature results	May produce false-mature results	Reliable at 20°C to 30°C range. Lower temperatures increase "maturity," and higher temperatures decrease "maturity" (bubble stability).	
Saturated phosphatidylcholine	Reliable	Reliable		

From Main DM, Main EK: *Obstetrics and gynecology: a pocket reference*, St Louis, 1984, Mosby.
L/S, Lecithin/sphingomyelin; *PG*, phosphatidylglycerol.

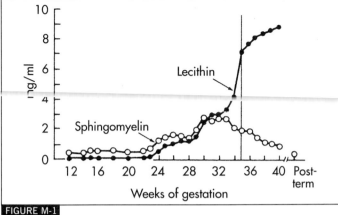

Phospholipid production versus gestational age in normal pregnancies. Changes in mean concentrations of lecithin and sphingomyelin in amniotic fluid during normal pregnancy. *(From Gluck L, Kulovich MV: Am J Obstet Gynecol 115:539, 1973.)*

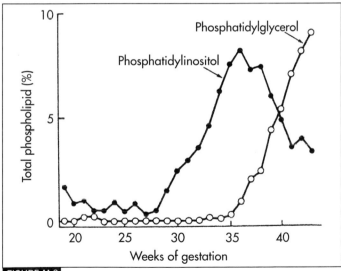

FIGURE M-2

Content of phosphatidylinositol and phosphatidylglycerol in amniotic fluid during normal gestation. Phospholipids were quantified by measuring phosphorus (P) content and expressed as percentages of total lipid phosphorus. Mean ± standard deviations of three to five samples are shown for each point. Phosphatidylglycerol appears to be important as a stabilizer for other lecithins, especially in the face of acidosis and maternal diabetes. Phosphatidylinositol's only clinical importance is to mark a sample as "not fully mature." *(From Hallman M et al: Am J Obstet Gynecol 125:613, 1976.)*

M

FETAL LUNG MATURITY

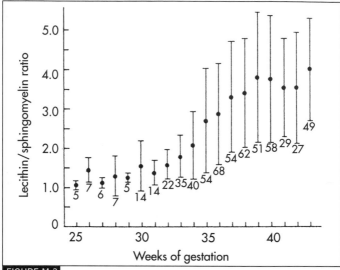

Lecithin/sphingomyelin (L/S) versus gestational age in 607 samples of amniotic fluid from 425 patients. Gestational age is given by the best antepartum estimate. One standard deviation is shown. Numbers immediately below standard deviation bars indicate number of amniotic fluid samples used for computation at each corresponding week of gestation. These results are comparable to Figure M-1. Note that in both graphs the mean age of a mature L/S ratio (2) is 34 to 35 weeks. *(From Donald IR et al: Am J Obstet Gynecol 115:547, 1973.)*

II. GLUCOCORTICOIDS FOR ACCELERATED FETAL LUNG MATURATION

A. Antenatal steroids have been demonstrated to reduce the incidence of RDS and neonatal deaths in infants delivered between 24 and 34 weeks' gestation.[1-8]

B. A comparison of corticosteroids is shown in Table M-4. The primary glucocorticoids used are as follows:

1. Betamethasone, 12 mg intramuscularly (IM) every 24 hours for two total doses

2. Dexamethasone, 5 mg IM every 12 hours for four total doses

C. Fetal and neonatal effects

1. Delivery must occur between 2 and 7 days after administration of the first dose of steroid for the beneficial effect to be present.

2. No increase in the incidence of neonatal infections has been noted except by a few investigators when a *premature rupture of membranes* was present before steroid administration.

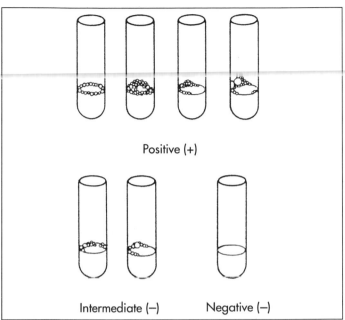

Positive (+)

Intermediate (−)   Negative (−)

FIGURE M-4

Foam stability, or "shake," test. *(From Main DM, Main EK: Obstetrics and gynecology: a pocket reference, St Louis, 1984, Mosby.)*

3. A reduction in intraventricular hemorrhage and the patent ductus arteriosus rate has been noted in premature babies (i.e., <30 weeks' gestation).
4. Follow-up of the children treated in utero demonstrates no physical, cognitive, or psychologic impairment.

D. Maternal effects

1. The maternal infection rate is not increased when glucocorticoids are used for fetal lung maturation, except possibly when premature rupture of membranes is present before steroid administration (Table M-5).
2. Glucose intolerance may develop temporarily.

III. THYROTROPIN-RELEASING HORMONE (TRH)[9,10]

A. In the early 1990s, TRH, when added to antepartum glucocorticoid treatment, appeared to reduce the incidence of RDS and improve infant survival in infants between 24 and 33 weeks' gestation. Studies over the past 5 years, however, have demonstrated a possibility of harm and definitely no benefit from TRH given to mothers before a premature delivery. Thus it is no longer recommended that TRH be administered to this group of patients.

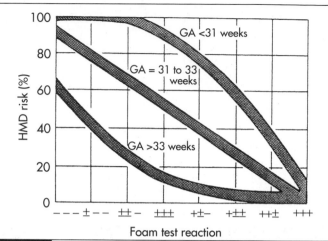

Risk of developing respiratory distress syndrome (RDS) based on "shake" test and gestational age. This graph allows for antenatal prediction of risk for hyaline membrane disease (HMD) from amniotic fluid foam test reaction at a given gestational age (GA). Foam test reaction is on longitudinal axis, and risk of HMD is on vertical axis. Risk is predicted from the shaded band appropriate for GA. Width of each band approximates error of estimate. For example, with foam test reaction of ± ± ±, risk of HMD is approximately 15% if GA is 33 weeks, 55% if GA is 31 to 33 weeks, and approximately 90% if it is 31 weeks. This figure is based on experience with 410 infants, 64 of whom developed HMD and all of whom had the "shake" test performed within 24 hours of delivery. *(From Schleuter MA et al: Am J Obstet Gynecol 134:761, 1979.)*

TABLE M-4

COMPARISON OF CORTICOSTEROIDS

Compounds	Equivalent Dose (mg)*	Antiinflammatory Potency†	Relative Sodium-Retaining Potency†	Maternal-Fetal Gradient†
Hydrocortisone (Cortisol)	20	1	1	5.8:1
Prednisone	5	4	0.8	10:1
Dexamethasone (Decadron)	0.75	25	0	
Betamethasone (Celestone)	0.75	25	0	3:1

From Main DM, Main EK: *Obstetrics and gynecology: a pocket reference,* St Louis, 1984, Mosby.
*Equivalent to 5 mg prednisone, usual adrenal replacement dose. (Note that 12 mg betamethasone or dexamethasone equals 80 mg of prednisone.)[2]
†Compared with hydrocortisone.[2]

Fetal Lung Maturity: Assessment Before Repeat Cesarean Delivery*

The assessment of fetal maturity is important in determining the timing of a repeat cesarean delivery. For patients being considered for elective repeat cesarean, fetal maturity may be assumed and amniocentesis need not be performed if one of the following criteria is met:

1. **Fetal heart tones** have been documented **for 20 weeks** by nonelectronic fetoscope or for 30 weeks by Doppler.
2. It has been **36 weeks** since a **positive serum or urine** human chorionic gonadotropin **pregnancy test** was performed by a reliable laboratory.
3. An ultrasound measurement of the **crown-rump length** obtained at 6 to 11 weeks' gestation supports a gestational age of >39 weeks.
4. An **ultrasound** obtained at **12 to 20 weeks' gestation confirms** the gestational age of >39 weeks determined by clinical history and physical examination.

These criteria are not intended to preclude the use of menstrual dating. If any one of the above criteria confirms gestational age assessment on the basis of menstrual dates in a patient with normal menstrual cycles and no immediately antecedent use of oral contraceptives, it is appropriate to schedule delivery at >39 weeks' gestation by the menstrual dates. Ultrasound may be considered confirmatory of menstrual dates if there is gestational age agreement within 1 week by crown-rump measurement obtained at 6 to 11 weeks' gestation or within 10 days by the average of multiple measurements obtained at 12 to 20 weeks' gestation.†

Awaiting the onset of spontaneous labor is another option.

*Committee on Obstetrics: *Maternal and fetal medicine.* Committee opinion No. 98, Washington, DC, 1991, American College of Obstetricians and Gynecologists.
†American College of Obstetricians and Gynecologists: *Ultrasound in pregnancy.* Tech Bull No. 116, Washington, DC, 1988, American College of Obstetricians and Gynecologists.

MEDICATION ADMINISTRATION
Medications in Pregnancy: FDA Guidelines

The Food and Drug Administration (FDA) has assigned risk factors (A, B, C, D, X) to all drugs based on the level of risk that a medication imparts to a fetus. These risk factors do not imply level of category with breast-feeding. Definitions for these risk factors are as follows:

Category A: Controlled studies in women fail to demonstrate a risk to the fetus in the first trimester (and there is no evidence of a risk in later trimesters), and the possibility of fetal harm appears remote.

Category B: Either animal-reproduction studies have not demonstrated a fetal risk but there are no controlled studies in pregnant women or animal-reproduction studies have shown an adverse effect (other than a decrease in fertility) that was not confirmed in controlled studies in women in the first trimester (and there is no evidence of a risk in later trimesters).

Category C: Either studies in animals have revealed adverse effects on the fetus (teratogenic, embryocidal, or other) and there are no controlled studies in women or studies in women and animals are not available. Drugs should be given only if the potential benefit justifies the potential risk to the fetus.

Category D: There is positive evidence of human fetal risk, but the benefits from use in pregnant women may be acceptable despite the risk (e.g., if the drug is needed in a life-threatening situation or for a serious disease for which safer drugs cannot be used or are ineffective).

Category X: Studies in animals or humans have demonstrated fetal abnormalities, or there is evidence of fetal risk based on human experience, or both, and the risk of the use of the drug in pregnant women clearly outweighs any possible benefit. The drug is contraindicated in women who are or may become pregnant.

Immunizations During Pregnancy

Ideally women would have preconceptual immunity to various diseases to which they are at risk of exposure. When this has not been accomplished, it is best to reduce exposure rather than vaccinate during pregnancy. At times, however, a pregnant woman may be exposed to a disease to which she has no natural immunity, and risks of infection to the mother and the fetus must be weighed against risks of vaccination. Table P-1 is useful in assessing these factors.

P

TABLE P-1

IMMUNIZATION DURING PREGNANCY

Immunobiologic Agent	Risk from Disease to Pregnant Woman	Risk from Disease to Fetus or Neonate	Type of Immunizing Agent	Risk from Immunizing Agent to Fetus	Indications for Immunization During Pregnancy	Dose Schedule	Comments
LIVE VIRUS VACCINES							
Measles	Significant morbidity, low mortality; not altered by pregnancy	Significant increase in abortion rate; may cause malforma- tions	Live attenuated virus vaccine	None confirmed	Contraindicated (see Immune globulins)	Single dose SC, preferably as measles-mumps-rubella*	Vaccination of susceptible women should be part of postpartum care
Mumps	Low morbidity and mortality; not altered by pregnancy	Probable increased rate of abor- tion in first trimester	Live attenuated virus vaccine	None confirmed	Contraindicated	Single dose SC, preferably as measles-mumps-rubella	Vaccination of susceptible women should be part of postpartum care
Poliomyelitis	No increased incidence in pregnancy but may be more severe if it does occur	Anoxic fetal damage reported; 50% mortality in neonatal disease	Live attenu- ated virus (oral polio vaccine [OPV]) and enhanced- potency	None confirmed	Not routinely recommended for women in United States except persons at increased risk of exposure	*Primary:* Two doses of e-IPV SC at 4- to 8- wk intervals and a third dose 6-12 mo after the	Vaccine indi- cated for sus- ceptible preg- nant women traveling in endemic areas or in

	Risk from disease to pregnant woman	Risk from disease to fetus or neonate	Type of immunizing agent	Risk from immunizing agent to fetus	Indications for immunization during pregnancy	Dose schedule	Comments
			inactivated virus (e-IPV) vaccine†			second dose *Immediate protection:* One dose OPV PO (in out-break setting)	other high-risk situations
Rubella	Low morbidity and mortality; not altered by pregnancy	High rate of abortion and congenital rubella syndrome	Live attenuated virus vaccine	None confirmed	Contraindicated	Single dose SC, preferably as measles-mumps-rubella	Teratogenicity of vaccine is theoretic, not confirmed to date; vaccination of susceptible women should be part of postpartum care
Yellow fever	Significant morbidity and mortality; not altered by pregnancy	Unknown	Live attenuated virus vaccine	Unknown	Contraindicated except if exposure is unavoidable	Single dose SC	Postponement of travel preferable to vaccination if possible

From American College of Obstetricians and Gynecologists: *Immunization during pregnancy.* Tech Bull No. 160, Washington, DC, 1991. The College.

SC, Subcutaneously; *PO,* orally; *IM,* intramuscularly; *ID,* Intradermally.

*Two doses necessary for adequate vaccination of students entering institutions of higher education, newly hired medical personnel, and international travelers.

†Inactivated polio vaccine recommended for nonimmunized adults at increased risk.

Continued

IMMUNIZATIONS DURING PREGNANCY

P

TABLE P-1
IMMUNIZATION DURING PREGNANCY—cont'd

Immunobiologic Agent	Risk from Disease to Pregnant Woman	Risk from Disease to Fetus or Neonate	Type of Immunizing Agent	Risk from Immunizing Agent to Fetus	Indications for Immunization During Pregnancy	Dose Schedule	Comments
INACTIVATED VIRUS VACCINES							
Influenza	Possible increase in morbidity and mortality during epidemic of new antigenic strain	Possible increased abortion rate; no malformations confirmed	Inactivated virus vaccine	None confirmed	Women with serious underlying diseases; public health authorities to be consulted for current recommendation	One dose IM every year	
Rabies	Near 100% fatality; not altered by pregnancy	Determined by maternal disease	Killed virus vaccine‡	Unknown	Indications for prophylaxis not altered by pregnancy; each case considered individually	Public health authorities to be consulted for indications, dosage, and route of administration	
Hepatitis B	Possible increased severity during third trimester	Possible increase in abortion rate and prematurity;	Recombinant vaccine	None reported	Preexposure and postexposure for women at risk of infection	Three- or four-dose series IM	Used with hepatitis B immune globulin for some exposures; exposed

	neonatal hepatitis can occur; high risk of newborn carrier state				

INACTIVATED BACTERIAL VACCINES

Cholera	Significant morbidity and mortality; more severe during third trimester	Increased risk of fetal death during third-trimester maternal illness	Killed bacterial vaccine	None confirmed	Indications not altered by pregnancy; vaccination recommended only in unusual outbreak situations	Single dose SC or IM, depending on manufacturer's recommendations when indicated
Plague	Significant morbidity and mortality; not altered by pregnancy	Determined by maternal disease	Killed bacterial vaccine	None reported	Selective vaccination of exposed persons	Public health authorities to be consulted for indications, dosage, and route of administration
Pneumococcus	No increased risk during pregnancy; no increase in severity of disease	Unknown	Polyvalent polysaccharide vaccine	No data available on use during pregnancy	Indications not altered by pregnancy; vaccine used only for high-risk individuals	In adults, one SC or IM dose only; consider repeat dose in 6 y for high-risk individuals

‡A human diploid cell vaccine against rabies is also available and has been used in pregnancy (Chabala S et al: Confirmed rabies exposure during pregnancy: treatment with human rabies immune globulin and human diploid cell vaccine. Am J Med 91: 423-424,1991).

IMMUNIZATIONS DURING PREGNANCY P

Continued

TABLE P-1

IMMUNIZATION DURING PREGNANCY—cont'd

Immunobiologic Agent	Risk from Disease to Pregnant Woman	Risk from Disease to Fetus or Neonate	Type of Immunizing Agent	Risk from Immunizing Agent to Fetus	Indications for Immunization During Pregnancy	Dose Schedule	Comments
INACTIVATED BACTERIAL VACCINES—cont'd							
Typhoid	Significant morbidity and mortality; not altered by pregnancy	Unknown	Killed or live attenuated oral bacterial vaccine	None confirmed	Not recommended routinely except for close, continued exposure or travel to endemic areas	*Killed:* *Primary:* Two injections SC at least 4 wk apart *Booster:* Single dose SC or ID (depending on type of product used) every 3 y *Oral:* *Primary:* Four doses on alternate days *Booster:* Schedule not yet determined	

TOXOIDS

Agent	Risk from disease to mother	Risk from disease to fetus/neonate	Risk from immunizing agent to fetus	Type of immunizing agent	Indications for immunization	Dose schedule	Comments
Tetanus-diphtheria	Severe morbidity; tetanus mortality 30%, diphtheria mortality 10%; unaltered by pregnancy	Neonatal tetanus mortality 60%	None confirmed	Combined tetanus-diphtheria toxoids preferred: adult tetanus-diphtheria formulation	Lack of primary series, or no booster within past 10 y	*Primary:* Two doses IM at 1- to 2-mo intervals with a third dose 6- to 12 mo after the second *Booster:* Single dose IM every 10 y, after completion of primary series	Updating of immune status should be part of antepartum care

SPECIFIC IMMUNE GLOBULINS

Agent	Risk from disease to mother	Risk from disease to fetus/neonate	Risk from immunizing agent to fetus	Type of immunizing agent	Indications for immunization	Dose schedule	Comments
Hepatitis B	Possible increased severity during third trimester	Possible increase in abortion rate and prematurity; neonatal hepatitis can occur; high risk of carriage in newborn	None reported	Hepatitis B immune globulin	Postexposure prophylaxis	Depends on exposure; consult Immunization Practices Advisory Committee recommendations (IM)	Usually given with HBV vaccine; exposed newborn needs immediate postexposure prophylaxis

Continued

IMMUNIZATIONS DURING PREGNANCY

P

IMMUNIZATION DURING PREGNANCY—cont'd

Immunobiologic Agent	Risk from Disease to Pregnant Woman	Risk from Disease to Fetus or Neonate	Type of Immunizing Agent	Risk from Immunizing Agent to Fetus	Indications for Immunization During Pregnancy	Dose Schedule	Comments
SPECIFIC IMMUNE GLOBULINS—cont'd							
Rabies	Near 100% fatality; not altered by pregnancy	Determined by maternal disease	Rabies immune globulin	None reported	Postexposure prophylaxis	Half dose at injury site, half dose in deltoid	Used in conjunction with rabies killed virus vaccine
Tetanus	Severe morbidity; mortality 21%	Neonatal tetanus mortality 60%	Tetanus immune globulin	None reported	Postexposure prophylaxis	One dose IM	Used in conjunction with tetanus toxoid
Varicella	Possible increase in severe varicella pneumonia	Can cause congenital varicella with increased mortality in neonatal period; very rarely causes congenital defects	Varicella-zoster immune globulin (obtained from the American Red Cross)	None reported	Can be considered for healthy pregnant women exposed to varicella to protect against maternal, not congenital, infection	One dose IM within 96 h of exposure	Indicated also for newborns of mothers who developed varicella within 4 d before delivery or 2 d following delivery; approximately

STANDARD IMMUNE GLOBULINS

Hepatitis A	Possible increased severity during third trimester	Probably increase in abortion rate and prematurity; possible transmission to neonate at delivery if mother is incubating the virus or is acutely ill at that time	Standard immune globulin	None reported	Postexposure prophylaxis	0.02 ml/kg IM in one dose of immune globulin	90%-95% of adults are immune to varicella; not indicated for prevention of congenital varcella Immune globulin should be given as soon as possible within 2 wk of exposure; infants born to mothers incubating the virus or who are acutely ill at delivery should receive one dose of 0.5 ml as soon as possible after birth

Continued

TABLE P-1

IMMUNIZATION DURING PREGNANCY—cont'd

Immunobiologic Agent	Risk from Disease to Pregnant Woman	Risk from Disease to Fetus or Neonate	Type of Immunizing Agent	Risk from Immunizing Agent to Fetus	Indications for Immunization During Pregnancy	Dose Schedule	Comments
STANDARD IMMUNE GLOBULINS—cont'd							
Measles	Significant morbidity, low mortality; not altered by pregnancy	Significant increase in abortion rate; may cause malformations	Standard immune globulin	None reported	Postexposure prophylaxis	0.25 ml/kg IM in one dose of immune globulin, up to 15 ml	Unclear if it prevents abortion; must be given within 6 d of exposure

Sexually Transmitted Disease Treatment Guidelines*

I. INTRODUCTION

A. Intrauterine or perinatally transmitted sexually transmitted disease (STD) can have fatal or severely debilitating effects on the fetus. Routine prenatal care should include an assessment for STD, which in most cases includes serologic screening for syphilis and hepatitis B, testing for chlamydia, and gonorrhea culture. Prenatal screening for human immunodeficiency virus (HIV) is indicated for all patients with risk factors for HIV or with a high-risk sexual partner; some authorities recommend HIV screening of all pregnant women.

B. Practical management issues are discussed in the sections pertaining to specific diseases. Pregnant women and their sexual partner(s) should be questioned about STDs and counseled about possible neonatal infections. Pregnant women with primary genital herpes infection, hepatitis B, primary cytomegalovirus (CMV) infection, or group B streptococcal infection may need to be referred to an expert for management. In the absence of lesions or other evidence of active disease, cesarean delivery and tests for herpes simplex virus (HSV) are *not* routinely indicated for pregnant women with a history of recurrent genital herpes infection. Routine human papillomavirus (HPV) screening is also not recommended. For a fuller discussion of these issues, as well as for infections not transmitted sexually, refer to *Guidelines for Perinatal Care,* ed 3, 1992, jointly written and published by the American Academy of Pediatrics and the American College of Obstetricians and Gynecologists.

II. ACQUIRED IMMUNODEFICIENCY SYNDROME AND HIV INFECTION IN THE GENERAL STD SETTING

A. The acquired immunodeficiency syndrome (AIDS) is a late manifestation of infection with HIV. Most people infected with HIV remain asymptomatic for long periods. HIV infection is most often diagnosed by using HIV antibody tests. Detectable antibody usually develops within 3 months after infection. Confirmed positive antibody test results mean that a person is infected with HIV and is capable of transmitting the virus to others. Although negative antibody test results usually mean a person is not infected, antibody tests cannot rule out infection from a recent exposure. If antibody testing is related to a specific exposure, the test should be repeated 3 and 6 months after the exposure.

*From Centers for Disease Control and Prevention: 1993 sexually transmitted diseases treatment guidelines. U.S. Department of Health and Human Services, Public Health Service, *MMWR Morb Mortal Wkly Rep* 42:RR-14, 1993.

B. Antibody testing for HIV begins with a screening test, usually an enzyme-linked immunosorbent assay (ELISA). If the screening test results are positive, it is followed by a more specific confirmatory test, most commonly the Western blot assay. New antibody tests are being developed and licensed that are either easier to perform or more accurate. Positive results from screening tests must be confirmed before being considered definitive.

C. The time between infection with HIV and development of AIDS ranges from a few months to >10 years. Most people who are infected with HIV eventually have some symptoms related to that infection. In one cohort study, AIDS developed in 48% of a group of gay men ≥10 years after infection, but additional AIDS cases are expected among those who have remained AIDS-free for >10 years.

D. Therapy with zidovudine (ZDV [previously known as Azidothymidine]) has been shown to benefit persons in the later stages of disease (AIDS or AIDS-related conditions along with a CD4 [T4] lymphocyte count <200/mm^3). Serious side effects, usually anemias and cytopenias, have been common during therapy with ZDV; therefore patients taking ZDV require careful follow-up in consultation with physicians who are familiar with ZDV therapy. Clinical trials are currently evaluating ZDV therapy for persons with asymptomatic HIV infection to see if it decreases the rate of progression to AIDS. Other trials are evaluating new drugs or combinations of drugs for persons with different stages of HIV infection, including asymptomatic infections. The complete therapeutic management of HIV infection is beyond the scope of this appendix.

E. **Perinatal infections.** Infants born to women with HIV infection may also be infected with HIV; this risk is estimated to be 30% to 40%. The mother in such a case may be asymptomatic and her HIV infection not recognized at delivery. Infected neonates are usually asymptomatic, and currently HIV infection cannot be readily or easily diagnosed at birth. (Positive antibody test results may reflect passively transferred maternal antibodies, and the infant must be observed over time to determine if neonatal infection is present.) Infection may not become evident until the child is 12 to 18 months of age. All pregnant women with a history of STD should be offered HIV counseling and testing. Recognition of HIV infection in pregnancy permits health care workers to inform patients about the risks of transmission to the infant and the risks of continuing pregnancy.

III. SYPHILIS

A. SEROLOGIC TESTS

1. Dark-field examinations and direct fluorescent antibody tests on lesions or tissue are the definitive methods for diagnosing early syphilis.
2. Presumptive diagnosis is possible by using two types of serologic tests for syphilis: treponemal (e.g., fluorescent treponemal antibody absorbed [FTA-ABS], microhemagglutination assay for antibody to

Treponema pallidum [MHATP]) and nontreponemal (e.g., Venereal Disease Research Laboratory [VDRL], rapid plasma reagin [RPR]).

   a. Neither test alone is sufficient for diagnosis. Treponemal antibody test results, once positive, usually remain so for life, regardless of treatment or disease activity. Treponemal antibody titers do not correlate with disease activity and should be reported as positive or negative. Nontreponemal antibody titers do tend to correlate with disease activity, usually rising with new infection and falling after treatment. Nontreponemal antibody test results should be reported quantitatively and titered out to a final end point rather than reported as greater than an arbitrary cutoff (e.g., 1:512). With regard to changes in nontreponemal test results, a fourfold change in titers is equivalent to a two-dilution change (e.g., from 1:16 to 1:4 or from 1:8 to 1:32).

   b. For sequential serologic tests, the same test (e.g., VDRL or RPR) should be used, and it should be run by the same laboratory. The VDRL and RPR are equally valid, but RPR titers are often slightly higher than VDRL titers and therefore are not comparable.

3. Neurosyphilis cannot be accurately diagnosed from any single test. Cerebrospinal fluid (CSF) tests should include cell count, protein, and VDRL (not RPR). The CSF leukocyte count is usually elevated (>5 WBCs/mm^3) when neurosyphilis is present and is a sensitive measure of the efficacy of therapy. VDRL is the standard test for CSF; **when results are positive,** it is considered **diagnostic** of neurosyphilis. However, results may be negative when neurosyphilis is present and cannot be used to rule out neurosyphilis. Some experts also order an FTA-ABS; this may be less specific (more false positives) but is highly sensitive. The positive predictive value of the CSF FTA-ABS is lower, but **when results are negative** this test provides evidence **against** neurosyphilis.

B. **TREATMENT**

1. **Penicillin therapy.** Penicillin is the preferred drug for treating patients with syphilis. Penicillin is the only proven therapy that has been widely used for patients with neurosyphilis, congenital syphilis, or syphilis during **pregnancy. For patients with penicillin allergy, skin testing with desensitization, if necessary,** is optimal.

2. The **Jarisch-Herxheimer reaction** is an acute febrile reaction, often accompanied by headache, myalgia, and other symptoms, that may occur after any therapy for syphilis, and patients should be so warned. Jarisch-Herxheimer reactions are more common in patients with early syphilis. Antipyretics may be recommended, but no proven methods exist for preventing this reaction. Pregnant patients, in particular, should be warned that early labor may occur.

3. **Persons sexually exposed** to a patient with early syphilis should be evaluated clinically and serologically. If the exposure occurred within the previous 90 days, the person may be infected yet seronegative and

therefore should be presumptively treated. (It may be advisable to presumptively treat persons exposed more than 90 days previously if serologic test results are not immediately available and follow-up is uncertain.) Patients who have other STDs may also have been exposed to syphilis and should have a serologic test for syphilis. The dual therapy regimen currently recommended for gonorrhea (ceftriaxone and doxycycline) is probably effective against incubating syphilis. If a different, nonpenicillin antibiotic regimen is used to treat gonorrhea, the patient should have a repeat serologic test for syphilis in 3 months.

4. **Early syphilis:** primary and secondary syphilis and early latent syphilis of less than 1 year's duration
   a. **Benzathine penicillin** G, 2.4 million units intramuscularly (IM), in one dose
   b. **Treatment failures** can occur with any regimen. Patients should be reexamined clinically and serologically at 3 months and 6 months. If nontreponemal antibody titers have not declined fourfold by 3 months with primary or secondary syphilis or by 6 months in early latent syphilis, or if signs or symptoms persist and reinfection has been ruled out, patients should have a CSF examination and be retreated appropriately.
   c. **HIV-infected patients** should have more frequent follow-up visits, including serologic testing at 1, 2, 3, 6, 9, and 12 months. In addition to the preceding guidelines for 3 and 6 months, any patient with a fourfold increase in titer at any time should have a CSF examination and be treated with the neurosyphilis regimen unless reinfection can be established as the cause of the increased titer.
   d. **Lumbar puncture** in early syphilis. CSF abnormalities are common in adults with early syphilis. Despite the frequency of these CSF findings, few patients develop neurosyphilis when the treatment regimens described previously are used. Therefore, unless clinical signs and symptoms of neurologic involvement (e.g., optic, auditory, cranial nerve, or meningeal symptoms) exist, lumbar puncture is not recommended for routine evaluation of early syphilis. This recommendation also applies to immunocompromised and HIV-infected patients because no clear data currently show that these patients need increased therapy.
   e. **All syphilis patients** should be counseled concerning the risks of HIV and should be encouraged to be tested for HIV.

5. **Late latent syphilis** of more than 1 year's duration, gummas, and cardiovascular syphilis
   a. All patients should have a thorough clinical examination. Ideally, all patients with syphilis of more than 1 year's duration should have a CSF examination; however, performance of lumbar puncture can be individualized. In older asymptomatic individuals, the yield of lumbar puncture is likely to be low; however, CSF examination is clearly indicated in the following specific situations:

(1) Neurologic signs or symptoms
(2) Treatment failure
(3) Serum nontreponemal antibody titer ≥32
(4) Other evidence of active syphilis (aortitis, gumma, or iritis)
(5) Nonpenicillin therapy planned
(6) Positive HIV antibody test results

b. If CSF examination is performed and reveals findings consistent with **neurosyphilis,** patients should be treated for neurosyphilis (see next section). Some experts also treat cardiovascular syphilis patients with a neurosyphilis regimen.

c. Recommended regimen. **Benzathine penicillin G,** 7.2 million units total, administered as three doses of 2.4 million units IM, given 1 week apart for 3 consecutive weeks.

d. **Quantitative nontreponemal serologic tests** should be repeated at 6 months and 12 months. If titers increase fourfold, if an initially high titer (≥1:32) fails to decrease, or if the patient has signs or symptoms attributable to syphilis, the patient should be evaluated for neurosyphilis and retreated appropriately.

6. All syphilis patients should be counseled concerning the risks of HIV and should be encouraged to be tested for HIV antibody.

7. Neurosyphilis. CNS disease may occur during any stage of syphilis. Clinical evidence of neurologic involvement (e.g., optic and auditory symptoms, cranial nerve palsies) warrants CSF examination. If present, treat with the following:

a. **Aqueous crystalline penicillin G,** 12 to 24 million U/d administered as 2 to 4 million units every 4 hours intravenously (IV), for 10 to 14 days.

b. Alternative regimen (if outpatient compliance can be ensured): **procaine penicillin,** 2.4 million U/d IM, **and probenecid,** 500 mg orally (PO) four times per day, both for 10 to 14 days. Many authorities recommend the addition of benzathine penicillin G, 2.4 million U/wk IM for three doses after completion of these neurosyphilis treatment regimens. No systematically collected data have evaluated therapeutic alternatives to penicillin. Patients who cannot tolerate penicillin should be skin tested and desensitized, if necessary, or managed in consultation with an expert.

c. If an initial CSF pleocytosis was present, CSF examination should be repeated every 6 months until the cell count is normal. If it has not decreased at 6 months or is not normal by 2 years, retreatment should be strongly considered.

8. Syphilis in pregnancy

a. Pregnant women should be **screened early** in pregnancy. Seropositive pregnant women should be considered infected unless treatment history and sequential serologic antibody titers are showing an appropriate response. In populations in which prenatal care utilization is not optimal, patients should be screened and, if necessary, treatment provided at the time pregnancy is detected. In areas of high syphilis prevalence or in patients at high risk, screening should be repeated in the third trimester and again at delivery.

b. **Treatment.** Patients should be treated with the **penicillin** regimen appropriate for the woman's stage of syphilis. Tetracycline and doxycycline are contraindicated in pregnancy. Erythromycin should not be used because of the high risk of failure to cure infection in the fetus. Pregnant women with histories of a penicillin allergy should first be carefully questioned regarding the validity of the history. If necessary, they should then be skin tested and either treated with penicillin or referred for desensitization. Women who are treated in the second half of pregnancy are at risk for **premature labor** or **fetal distress** (or both) if their treatment precipitates a Jarisch-Herxheimer reaction. They should be advised to seek medical attention after treatment if they notice any change in fetal movements or have any contractions. Stillbirth is a rare complication of treatment; however, because therapy is necessary to prevent further fetal damage, this concern should not delay treatment.

c. Monthly follow-up is mandatory so that retreatment can be given if needed. The antibody response should be the same as for nonpregnant patients.

9. **Congenital syphilis**

a. Infants should be evaluated if they were born to seropositive (nontreponemal test confirmed by treponemal test) women to whom any of the following pertain:

   (1) Have untreated syphilis

   (2) Were treated for syphilis less than 1 month **before** delivery

   (3) Were treated for syphilis during pregnancy with a nonpenicillin regimen

   (4) Did not have the expected decrease in nontreponemal antibody titers after treatment for syphilis

   (5) Do not have a well-documented history of treatment for syphilis

   (6) Were treated but had insufficient serologic follow-up during pregnancy to assess disease activity

b. **An infant should not be released from the hospital until the serologic status of the infant's mother is known.**

c. The **clinical and laboratory** evaluation of infants born to women described should include the following:

   (1) A thorough physical examination for evidence of congenital syphilis

   (2) Nontreponemal antibody titer

   (3) CSF analysis for cells, protein, and VDRL

   (4) Long-bone x-ray examination

   (5) Other tests as clinically indicated (e.g., chest x-ray examination)

   (6) If possible, obtain an FTA-ABS on the purified 19S-IgM fraction of serum (e.g., separation by Isolab columns)

d. **Infants should be treated** if they have any of the following:
   (1) Any evidence of active disease (physical or x-ray examination)
   (2) A reactive CSF VDRL
   (3) An abnormal CSF finding (white blood cell count >5/mm^3 or protein >50 mg/dl), regardless of CSF serology; **or**
   (4) Quantitative nontreponemal serologic titers that are fourfold (or greater) higher than their mother's
   (5) **Positive FTA-ABS 19S-IgM** antibody (if performed)
      (a) Even if the evaluation is normal, infants should be treated if their mothers have untreated syphilis or evidence of relapse or reinfection after treatment. Infants who meet the criteria listed in section IIIB9a but are not fully evaluated should be assumed to be infected and should be treated.
      (b) Treatment should consist of **aqueous crystalline penicillin G daily,** 100,000 to 150,000 U/kg of body weight (administered as 50,000 U/kg IV every 8 to 12 hours), or **procaine penicillin daily,** 50,000 U/kg (administered once IM) for 10 to 14 days. If more than 1 day of therapy is missed, the entire course **should** be restarted. All symptomatic neonates should also have an ophthalmologic examination.
e. Infants who meet the criteria listed in section IIIB9a but who, after evaluation, do not meet the criteria listed in section IIIB9d **are at low risk for congenital syphilis. If their mothers were treated with erythromycin during pregnancy** or if close follow-up cannot be **ensured,** they should be treated with **benzathine penicillin G,** 50,000 U/kg IM as a one-time dose.
f. Follow-up
   (1) Seropositive untreated infants must be closely followed at 1, 2, 3, 6, and 12 months of age. In the absence of infection, nontreponemal antibody titers should be decreasing by 3 months of age and should have disappeared by 6 months of age. If these titers are found to be stable or increasing, the child should be reevaluated and fully treated. In addition, in the absence of infection, treponemal antibodies may be present up to 1 year. If they are present beyond 1 year, the infant should be treated for congenital syphilis.
   (2) Treated infants should also be observed to ensure decreasing nontreponemal antibody titers; these should have disappeared by 6 months of age. Treponemal tests should not be used because they may remain positive despite effective therapy if the child was infected. Infants with documented CSF pleocytosis should be reexamined every 6 months or until the cell count is normal. If the cell count is still abnormal after 2 years or if a downward trend is not present at each examination, the infant should be retreated. The CSF VDRL should also be checked at 6 months; if it is still reactive, the infant should be retreated.

10. Management of patients with histories of penicillin allergy. Currently, no proven alternative therapies to penicillin are available for treating patients with neurosyphilis, congenital syphilis, or syphilis in pregnancy. Therefore skin testing with desensitization, if indicated, is recommended for these patients.

IV. GENITAL HERPES SIMPLEX VIRUS INFECTIONS

A. Genital herpes is a viral disease that may be chronic and recurring and for which no known cure exists. Systemic acyclovir treatment provides partial control of the symptoms and signs of herpes episodes; it accelerates healing but does not eradicate the infection nor affect the subsequent risk, frequency, or severity of recurrences after the drug is discontinued. Topical therapy with acyclovir is substantially less effective than therapy with the oral drug.

B. First clinical episode of genital herpes

1. The recommended regimen in a nonpregnant patient is either of the following:

  a. Valacyclovir (Valtrex) (pregnancy category B), 500 mg PO twice daily for 5 days

  b. Acyclovir (pregnancy category B), 200 mg PO five times per day for 7 to 10 days or until clinical resolution occurs.

2. Pregnancy

  a. The safety of systemic acyclovir therapy among pregnant women has not been established. Burroughs-Wellcome, in cooperation with the Centers for Disease Control and Prevention, maintains a registry to assess the effects of the use of acyclovir during pregnancy. Women who receive acyclovir during pregnancy should be reported to this registry (1-800-722-9292, ext. 58456).

  b. Current registry findings do not indicate an increase in the number of birth defects identified among the prospective reports when compared with those expected in the general population. Moreover, no consistent pattern of abnormalities emerges among retrospective reports. These findings provide some assurance in counseling women who have had inadvertent prenatal exposure to acyclovir. However, accumulated case histories comprise a sample of insufficient size for reaching reliable and definitive conclusions regarding the risks of acyclovir treatment to pregnant women and to their fetuses.

  c. In the presence of life-threatening maternal HSV infection (e.g., disseminated infection that includes encephalitis, pneumonitis, or hepatitis), acyclovir administered IV is indicated. Among pregnant women without life-threatening disease, systemic acyclovir should not be used to treat recurrences nor should it be used as suppressive therapy near term (or at other times during pregnancy) to prevent reactivation.

C. The recommended regimen for patients with **severe disease** or complications requiring hospitalization is acyclovir, 5 mg/kg body weight IV every 8 hours for 5 to 7 days or until clinical resolution (i.e., resolution of encephalitis, pneumonitis, or hepatitis) occurs. Among pregnant women without life-threatening disease, systemic acyclovir treatment **should not** be used for recurrent genital herpes episodes or as suppressive therapy to prevent reactivation near term.

D. Perinatal infections

1. Most mothers of infants who acquire neonatal herpes lack histories of clinically evident genital herpes. The risk for transmission to the neonate from an infected mother appears highest among women with first-episode genital herpes near the time of delivery and is low ($\leq 3\%$) among women with recurrent herpes. The results of viral cultures during pregnancy do not predict viral shedding at the time of delivery, and such cultures are not routinely indicated.

2. At the onset of labor, all women should be carefully questioned about symptoms of genital herpes and should be examined. Women without symptoms or signs of genital herpes infection (or prodrome) may deliver their babies vaginally. Among women who have a history of genital herpes or who have a sex partner with genital herpes, cultures of the birth canal at delivery may aid in decisions relating to neonatal management.

3. Infants delivered through an infected birth canal (proven by virus isolation or presumed by observation of lesions) should be observed carefully, including virus cultures obtained 24 to 48 hours after birth. Available data do not support the routine use of acyclovir as anticipatory treatment of asymptomatic infants delivered through an infected birth canal. Treatment should be reserved for infants who develop evidence of clinical disease and for those with positive postpartum cultures.

4. All infants with evidence of neonatal herpes should be treated with systemic acyclovir or vidarabine; refer to the *Report of the Committee on Infectious Diseases, American Academy of Pediatrics.* For ease of administration and to lower toxicity, acyclovir (30 mg/kg/d for 10 to 14 days) is the preferred drug. The care of these infants should be managed in consultation with an expert.

E. Counseling and management of sex partners. Patients with genital herpes should be told about the natural history of their disease with emphasis on the potential for recurrent episodes. Patients should be advised to abstain from sexual activity while lesions are present. Sexual transmission of HSV has been documented during periods without recognized lesions. Suppressive treatment with oral acyclovir reduces the frequency of recurrences but does not totally eliminate viral shedding. Genital herpes and other diseases causing genital ulcers have been associated with an increased risk of acquiring HIV infections; therefore condoms should be used during all sexual exposures. If sex partners of patients with genital herpes have genital lesions, they may benefit from evaluation; however, evaluation of asymptomatic partners is of little value in preventing transmission of HSV.

F. Office and hospital testing for herpes is available from Diagnology. This is a gG-2 absorption test that appears to give valid results in 10 minutes using a finger stick blood test.

V. GENITAL WARTS

A. Exophytic genital and anal warts are caused by certain types (most frequently types 6 and 11) of HPV. Other types that are sometimes present in the anogenital region (most commonly types 16, 18, and 31) have been found to be strongly associated with genital dysplasia and carcinoma. For this reason, biopsy is needed in all instances of atypical, pigmented, or persistent warts. All women with anogenital warts should have an annual Papanicolaou (Pap) smear. Some subclinical human papillomavirus infections may be detected by Pap smear and colposcopy. Application of diluted acetic acid may also indicate otherwise subclinical lesions, but false-positive test results occur.

B. No therapy has been shown to eradicate human papillomavirus. Human papillomavirus has been demonstrated in adjacent tissue after laser treatment of human papillomavirus–associated cervical intraepithelial neoplasia and after attempts to eliminate subclinical human papillomavirus by extensive laser vaporization of the anogenital area. The benefit of treating patients with subclinical human papillomavirus infection has not been demonstrated, and recurrence is common. The effect of genital wart treatment on human papillomavirus transmission and its natural history is unknown. **Therefore the goal of treatment is removal of exophytic warts and the amelioration of signs and symptoms, not the eradication of human papillomavirus.**

C. Sex partners should be examined for evidence of warts. Patients with anogenital warts should be made aware that they are contagious to uninfected sex partners. The use of condoms is recommended to help reduce transmission.

D. Pregnant patients and perinatal infections

1. Cesarean delivery for prevention of transmission of human papillomavirus infection to the neonate is not indicated. In rare instances, however, cesarean delivery may be indicated for women with genital warts if the pelvic outlet is obstructed or if vaginal delivery would result in excessive bleeding.

2. Genital papillary lesions have a tendency to proliferate and to become friable during pregnancy. Many experts advocate removal of visible warts during pregnancy, although data on this subject are limited.

3. Human papillomavirus types 6 and 11 can cause laryngeal papillomatosis in infants. The route of transmission (transplacental, birth canal, or postnatal) is unknown; therefore the preventive value of cesarean delivery is unknown. The perinatal transmission rate is also unknown, although it must be low, given the relatively high prevalence of genital warts and the rarity of laryngeal papillomas. Neither routine human papillomavirus screening tests nor cesarean delivery is indicated to prevent transmission of infection to the neonate.

4. Treatment recommendations (Table Q-1). In most clinical situations, cryotherapy with liquid nitrogen or a cryoprobe is the treatment of choice for external genital and perianal warts. Cryotherapy is nontoxic, does not require anesthesia, and, if used properly, does not result in scarring. Podophyllin (contraindicated in pregnancy), trichloroacetic acid, and electrodesiccation or electrocautery are alternative therapies. Treatment with interferon is not recommended because of its relatively low efficacy, high incidence of toxicity, and high cost. The carbon dioxide laser and conventional surgery are useful in the management of extensive warts, particularly for patients who have not responded to cryotherapy; these alternatives are inappropriate for limited lesions. Like more cost-effective treatments, these therapies do not eliminate human papillomavirus and often are associated with the recurrence of clinical cases.

   a. External genital and perianal warts
      (1) **Cryotherapy with liquid nitrogen or cryoprobe**
      (2) Trichloroacetic acid (80% to 90%). Apply only to warts; powder with talc or sodium bicarbonate (baking soda) to remove unreacted acid. Repeat application at weekly intervals.
      (3) Electrodesiccation or electrocautery. Electrodesiccation is contraindicated in patients with cardiac pacemakers or for lesions proximal to the anal verge. Extensive or refractory disease should be referred to an expert.

   b. For women with cervical warts, dysplasia must be excluded before treatment is begun. Management should therefore be carried out in consultation with an expert.

   c. Vaginal warts
      (1) Cryotherapy with liquid nitrogen. The use of a cryoprobe in the vagina is not recommended because of the risk of vaginal perforation and fistula formation.
      (2) Trichloroacetic acid (80% to 90%). Apply only to warts; powder with talc or sodium bicarbonate (baking soda) to remove unreacted acid. Repeat application at weekly intervals.

   d. Treatment for urethral meatus warts is **cryotherapy** with liquid nitrogen.

   e. Treatment for anal warts is cryotherapy with liquid nitrogen. Extensive or refractory disease should be referred to an expert.

Q

STD TREATMENT GUIDELINES

TABLE Q-1

TREATMENT OPTIONS FOR CONDYLOMA ACUMINATA (GENITAL WARTS)*

Location	Few, Small	Bulky	Extensive or Resistant
		Lesions	
Vulva, perianal, urethral meatus	Imiquimod 5% (Aldara)	Excision	5-FU
	TCA		Laser
	Podophyllin		Interferon
	Cryotherapy		
	Electrocautery		
	Local excision		
Vagina	TCA	Excision	5-FU
	Cryotherapy		Laser
			Interferon
Cervix	Cryotherapy	Excision	5-FU
	Electrocautery		Laser
	TCA		Interferon
Anorectal	TCA	Excision	5-FU
	Podophyllin		Laser
	Cryotherapy		Interferon
	Electrocautery		

TCA, Trichloroacetic acid; 5-FU, 5-fluorouracil.
*Podophyllin, 5-FU, and interferon should not be used during pregnancy.

VI. GONOCOCCAL INFECTIONS

A. Cultures of pregnant women should be taken and tested for *Neisseria gonorrhoeae* (and also for *Chlamydia trachomatis* and syphilis) at the first prenatal care visit. For women at high risk of STD, a second culture for gonorrhea (as well as tests for chlamydia and syphilis) should be obtained late in the third trimester.

B. Uncomplicated infections may be treated with the following:

1. A single dose of either of the following (all provide 98% efficacy)

  a. Ceftriaxone, 125 mg IM

  b. Cefixime, 400 mg PO

  c. Sexual partners may be treated with either of the above or either of the following:

    (1) Ciprofloxacin, 500 mg PO

    (2) Norfloxacin (Ofloxacin), 400 mg PO

2. In addition, provide treatment effective against coinfection with *C. trachomatis* (erythromycin base, 500 mg PO, four times per day for 7 days) because 40% of people infected with gonorrhea are also infected with *C. trachomatis.*

C. Pregnant women allergic to β-lactams should be treated with **spectinomycin,** 2 g IM once **(followed by erythromycin).** Follow-up cervical and rectal cultures for *N. gonorrhoeae* should be obtained 4 to 7 days after treatment is completed.

D. Gonococcal infections of infants

1. Infants born to mothers with untreated gonorrhea are at high risk of infection (e.g., ophthalmia and disseminated gonococcal infection [DGI]) and should be treated with a single injection of ceftriaxone (50 mg/kg IV or IM; not to exceed 125 mg). Ceftriaxone should be given cautiously to hyperbilirubinemic infants, especially premature infants. Topical prophylaxis for neonatal ophthalmia is not adequate treatment for documented infections of the eye or other sites.

2. Infants with documented gonococcal infections at any site (e.g., eye) should be evaluated for DGI. This evaluation should include a careful physical examination, especially of the joints, as well as blood and CSF cultures. Infants with gonococcal ophthalmia or DGI should be treated for 7 days (10 to 14 days if meningitis is present) with either one of the following regimens:

    a. Ceftriaxone, 25 to 50 mg/kg/d IV or IM in a single daily dose

    b. Cefotaxime, 25 mg/kg IV or IM every 12 hours

    c. Limited data suggest that uncomplicated gonococcal ophthalmia among infants may be cured with a single injection of ceftriaxone (50 mg/kg up to 125 mg/kg). A few experts use this regimen for children who have no clinical or laboratory evidence of disseminated disease.

    d. If the gonococcal isolate is proven to be susceptible to penicillin, **crystalline penicillin G** may be given. The dose is 100,000 U/kg/d given in two equal doses (four equal doses per day for infants more than 1 week old). The dose should be increased to 150,000 U/kg/d for meningitis.

    e. Infants with gonococcal ophthalmia should receive eye irrigations with buffered saline solutions until discharge has cleared. Topical antibiotic therapy alone is inadequate. Simultaneous infection with *C. trachomatis* has been reported and should be considered for patients who do not respond satisfactorily. Therefore the mother and the infant should be tested for chlamydial infection.

3. Prevention of ophthalmia neonatorum. Instillation of a prophylactic agent into the eyes of all newborn infants is recommended to prevent gonococcal ophthalmia neonatorum and is required by law in most states. Although all regimens listed below effectively prevent gonococcal eye disease, their efficacy in preventing chlamydial eye disease is unclear. Further, they do not eliminate nasopharyngeal colonization with *C. trachomatis*. Treatment of gonococcal and chlamydial infections in pregnant women is the best method for preventing neonatal gonococcal and chlamydial disease.

    a. Erythromycin (0.5%) ophthalmic ointment (once), tetracycline (1%) ophthalmic ointment (once), **or** silver nitrate (1%) aqueous solution (once).

    b. One of these should be instilled into the eyes of every neonate as soon as possible after delivery and definitely within 1 hour after birth. Single-use tubes or ampules are preferable to multiple-use tubes.

c. The efficacy of tetracycline and erythromycin in the prevention of tetracycline-resistant *N. gonorrhoeae* and penicillinase-producing *N. gonorrhoeae* ophthalmia is unknown, although both are probably effective because of the high concentrations of drug in these preparations. Bacitracin is **not** recommended.

VII. CHLAMYDIAL INFECTIONS

A. Pregnant women should undergo diagnostic testing for *C. trachomatis, N. gonorrhoeae,* and syphilis, if possible, at their first prenatal visit and, for women at high risk, during the third trimester. Risk factors for chlamydial disease during pregnancy include young age (<25 years old), history or presence of another STD, a new sex partner within the preceding 3 months, and multiple sex partners. Ideally, pregnant women with gonorrhea should be treated for chlamydia on the basis of diagnostic studies, but if chlamydial testing is not available, treatment should be given because of the high likelihood of coinfection.

B. Results of chlamydial tests should be interpreted with care. The sensitivity of all currently available laboratory tests for *C. trachomatis* is substantially less than 100%; thus false-negative tests are possible. Although the specificity of nonculture tests has improved substantially, false-positive test results may still occur with nonculture tests. Persons with chlamydial infections may remain asymptomatic for extended periods.

C. Treatment of uncomplicated infection in pregnancy

1. Erythromycin base, 500 mg PO four times per day for 7 days. If this regimen is not tolerated, the following regimens are recommended:

a. Erythromycin base, 250 mg PO four times per day for 14 days

b. Erythromycin ethylsuccinate, 800 mg PO four times per day for 7 days

c. Erythromycin ethylsuccinate, 400 mg PO four times per day for 14 days

d. Zithromax (azithromycin), single 1-g PO dose (not as well studied in pregnancy as erythromycin, risk factor B)

2. If erythromycin cannot be tolerated, an alternative is amoxicillin, 500 mg PO three times per day for 7 days (limited data exist concerning this regimen). Erythromycin estolate is contraindicated during pregnancy because of drug-related hepatoxicity can result.

D. Sex partners of patients who have *C. trachomatis* infection should be tested and treated for *C. trachomatis* if their contact was within 30 days of onset of symptoms. If testing is unavailable, they should be treated with the appropriate antimicrobial regimen.

E. **Chlamydial infections among infants.** *C. trachomatis* infection of neonates results from perinatal exposure to the mother's infected cervix.

The prevalence of *C. trachomatis* infection generally exceeds 5% among pregnant women, regardless of race or ethnicity or socioeconomic status. Neonatal ocular prophylaxis with silver nitrate solution or antibiotic ointments is ineffective in preventing perinatal transmission of chlamydial infection from the mother to the infant. However, ocular prophylaxis with those agents does prevent gonococcal ophthalmia and should be continued for that reason (see section VID3). Initial *C. trachomatis* perinatal infection involves mucous membranes of the eye, oropharynx, urogenital tract, and rectum. *C. trachomatis* infection among neonates can most often be recognized because of conjunctivitis developing 5 to 12 days after birth. Chlamydia is the most frequent identifiable infectious cause of ophthalmia neonatorum. *C. trachomatis* is also a common cause of subacute, afebrile pneumonia with onset from 1 to 3 months of age. Asymptomatic infections of the oropharynx, genital tract, and rectum among neonates also occur.

1. **Ophthalmia neonatorum caused by *C. trachomatis*.** A chlamydial etiology should be considered for all infants with conjunctivitis through 30 days of age.
   a. **Diagnostic considerations.** Sensitive and specific methods to diagnose chlamydial ophthalmia for the neonate include isolation by tissue culture and nonculture tests, direct fluorescent antibody tests, and immunoassays. Giemsa-stained smears are specific for *C. trachomatis* but are not sensitive. Specimens must contain conjunctival cells, not exudate alone. Specimens for culture isolation and nonculture tests should be obtained from the everted eyelid using a Dacron-tipped swab or the swab specified by the manufacturer's test kit. A specific diagnosis of *C. trachomatis* infection confirms the need for chlamydial treatment not only for the neonate, but also for the mother and her sex partner or partners. Ocular exudate from infants being evaluated for chlamydial conjunctivitis should also be tested for *N. gonorrhoeae*.
   b. **Recommended regimen. Erythromycin,** 50 mg/kg/day PO divided into four doses for 10 to 14 days. Topical antibiotic therapy alone is inadequate for treatment of chlamydial infection and is unnecessary when systemic treatment is undertaken.
   c. **Follow-up.** The possibility of chlamydial pneumonia should be considered. The efficacy of erythromycin treatment is approximately 80%; a second course of therapy may be required. Follow-up of infants to determine resolution is recommended.
   d. **Management of mothers and their sex partners.** The mothers of infants who have chlamydial infection and the mothers' sex partners should be evaluated and treated following the treatment recommendations for adults with chlamydial infections (see recommendations listed in section VIIC).
2. **Infant pneumonia caused by *C. trachomatis*.** Characteristic signs of chlamydial pneumonia among infants include a repetitive staccato

cough with tachypnea, and hyperinflation and bilateral diffuse infiltrates on chest roentgenogram. Wheezing is rare, and infants are typically afebrile. Peripheral eosinophilia, documented in a complete blood count, is sometimes observed among infants with chlamydial pneumonia. Because variation from this clinical presentation is common, initial treatment and diagnostic tests should encompass *C. trachomatis* for all infants 1 to 3 months of age who have possible pneumonia.

VIII. BACTERIAL VAGINOSIS

A. Bacterial vaginosis (BV) (formerly called nonspecific vaginitis, *Haemophilus*-associated vaginitis, or *Gardnerella*-associated vaginitis) is the clinical result of alterations in the vaginal microflora. Clinical diagnosis is made when three or four criteria (homogeneous discharge, pH >4.5, positive amine odor test, or presence of clue cells) are present. Diagnosis can also be made from Gram's stain or culture. However, the most accurate method of diagnosis is DNA testing (office testing for this is available from Becton Dickinson & Co., Affirm VPIII microbial identification test). Asymptomatic infections are common.

B. Treatment of male partners. No clinical counterpart of BV is recognized in the male, and treatment of the male sex partner has not been shown to be beneficial for the patient or the male partner.

C. In pregnancy, recent studies suggest that BV may be a factor in premature rupture of membranes and premature delivery; thus close clinical follow-up of pregnant women with BV is essential. Random and controlled trials have not been performed. Until such studies have been conducted, treatment of pregnant women with BV should be at the option of the physician.

D. Clindamycin vaginal cream is the treatment of choice in the first trimester.

E. During the second and third trimesters, oral metronidazole may be used (2 g PO in a single dose or 500 mg PO twice daily for 7 days), although the vaginal clindamycin cream (2%, one full applicator [5 g] in the vagina at bedtime for 7 days) or metronidazole gel (0.75%, one full applicator [5 g] in the vagina twice daily for 5 days) may be preferred.

IX. ECTOPARASITIC INFECTIONS

A. PEDICULOSIS PUBIS

1. Permethrin cream rinse (1%) applied to affected area and washed off after 10 minutes

2. Pyrethrins and piperonyl butoxide applied to the affected area and washed off after 10 minutes or lindane shampoo (1%) applied for 4 minutes and then thoroughly washed off (not recommended for pregnant or lactating women)

3. Patients should be reevaluated after 1 week if symptoms persist. Retreatment may be necessary if lice are found or eggs are observed at the hair-skin junction.

4. **Sex partners should be treated as previously mentioned.**

5. Special considerations. Pediculosis of the eyelashes should be treated by the application of occlusive ophthalmic ointment to the eyelid margins two times per day for 10 days to smother lice and nits. Lindane or other drugs should not be applied to the eyes. Clothing or bed linen that may have been contaminated by the patient within the preceding 2 days should be washed and dried by machine (hot cycle in each) or dry cleaned.

B. Scabies. Lindane lotion may not be used in pregnant or lactating women but may be used in sexual contacts.

1. Lindane (1%), 1 oz of lotion or 30 g of cream applied thinly to all areas of the body from the neck down and washed off thoroughly after 8 hours

2. Crotamiton (10%), applied to the entire body from the neck down for two nights and washed off thoroughly 24 hours after the second application

3. Pruritus may persist for several weeks after adequate therapy. A single retreatment after 1 week may be appropriate if no clinical improvement occurs. Additional weekly treatments are warranted only if live mites can be demonstrated. Clothing or bed linen that may have been contaminated by the patient within the preceding 2 days should be washed and dried by machine (hot cycle in each) or dry cleaned.

Q

STD TREATMENT GUIDELINES

Drugs of Abuse:
Urine Drug Screens

Various screening techniques are available to detect the presence of medications in a patient. The qualitative thin-layer chromatography (TLC) with enzyme-multiplication immunoassay technique (EMIT) confirmation of opiates, cocaine, and benzodiazepines (three areas of TLC weakness) is the most commonly ordered initial urine drug test in university and large private hospitals. The comprehensive quantitative drug test is useful once the qualitative test identifies a particular substance in the patient's urine sample. Alcohol and marijuana are not routinely analyzed on these tests. Alcohol is detected best in the blood. Both these chemicals may be requested and added to the standard TLC-EMIT panel used at your hospital.

R

TABLE R-1
SCREENING CRITERIA FOR DRUGS OF ABUSE

Antepartum hemorrhage

History of intravenous drug use

Preterm labor

Preterm premature rupture of membranes

Pregnancy-induced hypertension

Bizarre behavior

No prenatal care

Tattoos

History of hepatitis

Unexplained seizure

Obtundation

DRUG OF ABUSE SCREEN, QUALITATIVE

Technique:	Screen: Thin-layer chromatography, enzyme-multiplied immunoassay
	Confirm: TLC, EMIT, HPLC, GLC, GCMS
Specimen required:	50 ml urine
Analytic time:	2-4 h
Day(s) test set up:	Daily
	Available stat
Normal test values:	None detected

This rapid qualitative analysis is performed on urine and is designed for the detection of drugs in the overdose situation. The drugs listed below are detected as either their parent compound or their urinary metabolite.

Analyses Performed

Amphetamines
  Amphetamine
  Methamphetamine
Antidepressants
  Amitriptyline (Elavil)
  Amoxepin
  Desipramine (Norpramin)
  Doxepin (Sinequan)
  Imipramine (Tofranil)
  Nortriptyline (Aventyl)
Antihistamines
  Diphenhydramine (Benadryl)
  Dimenhydrinate
    (Dramamine)
  Ephedrine (Isupres)
  Pseudoephedrine
  Phenylpropanolamine
    (Dietac)
Barbiturates
  Amobarbital (Amytal)
  Butabarbital (Butabarb)
  Butalbital
  Pentobarbital (Nembutal)
  Phenobarbital (Luminal)
  Secobarbital (Seconal)
Benzodiazepines
    (undifferentiated)
Cardiacs
Lidocaine (Xylocaine)
Quinidine/quinine

Narcotics
  Codeine
  Hydrocodone
  Hydromorphone
  Meperidine (Demerol)
  Methadone (Dolophine)
  Morphine (heroin)
  Norpropoxyphene
  Pentazocine (Talwin)
  Propoxyphene (Darvon)
Phenothiazines
    (undifferentiated)
Sedatives and hypnotics
  Ethchlorvynol
    (Placidyl)
  Glutethimide (Doriden)
  Meprobamate (Equanil)
  Methaqualone
    (Quaalude)
Miscellaneous Agents
  Cocaine (as
    benzoylecgonine)
  Dextromethorphan
  Phencyclidine (PCP)
  Phentermine
  Phenytoin (Dilantin)
  Strychnine

R

DRUGS OF ABUSE: URINE DRUG SCREENS

Test code: DAUSC.
EMIT, Enzyme-multiplication immunoassay technique; *GCMS,* gas chromatography–mass spectrometry; *GLC,* gas-liquid chromatography; *HPLC,* high-pressure liquid chromatography; *TLC,* thin-layer chromatography.

TABLE R-3

DRUG COMPREHENSIVE PANEL, QUANTITATIVE

Technique:	Screen: Thin-layer chromatography, spectrophotometric, EMIT
	Confirm: TLC, EMIT, HPLC, GLC, GCMS
Specimen required:	75 ml random urine; 15 ml serum and gastric contents
	(if available). *Do not use serum separator tubes.*
	Consultation with the attending physician is desirable. Blood
	and urine are required for complete analysis. If only blood
	is submitted, only the drugs marked by an asterisk can be
	detected. If only urine is submitted, all classes of drugs will
	be detected as either the parent compound or its urinary
	metabolite.
Analytic time:	Positive result: dependent on the number of drugs detected
	None detected: results within 3 h
Day(s) test set up:	Daily
	Available stat
Normal test values:	None detected
	This analysis is particularly valuable when drug overdose is
	possible or suspected but the causative agent is unknown
	and other data available to the physician are insufficient to
	permit definite treatment. The study includes qualitative
	analysis for the drugs listed below and blood quantitations
	of the drugs marked with an asterisk (*).

Analyses Performed

Amphetamines
  Amphetamine
  Methamphetamine

Analgesics
  *Acetaminophen (Tylenol)
  *Salicylate (aspirin)

Antidepressants
  Amitriptyline (Elavil)
  Amoxepin
  Desipramine (Norpramin)
  Doxepin (Sinequan)
  Imipramine (Tofranil)
  Maprotiline (Ludiomil)
  Nortriptyline (Aventyl)

Antihistamines
  Diphenhydramine (Benadryl)
  Dimenhydrinate (Dramamine)
  Ephedrine (Isupres)/
    pseudoephedrine
  Methapyrilene
  Phenylpropanolamine
    (Dietac)
  Pyrilamine

Barbiturates
  *Amobarbital (Amytal)
  *Butabarbital (Butabarb)/
    butalbital
  *Pentobarbital (Nembutal)
  *Phenobarbital (Luminal)
  *Secobarbital (Seconal)

Benzodiazepines
  *Chlordiazepoxide (Librium)
  *Diazepam (Valium) and
    metabolite
  Oxazepam

Cardioactive agents
  Lidocaine (Xylocaine)
  Quinidine/quinine

TABLE R-3

DRUG COMPREHENSIVE PANEL, QUANTITATIVE—cont'd

Narcotics	Sedatives and hypnotics
Codeine	*Carisoprodol (Soma)
Hydrocodone	*Ethchlorvynol (Placidyl)
Hydromorphone	Ethinamate (Valmid)
Meperidine (Demerol)	*Glutethimide (Doriden)
Methadone (Dolophine)	Mebutamate
Morphine (heroin)	*Meprobamate (Equanil)
Norpropoxyphene	*Methaqualone
Pentazocine (Talwin)	(Quaalude)
Propoxyphene (Darvon)	*Methocarbamol
and metabolite	(Robaxin)
Phenothiazines	*Methyprylon (Noludar)
(undifferentiated unless	**Miscellaneous agents**
parent chemical present)	Cocaine (as
Chlorpromazine (Thorazine)	benzoylecgonine)
Thioridazine (Mellaril)	Dextromethorphan
Trifluoperazine	(Nyquil)
(Stelazine)	*Ethanol
Trifluorpromazine	Phencyclidine (PCP)
Trimeprazine	Phentermine
	Strychnine

Modified from *Toxicology Laboratory Handbook*, Irvine, Calif, University of California at Irvine Medical Center.

Test Code: COMADS.

EMIT, Enzyme-multiplication immunoassay technique; *GCMS*, gas chromatography–mass spectrometry; *GLC*, gas-liquid chromatography; *HPLC*, high-pressure liquid chromatography; *TLC*, thin-layer chromatography.

R

TABLE R-4

DETECTION TIME GUIDE FOR DRUGS IN URINE

Interpretation of detection time must take into account variability of urine specimens, drug metabolism and half-life, the patient's physical condition, fluid intake, and method and frequency of ingestion. The following are only general guidelines and apply to the commonly used TLC and EMIT confirmation screens for drugs of abuse.

Drug	Sensitivity Cutoff Values	Approximate Detection Time
Alcohol	20 mg/dl	
Amphetamines	300 ng/dl	2 d
Barbiturates	300 ng/ml	Short-acting (i.e., secobarbital), 1 d
		Long-acting (i.e., phenobarbital), 2-3 wk
Benzodiazepines	300 ng/ml	3 d if therapeutic dose ingested
Cocaine	300 ng/ml	Metabolite detectable for 2-4 d
Methadone	300 ng/ml	Approximately 3 d
Methaqualone	300 ng/ml	14 d
Opiates	300 ng/ml	2 d
Phencyclidine	75 ng/ml	Approximately 8 d
Propoxyphene	300 ng/ml	6 h to 2 d
Marijuana (THC)	100 ng/ml	

Modified from *Toxicology Laboratory Handbook*, Irvine, Calif, University of California at Irvine Medical Center.

TLC, Thin-layer chromatography; *EMIT*, enzyme-multiplication immunoassay technique.

Drug Use During Pregnancy: Maternal and Embryonic Effects

S

TABLE S-1		
FREQUENCY OF COCAINE AND ALCOHOL USE WITH OTHER SUBSTANCES		
Alcohol use with other substances listed		
T's and blues		53%
Heroin		29%
Cocaine		19%
Methamphetamine		7%
TOTAL (AVERAGE)		19%
Cocaine use with other substances listed		
Heroin		54%
Methamphetamine		12%
T's and blues		12%
TOTAL (AVERAGE)		21%

Modified from Cunningham FG, MacDonald PC, Gant NF, editors: *Williams' obstetrics,* ed 17, Norwalk, Conn, 1989, Appleton & Lange.
T's and blues, Pentazocine (Talwin) and tripelennamine citrate (pyribenzamine citrate).

TABLE S-2

SUMMARY OF SOME MATERNAL EFFECTS OF SOCIAL AND ILLICIT SUBSTANCE
USE DURING PREGNANCY

Substance	Placental Abruption	Central Nervous System Damage	Intracranial Hemorrhage	Hepatic or Renal Damage
Alcohol	+	+		+
Amphetamines	(+)	+	+	?
Barbiturates	−	+	+	?
Benzodiazepines	−	+	−	?
Cocaine*	+	+	+	+
Codeine	−	+	−	?
Heroin	+	+	+	+
Inhalants	?	+	−	+
LSD	?	+	—	?
Marijuana	−	(−)	—	−
Methadone	+	+	−	+
Methamphetamine	(+)	+	?	?
Morphine	(+)	+	−	+
PCP	?	(+)	(+)	+
Tobacco	+	(−)	−	+
T's and blues*	(+)	(+)	(+)	+

From Cunningham FG, MacDonald PC, Gant NF, editors: *Williams' obstetrics*, ed 17, Norwalk, Conn, 1989, Appleton & Lange.

T's and blues, Pentazocine (Talwin) and tripelennamine citrate (pyribenzamine citrate); *LSD,* lysergic acid diethylamide; *PCP,* phencyclidine.

+, Data conclusive of positive findings.

−, Data conclusive of negative findings.

(+), Data inconclusive but suggestive of positive findings.

(−), Data inconclusive but suggestive of negative findings.

?, Risks are unknown.

*May cause infarction/embolism.

TABLE S-3

SUMMARY OF SOME EMBRYOFETAL EFFECTS OF SOCIAL AND ILLICIT
SUBSTANCE USE DURING PREGNANCY

Substance	Growth Retardation	Congenital Anomalies	Withdrawal Syndrome
Alcohol	+	+	+
Amphetamines	+	?(−)	+
Barbiturates	+	?(−)	+
Benzodiazepines	?(+)	?(−)	?(+)
Cocaine	+	+	+
Codeine	?(+)	(−)	+
Heroin	+	−	+
Inhalants	+	+	?(−)
LSD	?	(−)	?(−)
Marijuana	+	−	−
Methadone	+	−	+
Methamphetamine	+	−	+
Morphine	+	(−)	+
PCP	+	?	+
Tobacco	+	−	−
T's and blues*	+	(−)	+

From Cunningham FG, MacDonald PC, Gant NF, editors: *Williams' obstetrics,* ed 17, Norwalk,
Conn, 1989, Appleton & Lange.
T's and blues, Pentazocine (Talwin) and tripelennamine citrate (pyribenzamine citrate); *LSD,* lysergic
acid diethylamide; *PCP,* phencyclidine.
+, Data conclusive of positive findings.
−, Data conclusive of negative findings.
(+), Data inconclusive but suggestive of positive findings.
(−), Data inconclusive but suggestive of negative findings.
?, Risks are unknown.
*May cause infarction/embolism.

Drug Use During Pregnancy: Perinatal Characteristics

TABLE T-1

PERINATAL CHARACTERISTICS OF OFFSPRING OF WOMEN WHO ABUSED
METHAMPHETAMINES COMPARED WITH CONTROL GROUP

Characteristics	Methamphetamine (n = 52)	Controls (n = 52)
Birth weight (g)	2957	3295*
Head circumference (cm)	48.1	49.8*
Gestational age (wk)	39.1	39.3*
Any congenital abnormality (%)†	12	14‡

From Cunningham FG, MacDonald PC, Gant NF, editors: *Williams' obstetrics*, ed 17, Norwalk,
Conn, 1989, Appleton & Lange.
*P <0.05.
†Major and minor.
‡P = Not significant.

TABLE T-2

PERINATAL CHARACTERISTICS OF OFFSPRING OF WOMEN WHO ABUSED T'S
AND BLUES COMPARED WITH CONTROL GROUP

Characteristics	T's and Blues (n = 23)	Controls (n = 100)
Birth weight (g)	2752	3295*
Head circumference (cm)	32	33.9*
Gestational age (wk)	38.9	39.3†
Congenital abnormalities (%)	13	6‡

From Cunningham FG, MacDonald PC, Gant NF, editors: *Williams' obstetrics*, ed 17, Norwalk,
Conn, 1989, Appleton & Lange.
T's and blues, Pentazocine (Talwin) and tripelennamine citrate (pyribenzamine citrate).
*P <0.05.
†P = Not significant.
‡This combination of drugs is a less expensive substitute for heroin.

Definition of Terms: Street Names of Drugs of Abuse

TABLE U-1	
Substance	**Street Names**
Amphetamine	AMT Hearts
(dextroamphetamine)	Barn Lid poppers
	B-bombs Peaches
	Bennies Pep pills
	Benz Purple hearts
	Bombita Roses
	Brain ticklers* Sparkle plenties
	Brownies Splash
	Cartwheels Speed
	Chalk Tens
	Copilots Thrusters
	Crossroads Uppers, uppies, or ups
	Crystal West coast turnarounds
	Dexies Whites
	Fives
Barbiturates	Blockbusters Nemmies
	Blues* Nimby
	Brain ticklers* Pinks
	Courage pills Rainbows
	Downers* Red birds
	Downie Red devils
	Gangster pills Reds
	G.B. Reds and blues
	Goofball Seggy
	Gorilla pills Tooies
	Idiot pills Yellow jackets
	King Kong pills
Benzodiazepines	Blues* Vals
	Downers*
Cocaine	Bernies Dust
	Burese Flake
	Candyman* Heaven dust
	Coke Lady snow
	Cola Snow
	Corrine Star dust
	Crack

Continued

TABLE U-1 —cont'd	
Substance	**Street Names**
Codeine	Blue velvet
Heroin	Bolsa — H-caps
	Boy — Henry
	Brown stuff — Him
	Caballo — Horse
	Candyman* — Junk
	Cura — Poison
	Duji — Scag
	Dogie — Smack
	Doojie — Tapita
	Dope — Tecata
	Harry — White lady
Lysergic acid diethylamide (LSD)	Acid — LSM
	Beast — Microdot (yellow, blue, white, etc.)
	Big D —
	Blue acid — Mind detergent
	Chief — Orange sunshine
	Deeda — Pellets
	Electric Kool-Ade — Purple haze
	Ghost — Tabs
	Hawk — Trips
	"L" — Window pane
Marijuana	Acapulco gold — Joints
	Baby — Juana
	Bhang — Kif
	Black gunion — Loco weed
	Duby or dooby — Maruamba
	Giggle weed — Mary Jane
	Grass — Pot
	Grefa, greta, grifa, or griffo — Rafe
	Gunjah — Reefer
	Hamp — Rosa Maria
	Hash, hashish, hash oil (extracted from marijuana) — Skunk
	— Smoke
	— Texas tea
	Herb — Yamba
	Hootch

Continued

TABLE U-1 —cont'd		
Substance	Street Names	
Methamphetamines	Adam	Ice
	Black beauties	MDA
	Crank	MDMA
	Crystal	MDEA
	Ectasy	Meth
	Eve	Methedrine
PCP	Angel dust	

From Cunningham FG, MacDonald PC. Gant NF, editors: *Williams' obstetrics,* ed 17, Norwalk, Conn, 1989, Appleton & Lange.
*Duplicate street terms are marked with an asterisk.

U

STREET NAMES OF DRUGS OF ABUSE

Definition of Terms: Vital Statistics

To aid in the reduction of the number of mothers and infants who die as the result of pregnancy and labor, it is important to know how many such deaths there are in the United States each year and in what circumstances. To evaluate these data correctly, a variety of events concerned with pregnancy outcomes have been defined by various agencies.

Birth. This is the complete expulsion or extraction from the mother of a fetus, irrespective of whether the umbilical cord has been cut or the placenta is attached. Fetuses weighing <500 g usually are not considered as births, but rather as *abortuses,* for purposes of perinatal statistics. In the absence of a birth weight, a body length of 25 cm, crown to heel, is usually equated with 500 g.

Approximately 20 weeks' gestational age is commonly considered to be equivalent to 500-g fetal weight; however, a 500-g fetus is more likely to be 22 (menstrual) weeks' gestational age.

Birth rate. The number of births per 1000 population is the birth rate, or crude birth rate. The birth rate in the United States for the year ending February 1999 was 14.5 (*National Vital Statistics Report* vol. 49, No. 1, 1999).

Fertility rate. This term refers to the number of live births per 1000 female population aged 15 through 44 years. In 1999 this was 65.9 (*National Vital Statistics Report* vol. 49, No. 1, 1999).

Live birth. Whenever the infant at or sometime after birth breathes spontaneously or shows any other sign of life, such as heartbeat or definite spontaneous movement of voluntary muscles, a live birth is recorded.

Stillbirth. None of the signs of life are present at or after birth.

Neonatal death. Early neonatal death refers to death of a live-born infant during the first 7 days after birth. Late neonatal death refers to death after 7 days but before 29 days.

Stillbirth rate. The number of stillborn infants per 1000 infants born.

Fetal death rate. This term is synonymous with stillbirth rate.

Neonatal mortality. The number of neonatal deaths per 1000 live births.

Perinatal mortality. This rate is defined as the number of stillbirths plus neonatal deaths per 1000 total births.

Low birth weight. If the first newborn weight obtained after birth is <2500 g, the infant is termed low birth weight.

Term infant. An infant born anytime after 37 completed (menstrual) weeks of gestation through 42 completed weeks of gestation (260 to 294

From Cunningham FG, MacDonald PC, Gant NF, editors: *Williams' obstetrics,* ed 17, Norwalk, Conn, 1989, Appleton & Lange.

days) is considered by most to be a term infant. Such a definition implies that birth at any time within this period is optimal, whereas birth before or afterward is not. Such an implication is not warranted. Some infants born between 37 and 38 weeks are at risk of functional prematurity, for example, the development of respiratory distress in the newborn infant of a diabetic mother. In the past, some considered gestation extending 41 weeks to be postterm; however, any risk to the fetus that might be imposed by remaining in utero until 42 weeks rather than 41 weeks does not appear to be appreciable. Consequently, there is no good reason for distorting the range for term birth to 3 weeks below the mean of 40 weeks but only 1 week beyond the mean.

Preterm or premature infant. An infant born before 37 completed weeks has been so classified, although born before 38 completed weeks would seem more appropriate for reasons stated above.

Postterm infant. An infant born anytime after completion of the 42 weeks' gestation has been classified by some as being postterm.

Abortus. A fetus or embryo removed or expelled from the uterus during the first half of gestation (20 weeks or less) weighing <500 g or measuring <25 cm is also referred to as an abortus.

Direct maternal death. Death of the mother resulting from obstetric complications of the pregnancy state, labor, or puerperium and from interventions, omissions, incorrect treatment, or a chain of events resulting from any of the above is considered a direct maternal death. An example is maternal death from exsanguination resulting from rupture of the uterus.

Indirect maternal death. An obstetric death not directly caused by obstetric causes, but resulting from previously existing disease or a disease that developed during pregnancy, labor, or the puerperium and that was aggravated by the maternal physiologic adaptation to pregnancy, is classified as an indirect maternal death. An example is maternal death from complications of mitral stenosis.

Nonmaternal death. Death of the mother resulting from accidental or incidental causes in no way related to the pregnancy may be classified as a nonmaternal death. An example is death from an automobile accident.

Maternal death rate or maternal mortality. The number of maternal deaths that result from the reproductive process per 100,000 live births.

Definition of Terms: Symbols

†	one
††	two, etc.
μl	microliter
±	plus or minus
>	greater than
<	less than
1°	primary
2°	secondary
Ψ	psychiatry
→	to, toward
≠	against, opposite
≅	approximately equal to
Δ	change
(x)	location of abdominal findings
+	positive
β	beta
@	at
↑	increased
↓	decreased
♀	female
♂	male
®	right
Ⓛ	left
m̂	murmur
x+	location of fetal heart tones
~	proportional to
♀x	location of pulses or reflexes
(°)	degree
1:1	one to one
−	negative

Definition of Terms: Abbreviations

A

a	before; arterial
aa	of each; arteries
Ab	abortion
abd	abdomen
ABE	acute bacterial endocarditis
ABG	arterial blood gas
ac	before meals
AC	acromioclavicular
A/C	assist control
ACA	anticardiolipin antibody
ACT	activated clotting time
ACTH	adrenocorticotropic hormone
a.d.	right ear
ad lib	freely, as desired
ADA	American Diabetic Association
ADH	antidiuretic hormone
ADL	activities of daily living
adm	admission
ADP	adenosine diphosphate
adx	adnexa
AF	atrial fibrillation
AFB	acid-fast bacillus
afeb	afebrile
AFI	amniotic fluid index
AFV	amniotic fluid volume
+A/G	albumin-to-globulin ratio
AGE	acute gastroenteritis
$AgNO_3$	silver nitrate
A/H	auditory hallucinations
AHF	antihemolytic factor
AHFS	American Hospital Formulary Service
AI	aortic insufficiency
AIDS	acquired immunodeficiency syndrome
AK	above the knee
aka	also known as
AKA	above-the-knee amputation
ALD	alcoholic liver disease
alk phos	alkaline phosphatase
ALL	acute lymphocytic leukemia
$AL(OH)_3$	aluminum hydroxide
ALT	alanine aminotransferase (SGPT)

AMA	against medical advice
amb	ambulate
AML	acute myeloblastic leukemia
amnio	amniocentesis
amp	amputation
amt	amount
ANA	antinuclear antibodies
angio	angiography
anx. neur.	anxiety neurosis
anx. reac.	anxiety reaction
AODM	adult-onset diabetes mellitus
AOM	acute otitis media
AP	anteroposterior
A&P	anterior and posterior
APA	antiphospholipid antibody
APAP	acetaminophen
APC-R	activated protein C resistance
Appy	appendectomy
APT	alum-precipitated toxoid
aq	water
AR	aortic regurgitation
ARDS	acute respiratory distress syndrome
ARF	acute renal failure
AROM	artificial rupture of membranes
ARV	alleged rape victim
a.s.	left ear
AS	aortic stenosis
ASA	aspirin
ASAP	as soon as possible
ASAV	alleged sexual assault victim
ASB	asymptomatic bacteriuria
ASCVD	arteriosclerotic cardiovascular disease
ASD	atrial septal defect
ASHD	arteriosclerotic heart disease
ASO	antistreptolysin O
AST	aspartate aminotransferase (SGOT)
at	atrial
ATN	acute tubular necrosis
ATP	adenosine triphosphate
a.u.	*aures uterque* (each ear)
AV	atrioventricular
A/V	auditory/visual
A/W	alive and well
ax	axillary

B

BBB	bundle branch block
BBBB	bilateral bundle branch block
B&C	board and care
BCC	basal cell carcinoma
BCG	bacillus Calmette-Guérin
BCP	birth control pills
BCS	battered child syndrome
be	base excess
BE	barium enema
BIB	brought in by
BIBPD	brought in by police department
BICU	burn intensive care unit
bid	*bis in die* (twice per day)
BK	below the knee
BKA	below-the-knee amputation
blbs	bilateral breath sounds
blk	block
BM	bowel movement
BMR	basal metabolic rate
BOA	born out of asepsis
BOE	bilateral otitis externa
BOM	bilateral otitis media
BOW	bag of water
BP	blood pressure
BPH	benign prostatic hypertrophy
bpm	beats per minute
BPP	biophysical profile
BR	bed rest
BRBPR	bright red blood per rectum
BRP	bathroom privileges
bs	blood sugar
BS	bowel sounds
B/S	breath sounds
BSA	body surface area
BSO	bilateral salpingo-oophorectomy
BSP	bromsulphalein
BTL	bilateral tubal ligation
btw	between
BU	burn unit
BUN	blood urea nitrogen
BV	bacterial vaginosis
BW	birth weight
BWS	battered wife syndrome
Bx	biopsy

C

$\overline{c}$	with
C	centrigrade or Celsius, degree of
C1-C2	first and second cervical vertebrae
Ca^{2+}	calcium ion
CA	cancer, carcinoma
CABG	coronary artery bypass graft
$CaCl_2$	calcium chloride
$CaCO_3$	calcium carbonate
CAD	coronary artery disease
CAH	congenital adrenal hyperplasia
cap	capsule
cath	catheterization
CBC	complete blood cell count
CBD	common bile duct
CBDE	common bile duct exploration
CBS	chronic brain syndrome
cc	cubic centimeter
CC	chief complaint
c/c/e	cyanosis, clubbing, edema
CCU	coronary care unit
CDC	Centers for Disease Control and Prevention
cf	count fingers
CF	cystic fibrosis
CHB	complete heart block
CHD	congenital heart disease
CHF	congestive heart failure
chr	chronic
chr ETOH	chronic alcoholism
circ	circumcision
cis Pt	*cis*-platinum
CK	creatine kinase
CLL	chronic lymphocytic leukemia
cm	centimeter
CML	chronic myelocytic leukemia
CMS	circulation, motion, and sensation
CMV	cytomegalovirus
CNS	central nervous system
CO	cardiac output
C/O	complaints of
CO_2	carbon dioxide
cocci	coccidioidomycosis
COM	chronic otitis media
comp	compound
COPD	chronic obstructive pulmonary disease
CP	cerebral palsy

CPAP	continuous positive airway pressure
CPD	cephalopelvic disproportion
Cpeak	peak compliance
CPK	creatinine phosphokinase; *see* CK
CPR	cardiopulmonary resuscitation
CRF	chronic renal failure
CRIT	hematocrit (hct)
CS	cesarean section
C&S	culture and sensitivity
CSF	cerebrospinal fluid
CST	contraction stress test
Cstat	static compliance
CT	computed tomography
CUS	chronic undifferentiated schizophrenia
CV	cardiovascular
CVA	cerebrovascular accident
CVAT	costovertebral angle tenderness
CVD	cardiovascular disease
CVP	central venous pressure
cx	cervix
CXR	chest x-ray

D

d	day
D/C	discontinue
D&C	dilation and curettage
DCR	dacryocystorhinotomy
DD	differential diagnosis
decel	deceleration
depr neur	depressive neurosis
DFA	diet for age
DGI	disseminated gonococcal infection
DI	diabetes insipidus
DIC	disseminated intravascular coagulation
diff	differential count
DIP	distal interphalangeal joint
DJD	degenerative joint disease
DKA	diabetic ketoacidosis
dl	deciliter
DL&B	direct laryngoscopy and bronchoscopy
D_5LR	dextrose in 5% lactated Ringer's solution
DM	diabetes mellitus
DMD	Doctor of Dental Medicine
DNA	deoxyribonucleic acid
DNR	do not resuscitate
D_5NS	5% dextrose in normal saline

$D_5\frac{1}{2}NS$	5% dextrose and 0.45% normal saline solution
DOA	dead on arrival
DOE	dyspnea on exertion
DPT	diphtheria-pertussis-tetanus immunization
DR	diabetic retinopathy
drsg	dressing
D/S	dextrose in saline
DSD	discharge summary dictated
DSPC	disaturated phosphatidylcholine
DSS	dioctyl sodium sulfosuccinate
DT	delerium tremens
DTR	deep tendon reflex
DU	duodenal ulcer
DUB	dysfunctional uterine bleeding
DVT	deep venous thrombosis
D/W	dextrose in water
D_5W	5% dextrose in water
Dx	diagnosis
DZ	dizygotic (twins)

E

E	esophoria (distance [i.e., 20 ft, 6 m])
E′	esophoria (near [i.e., 14 in, 33 cm])
EBL	estimated blood loss
ECCE	extracapsular cataract extraction
ecf	extracellular fluid
ECF	extended care facility
ECG	electrocardiogram
ECT	electroconvulsive therapy
EDC	estimated date of confinement (due date)
EDTA	ethylenediamine tetraacetic acid
EEG	electroencephalogram
EENT	eyes, ears, nose, and throat
EFW	estimated fetal weight
e.g.	for example
EGA	estimated gestational age; echogenic area
EICT	external isometric contraction
e-IPV	enhanced-potency inactivated virus
EKG	electrocardiogram
ELISA	enzyme-linked immunosorbent assay
elix	elixir
EMG	electromyogram
EMI	electromagnetic interference
EMIT	enzyme-multiplication immunoassay technique
ENG	electronystagmogram
ENT	ear, nose, and throat

EOMI	extraocular movements intact
EOMs	extraocular movements
eos	eosinophils
EPS	extrapyramidal symptoms
ER	Emergency Room
E&R	equal and reactives
ERE	Emergency Room Emergent
ERN	Emergency Room Nonemergent
ERU	Emergency Room Urgent
ERV	expiratory reserve volume
ESR	erythrocyte sedimentation rate
et	and
ET	esotropia (distance); endotracheal
(ET)	intermittent esotropia
eth	ether
ETI	endotracheal intubation
ETOH	ethyl alcohol
EUA	examination under anesthesia
Exc	excision
expl	exploration
ext	external

F

F	Fahrenheit, degree of
FB	foreign body
FBS	fasting blood sugar
FDA	Food and Drug Administration
FDP	fibrinogen degradation products
Fe	iron
FEF	forced expiratory flow
$FeSO_4$	ferrous sulfate
FEV	forced expiratory volume
FEV_1	first second of expiration
FFA	free fatty acids
FH	fundal height
FHR	fetal heart rate
FHTs	fetal heart tones
fib	fibrillation
fld ext	fluid extract
FLM	fetal lung maturity
FMC	fetal movement count
FRC	functional residual capacity
FSH	follicle-stimulating hormone
FSI	foam stability index
FTA-ABS	fluorescent treponemal antibody, absorbed
FTP	failure to progress

FTSG	full-thickness skin graft
FTT	failure to thrive
F/U	follow-up
FUO	fever of unknown origin
FVC	forced vital capacity
FWB	full weight bearing
fx	fracture

G

g	gram
G	gravida
GA	gestational age; general anesthesia
GB	gallbladder
GBS	group B streptococcus
GC	*Neisseria gonorrhoeae* (also known as gonococcus)
GCMS	gas chromatography–mass spectroscopy
GE	gastroenteritis
gen	general
GET	general endotracheal intubation
GFR	glomerular filtration rate
GH	growth hormone
GI	gastrointestinal
GLC	gas-liquid chromatography
GME	graduate medical education
G-6-P	glucose-6-phosphate
G-6-PD	glucose-6-phosphate dehydrogenase
gr	grain
GSW	gunshot wound
gtt	drops
GTT	glucose tolerance test
GU	genitourinary
Gy	gray
GYN	gynecology

H

h	hour
HA	headache; hepatitis A
H/A	heated aerosol
HAA	hepatitis-associated antigen
HAL	hyperalimentation
Hb	hemoglobin
HB	heart block (first, second or third degree); hepatitis B
HbA_{1c}	hemoglobin A_{1c}, glycosylated hemoglobin A
HBAg	hepatitis B antigen
HBcAb	hepatitis B core antibody
HBcAg	hepatitis B core antigen

HBeAg	hepatitis B e antigen
HBIg	hepatitis B immunoglobulin
HBP	high blood pressure
HBsAb	hepatitis B surface antibody
HBsAg	hepatitis B surface antigen
HBV	hepatitis B virus
HCAb	hepatitis C antibody
HCC	home care coordinator
hCG	human chorionic gonadotropin
HCl	hydrochloric acid
HCO_3^-	bicarbonate
Hct	hematocrit
HCTZ	hydrochlorothiazide
HCVD	hypertensive cardiovascular disease
HEENT	head, eyes, ears, nose, and throat
HELLP	hemolysis, elevated liver enzymes, and low platelet count
H-flu	*Haemophilus influenzae*
Hgb	hemoglobin
HGH	human growth hormone
H/H	hemoglobin/hematocrit
H/I	homicidal ideation
Histo	histoplasmosis
HIV	human immunodeficiency virus
HIVD	herniated interventricular disk
hm	hand motions
HMD	hyaline membrane disease
HNO_3	nitric acid
HNP	herniated nucleus pulposus
H_2O	water
H_2O_2	hydrogen peroxide
HO	house officer
HOB	head of bed
H&P	history and physical
hpf	high-power field
HPI	history of present illness
HPLC	high-pressure liquid chromatography
HPV	human papillomavirus
hr	hour
HR	heart rate
hs	at bedtime
H_2SO_4	sulfuric acid
HSV	herpes simplex virus
Ht	height
HTLV	human T-cell leukemia-lymphoma virus
HTN	hypertension

HVD	hypertensive vascular disease
HW	housewife
Hx	history
hyst	hysterectomy

I

I$_{131}$	radioactive iodine
IAM	internal auditory meatus
IBC	iron-binding capacity
IC	inspiratory capacity
ICBG	iliac crest bone graft
ICCP	intracapsular cataract pressure
ICF	intracellular fluid
ICU	intensive care unit
ID	identification; intradermal
I&D	incision and drainage
IDL	intraocular lens
IDU	idoxuridine
IFA	indirect fluorescent antibody
Ig	immunoglobulin
IgG	immunoglobulin G
IgM	immunoglobulin M
IHA	indirect hemagglutination
IHSS	idiopathic hypertrophic subaortic stenosis
IJ	ileojejunal
IM	intramuscular
IMF	inferior maxillary fracture
Imp	impression
IMV	intermittent mandatory ventilation
Ing	inguinal
INH	isoniazid
I&O	intake and output
IOCG	interoperative cholangiography
IOP	intraocular pressure
ip	interim permitte
IP	intraperitoneal
IPPB	intermittent positive pressure breathing
IRV	inspiratory reserve volume
IS	incentive spirometer
IT	intrathecal
ITP	immunologic thrombocytopenia
IU	international units
IUD	intrauterine device
IUG	intrauterine gestation
IUGR	intrauterine growth retardation
IUP	intrauterine pregnancy

IUT	intrauterine transfusion
IV	intravenous
IVC	inferior vena cava
IVH	intraventricular hemorrhage
IVP	intravenous pyelogram; intravenous push
IVPB	intravenous piggyback
IVS	intraventricular septum

J

JODM	juvenile-onset diabetes mellitus
JRA	juvenile rheumatoid arthritis
jt	joint
JVD	jugular venous distention
JVP	jugular venous pressure

K

K^+	potassium
KCl	potassium chloride
kg	kilogram
KP	keratic precipitates
KPE	Kelmas phacoemulsification
KUB	kidneys, ureter, and bladder

L

L	liter
L1-L2	first and second lumbar vertebrae
LA	local anesthesia
LAC	long arm cast; lupus anticoagulant
LAD	left axis deviation
LAH	left axial hypertrophy
lap	laparotomy
LATS	long arm thumb spica
lb	pound
LB	lower back
LBBB	left bundle branch block
LBP	lower back pain
LBW	low birth weight
LC	living children
LCD	liquor carbonis detergens
LCS	lichen chronicus simplex
LD	lethal dose
LD_{50}	median lethal dose
LDH	lactic dehydrogenase
L-dopa	levodopa
le	left extremity
LE	lupus erythematosus

LFT	liver function test
lg	large
LGA	large for gestational age
LGL	Lown-Ganong-Levine
LH	luteinizing hormone
lig	ligation
lih	left inguinal hernia
liq	liquid
LL	left lung
LLC	long leg cast
LLE	left lower extremity
LLL	lower left lobe
LLQ	left lower quadrant
LMD	local medical doctor
LMP	last menstrual period
LMW	low molecular weight
LOA	left occiput anterior
LOC	loss of consciousness
LOP	left occiput posterior
LOT	left occiput transverse
LP	lumbar puncture
LPD	luteal phase defect
LPT	licensed psychiatric technician
LR	lactated Ringer's solution
LS	lumbosacral
L/S	lecithin/sphingomyelin
LSD	lysergic acid diethylamide
LSW	licensed social worker
LTB	laryngotracheobronchitis
LUD	left upper decubitus
LUE	left upper extremity
LUL	left upper lobe
LUQ	left upper quadrant
LVD	left ventricular dysfunction
LVET	left ventricular ejection time
LVH	left ventricular hypertrophy
LVID	left ventricular internal dimension
LVN	licensed vocational nurse
LVP	left ventricular pressure
L&W	living and well

M

m	meter
MA	mental age
M/A	Mexican American
MAV	minute alveolar volume

mca	middle cerebral artery
MCA	motorcycle accident
μg	microgram
mch	mean corpuscular hemoglobin
MCH	Mission Community Hospital
MCHC	mean corpuscular hemoglobin count
MCP	metacarpophalangeal
MCV	mean corpuscular volume
M.D.	medical doctor
mEq	milliequivalents
MER	medical emergency room
met	metastasis
MG	myasthenia gravis
Mg^{++}	magnesium
mg/dl	milligram/deciliter
$Mg(OH)_2$	magnesium hydroxide
$MgSO_4$	magnesium sulfate
MH	mental health
MHATP	microhemagglutination assay for antibody to *Treponema pallidum*
MHC	mental health crisis
MI	myocardial infarction
MIC	minimal inhibitory concentration
min	minute
ml	milliliter
ML	midline
MLH	Martin Luther Hospital
mm	millimeter
mm Hg	millimeters of mercury
mmol	millimoles
MMR	maternal mortality rate; mumps, measles, rubella immunizations
mo	month
MOA	monoamine oxidase
mod	moderate
MOM	milk of magnesia
MR	mitral regurgitation
MR ×___	may repeat ___ times
MRI	magnetic resonance imaging
ms	mitral stenosis
MS	morphine sulfate
MTX	methotrexate
mv	multivitamins
MV	minute volume
MVA	motor vehicle accident
MVP	mitral valve prolapse

X

DEFINITION OF TERMS: ABBREVIATIONS

MVV	maximal voluntary ventilation
MZ	monozygotic (twins)

N

Na^{2+}	sodium
NA	nurse's aide
N/A	not applicable
NaCl	sodium chloride
NAD	no acute distress
$NaHCO_3$	sodium bicarbonate
NB	newborn
Neb meds	nebulized medications
NEC	necrotizing enterocolitis
neg	negative
NG	nasogastric
NH_4Cl	ammonium chloride
NICU	neonatal intensive care unit
NIL	not in active labor
NK	not known
NKA	no known allergies
nl	normal
NLP	no light perception
nm	neuromuscular
NMR	nuclear magnetic resonance
noc	night
NOS	not otherwise specified
NP	nasopharynx
NPC	near point of convergence
NPDR	nonproliferative diabetic retinopathy
NPH	neutral protamine Hagedorn (insulin)
NPN	nonprotein nitrogen
NPO	*nil per os* (nothing by mouth)
NS	normal saline
NSAID	nonsteroidal antiinflammatory drug
NSR	normal sinus rhythm
NST	nonstress test
NSVD	normal spontaneous vaginal delivery
NT	nasotracheal
NTG	nitroglycerin
N&V	nausea and vomiting

O

O	negative
O_2	oxygen
OA	occiput anterior
OB	obstetric

OB+	occult blood positive
OBS	organic brain syndrome
OCG	oral cholecystogram
OCP	oral contraceptive pills
OCT	oxytocin challenge test
o.d.	right eye
OD	overdose
OM	otitis media
OMFS	oral and maxillofacial surgery
OOB	out of bed
OOP	out of plaster
op	operation
OP	occiput posterior
OPC	outpatient clinic
OPD	outpatient department
OPV	oral poliovirus vaccine
OR	operating room
ORIF	open reduction and internal fixation
o.s.	left eye
osm	osmolar
OT	occupational therapy
otc	over the counter
o.u.	each eye, both eyes
oz	ounce

P

p	after; pressure
P	pulse
PA	posteroanterior; pernicious anemia
P&A	percussion and auscultation
PAC	premature atrial contractions
PAP	Papanicolaou smear
Par	paranoid
Para I	primipara
PARR	postanesthesia recovery room
PAS	paraaminosalicylic acid
PAT	paroxysmal atrial tachycardia
path	pathology
Pb	barometric pressure; phenobarbital
PB	piggyback
PBI	protein-bound iodine
pc	after meals
PCC	patient care coordinator
PCN	penicillin
P_{CO_2}	partial pressure of carbon dioxide
PCP	phencyclidine

PCWP	pulmonary capillary wedge pressure
PD	interpupillary distance
PDA	patent ductus arteriosus
PD&P	postural drainage and percussion
PDR	*Physicians' Desk Reference*
PE	physical examination; pulmonary embolus
PEAU	psychiatric emergency admitting unit
Ped	pediatrician
Peds	pediatrics
PEEP	positive end-expiratory pressure
PEFR	peak expiratory flow rate
PEP	peak expiratory pressure
perf	perforation
PERLA	pupils equal, reactive to light and accommodation
PERRLA	pupils equal, round, reactive to light and accommodation
PET	positron emission tomography
PETs	pressure equalization tubes
PEU	protected environment unit
PFR	peak flow rate
PFT	pulmonary function test
Pg	pregnant
PG	phosphatidylglycerol
1° PG	1 hour post-Glucola
pH	hydrogen ion concentration (pH = 7, neutral; pH <7, acidic; pH >7, alkaline)
PH	past history
PHA	phytohemagglutinin
PharmD	doctor of pharmacy
PhD	doctor of philosophy
PHN	public health nurse
PI	present illness
P/I	paranoid ideation
PICU	pediatric intensive care unit
PID	pelvic inflammatory disease
PIH	pregnancy-induced hypertension
PIP	proximal interphalangeal (joint)
PK	psychokinesis
PKU	phenylketonuria
PL	pediatric level
PMD	private medical doctor
PMH	past medical history
PMI	point of maximal impulse
PMP	previous menstrual period
PM&R	physical medicine and rehabilitation
PNB	prostatic needle biopsy
PND	paroxysmal nocturnal dyspnea

PNM	perinatal mortality
PNMR	perinatal mortality rate
PO	*per os* (by mouth); postoperative
Po$_2$	partial pressure of oxygen
post	posterior
postop	postoperative
POV	privately owned vehicle
pp	postpartum
PP	postprandial
PPD	purified protein derivative (tuberculin)
Ppeak	postoperative peak pressure
PPP	palatopharyngoplasty
pPROM, PPROM	preterm premature rupture of membranes
PR	per rectum
PRBC	packed red blood cell
preg	pregnancy
preop	preoperative
prep	preparation
prn	whenever necessary
prob	problem
prog	prognosis
PROM	premature rupture of fetal membranes
Protime (PT)	prothrombin time
prox	proximal
PS	pulmonary stenosis
PSP	phenolsulfonphthalein
Pstat	static pressure
pt	patient
PT	physical therapy; prothrombin time
PTA	prior to admission
PTB	patella tendon bearing
PTH	parathyroid hormone
PTL	preterm labor
PTT	partial thromboplastin time
PTU	propylthiouracil
PUBS	percutaneous umbilical vein blood sampling
PUD	peptic ulcer disease
PVC	premature ventricular contractions
PWB	partial weight bearing
px	pneumothorax
PX	physical examination
PZI	protamine zinc insulin

Q

q	every (e.g., q8h)
qam	every morning
qd	every day, once per day

qh	every hour
qhs	every night at bedtime
qid	four times per day
qod	every other day
qs	quantity sufficient to make

R

R	respiration; roentgen
ra	room air
RA	rheumatoid arthritis
rad	radiation absorbed dose
RAD	right axis deviation
RAE	right atrial enlargement
RAF	rheumatoid arthritis factor
RAH	right atrial hypertrophy
RAI	radioactive iodine
RAIU	radioactive iodine uptake
RAO	right anterior oblique
RAP	right atrial pressure
RAS	renal artery stenosis
RBBB	right bundle branch block
rbc	red blood cell
RBC	red blood count
RBF	renal blood flow
RCA	right coronary artery
RCD	relative cardiac dullness
RCS	reticulum cell sarcoma
RD	respiratory disease
rda	right dorsoanterior
RDA	recommended daily allowance
rdp	right dorsoposterior
RDS	respiratory distress syndrome
RE	regional enteritis
re	right extremity
rehab	rehabilitation
rem	roentgen equivalent man
req	request
retic	reticulocyte
RFS	renal function study
Rh	Rhesus (factor)
RHD	rheumatic heart disease
RI	respiratory illness
RIA	radioimmunoassay
RICU	respiratory intensive care unit
RJ	Robert Jones dressing
RL	right lung

RLC	residual lung capacity
RLE	right lower extremity
RLF	retrolental fibroplasia
RLL	right lower lobe
RLQ	right lower quadrant
RML	right middle lobe
RN	registered nurse
RND	radical neck dissection
R/O	rule out
ROA	right occiput anterior
ROAD	reversible obstructive artery disease
ROM	rupture of membranes; range of motion
ROP	right occiput posterior
ROS	review of systems
ROT	right occiput transverse
rpr	reactive protein reagent
RPR	rapid plasma reagin (syphilis screen)
RQ	respiratory quotient
rr	respiratory rate
RR	recovery room
RRR	regular rate and rhythm
R/S	restraint and seclusion
RSR	regular sinus rhythm
Rt	right
RT	radiation therapy
RTA	renal tubular acidosis
RTC	return to clinic
RTO	return to office
RUE	right upper extremity
RUL	right upper lobe
RUQ	right upper quadrant
RV	residual volume
RVE	right ventricular enlargement
RVID	right ventricular internal dimension
RVT	renal vein thrombosis
rx	treatment, therapy
Rx	prescription

S

s	second; without
S1 & S2	heart sounds, first and second
S3 & S4	heart sounds, third and fourth
S/A	suicide attempt
S&A	sugar and acetone
SAB	spontaneous abortion
SAC	short arm cast

SAH	subarachnoid hemorrhage
SAP	systemic arterial pressure
sat	saturated
SATS	short arm thumb spica
SB	standby
SBE	subacute bacterial endocarditis
SBO	small bowel obstruction
SC	subcutaneous
SCUT	schizophrenia, chronic undifferentiated type
SE	southeast
SEM	systolic ejection murmur
SG	Swan-Ganz; specific gravity
SGA	small for gestational age
SGOT	serum glutamic oxaloacetic transaminase (AST)
SGPT	serum glutamic pyruvic transaminase (ALT)
SIADH	syndrome of inappropriate secretion of antidiuretic hormone
sig	let it be labeled, write
SIMV	synchronized intermittent mandatory ventilation
SL	sublingual
SLC	short leg cast
SLE	systemic lupus erythematosus
SLWC	short leg walking cast
SMR	submucosal resection
SNF	skilled nursing facility
S&O	salpingo-oophorectomy
So_1	oxygen saturation
SOAP	subjective, objective assessment plan
SOAPE	subjective, objective assessment plan, evaluation
sob	side of bed
SOB	shortness of breath
sol	solution
SOM	serous otitis media
sos	if necessary
S/P	status post
SPA	salt-poor albumin
spec	specimen
SPECT	single photon emission computed tomography
SPT	senior psychiatric technician
SQ	subcutaneous
SR	sedimentation rate
SROM	spontaneous rupture of membranes
ss	one half
SSE	soap suds enema; sterile speculum examination
SSKI	saturated solution potassium iodide
SSS	sick sinus syndrome

S/T	suicide ideation
stat	immediately
STD	sexually transmitted disease
STSG	split-thickness skin graft
suct	suction
SUN	serum urea nitrogen
supp	suppository
Sv	sievert
SV	supraventricular
sx	symptoms
syr	syrup

T

T	temperature
T1, T2	first, second thoracic vertebrae
T3	triiodothyronine
T4	thyroxine
TA	trained aide
T&A	tonsillectomy and adenoidectomy
tab	tablet
TAB	therapeutic abortion
TAH	total abdominal hysterectomy
TAL	tendon Achilles lengthening
TAT	tetanus antitoxin
TB	tuberculosis
tbsp	tablespoon
TBW	total body water
tc	total capacity
TC	temporary custody
T&C	type and crossmatch
TCDB	turn, cough, deep breathe
TCI	transient cerebral ischemia
TCN	tetracycline
Td	tetanus and diphtheria toxins
TDX	test for surfactant/albumin ratio
TEF	tracheoesophageal fistula
TGT	thromboplastin generation test
T&H	type and hold
TIA	transient ischemic attack
TIBC	total iron-binding capacity
tid	*ter in die* (three times per day)
TIE	transient ischemic episode
TKO	to keep open
TL	tubal ligation
tlc	total lung capacity
TLC	tender loving care; thin-layer chromatography

tm	temporomandibular
TM	tympanic membrane
TMJ	temporomandibular joint
TMP/SMX	trimethoprim-sulfamethoxazole
TMST	treadmill stress test
TND	term normal delivery
TO	telephone order
TOA	tuboovarian abscess
toco	tocodynamometer
t-PA	tissue-type plasminogen activator
TPN	total parenteral nutrition
TPR	temperature, pulse, and respiration
tr	tincture
Tr	trace
TR	tricuspid regurgitation
TRC	therapeutic residential center
Trend	Trendelenburg
TRH	thyrotropin-releasing hormone
TRIS	tris (hydroxymethyl) aminomethane
TS	tricuspid stenosis
TSH	thyroid-stimulating hormone
tsp	teaspoon
TTN	transient tachypnea of newborn
TURB	transurethral resection of the bladder
TURBT	transurethral resection of the bladder tumor
TURP	transurethral resection of the prostate
TV	tidal volume
TVC	total volume capacity
TVH	total vaginal hysterectomy
TWE	tap water enema
Tx	treatment

U

U	unit
UA	uric acid; urinalysis
UC	uterine contractions
UCHD	usual childhood diseases
UCHI	usual childhood illnesses
UCI (MC)	University of California, Irvine (Medical Center)
ud	as directed
UGI	upper gastrointestinal
UL	upper lobe
U&L	upper and lower
ULQ	upper left quadrant
UMB	umbilicus
UMN	upper motor neuron

UMNB	upper motor neurogenic bladder
UN	urea nitrogen
ung	ointment
uni	one
UO	urinary output
UOQ	upper outer quadrant
UPI	uteroplacental insufficiency
UPJ	ureteropelvic junction
URD	upper respiratory disease
URI	upper respiratory infection
Urol	urology
URQ	upper right quadrant
US	sonogram (ultrasound)
UTI	urinary tract infection
UVJ	ureterovesical junction

V

v	venous
V	ventricular
Va	visual acuity
VA	ventriculoatrial
Vac C	visual acuity without correction
Vac CC	visual acuity with correction
vasc	vascular
VB	viable birth
VC	vital capacity
VCG	vector cardiogram
VCR	vincristine
VCUG	voiding cystourethrogram
VD	venereal disease
VDRL	Venereal Disease Research Laboratories (syphilis screen)
Vds	volume of dead space
VE	vaginal examination
Vevent	expired gas volume ventilator
vf	visual field
VF	ventricular fibrillation
VH	ventricular hypertrophy
V/H	visual hallucinations
Vits	vitamins
VMA	vanillylmandelic acid
VNA	Visiting Nurses Association
VO	verbal order
vol	volume
VP	vasa previa; ventriculoperitoneal
V&P	vagotomy and pyloroplasty

VPC	ventricular premature contractions
$\dot{V}/\dot{Q}$	ventilation/perfusion
VS	vital signs
VSD	ventricular septal defect
Vt	tidal volume
VTE	venous thromboembolism
Vtx	vertex

W

warming blk	hypothermia mattress
W/B	waist belt
WBC	white blood cells, white blood cell count
WBTT	weight bearing to tolerance
W/C	wheelchair
WD/WN	well developed/well nourished
wk	week
WNL	within normal limits
WO	without
WPF	Wright peak flow
wr	weakly reactive
WR	Wassermann reaction
wt	weight
Wt	weakly positive
w/u	workup

X

x	mean value
'	times
X^1	exophoria (near)
XM	crossmatch
XR	x-ray
XT	exotropia (distance)
X(T)	intermittent exotropia (distance)
XT^1	exotropia (near)

Y

y	year
yo	years old; years of
YS	yellow spot (retina)

Z

Z	zero
ZDV	zidovudine
ZIG	zoster immune globulin
Zno	zinc oxide

Useful Telephone Numbers

The columns below are for the telephone numbers of the two hospitals most commonly used.

	Hospital A	Hospital B
Hospital		
Information	_____	_____
Paging	_____	_____
Laboratories		
Arterial Blood Gas Laboratory	_____	_____
Blood Bank	_____	_____
Chemistry	_____	_____
Hematology	_____	_____
Microbiology	_____	_____
Special Chemistry	_____	_____
Services		
Center for Fetal Evaluation	_____	_____
Genetics		
Counseling	_____	_____
Laboratory	_____	_____
Medical Social Work	_____	_____
Wards		
Antepartum	_____	_____
Labor and Delivery	_____	_____
Postpartum	_____	_____
Emergency Room	_____	_____
Surgery	_____	_____
Physician Consult		
Perinatology	_____	_____
Cardiology	_____	_____
Infectious Disease	_____	_____
Internal Medicine	_____	_____
Neurology	_____	_____
Pulmonary	_____	_____
Surgery	_____	_____

Y

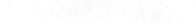

INDEX

Note: Page numbers followed by f refer to figures; page numbers followed by t refer to tables.

A

Abbreviations, 339-362
Abdominal pain
    appendicitis and, 17-20, 18t, 20f
    gallbladder disease and, 20-22, 22f
    pancreatitis and, 23-25
    peptic ulcer and, 25-27, 26t
    pyelonephritis and, 28
ABO blood type testing, 112
Abortion
    complete, 198
    Incomplete, 198
    inevitable, 197
    isoimmunization and, 112
    missed, 198
    recurrent, 198-199
    spontaneous, 195
    threatened, 197
Abortus, 336
Abruptio placentae, 168-179
    blood replacement in, 177t, 178t
    classification of, 175t
    coagulation studies in, 174t
    definition of, 168
    evaluation of, 172-173
    fetal death and, 203
    incidence of, 169
    management of, 174-179, 176f
    morbidity and mortality with, 170-172
    pathophysiology of, 170
Accelerated fetal lung maturation, 282-
        283, 283t, 284f, 284t, 285,
        285t
Acid-base balance asthma, 31t
Acidemia, neonatal, 238t
Acidosis in asthma, 31t
Acoustic stimulation, 266
Acquired immunodeficiency disease,
        301-302
Activated protein C resistance, 187
Acute abdominal pain, 17-28. See also
        Abdominal pain.

Acute appendicitis, 17-20, 18t, 20f
Acute pancreatitis, 23-25
Acyclovir, 308
Admission note, 11-13
Aerosolized bronchodilator, 33-34
Airway resistance, 33t
Albumin
    isoimmunization and, 101
    surfactant/albumin ratio and, 277
Algorithm for isoimmunization, 110f-
        111f
Alkalosis in asthma, 31t
Allergic asthma, 29
Alum-precipitated toxoid test in abruptio
        placentae, 172, 175t
Aluminum hydroxide, 26, 26t
Alupent, 33, 35
American Diabetes Association diet, 40
Amide local anesthetic, 221, 222t, 223
Aminophylline, 34-35
Amniocentesis
    chorioamnionitis and, 124
    in isoimmunization, 112
    premature rupture of membranes
        and, 129
    preterm labor and, 137
Amniostat-FLM, 278t, 279t
Amniotic fluid
    fetal surveillance and, 274t
    in fetal lung maturity testing, 277,
        278t-280t, 281f, 282f
    in isoimmunization, 106, 107
    perinatal mortality and, 274t
    volume of, 247t-249t, 250f, 251f
Amniotic membrane
    infection of, 119, 123-126
    premature rupture of, 119, 127-131
Amphetamine
    abuse screen for, 321t, 322t
    street names of, 331t
Ampicillin
    for chorioamnionitis, 125

Ampicillin—cont'd
for group B streptococcus, 118
for pyelonephritis, 87
Amylase/creatinine clearance ratio
formula for, 22f
in pancreatitis, 24
Amylase in pancreatitis, 23
Analgesia/anesthesia, 215-224
abuse screen for, 322t
complications of, 223-224
considerations in, 220
dissociative drugs for, 216
for cesarean delivery, 219
inhalation, 219
local, 220-221, 222t, 223
narcotic, 215
regional, 216-219, 217f, 218f
sedative tranquilizers for, 215
Anemia, 101, 108
Anesthesia, 215-224. See also
Analgesia/anesthesia.
Angiography
in peptic ulcer disease, 27
in pulmonary embolism, 191t
Anomaly, risk factors for, 7
Antacid, 26, 26t
Antepartum fetal death, 3-4
Antepartum fetal surveillance, 265-275.
See also Fetal surveillance.
Antepartum hemorrhage, 167-185. See
also Hemorrhage, antepartum.
Antepartum testing for hypertension,
66-67
Antibiotic
cervical cerclage and, 99
chorioamnionitis and, 125, 126
group B streptococcus and, 118-119
in appendicitis, 20
in pancreatitis, 24
in pyelonephritis, 86
premature rupture of membranes
and, 130
Antibody
anticardiolipin, 199, 200, 203
antiplatelet, 77

Antibody—cont'd
hepatitis B, 54, 57
isoimmunization and, 101, 102t-
103t, 103
maternal titers of, 105
Anticardiolipin antibody, 199, 200, 203
Anticholinergic drug, 27
Anticoagulant, lupus, 199, 200
Anticonvulsant drug, 80-81
Antidepressant, 321t, 322t
Antigen, hepatitis B, 54
Antihistamine
abuse screen for, 321t
for hyperemesis gravidarum, 92
Antiplatelet antibody, 77
Antiviral therapy for herpes infection, 308
Appendicitis, acute, 17-20, 18t, 20f
Arterial blood gases asthma, 30
Ascites, 106
Asphyxia, risk factors for, 6
Asthma, 28-36
definition of, 29
etiology of, 29
evaluation of, 30-31, 31t, 32t, 33,
33t
incidence of, 29
management of, 33-36
maternal morbidity/mortality from, 30
perinatal morbidity/mortality from,
29-30
Atenolol, 67
Auscultation in hypertension, 66t
Autosomal trisomy, 196

B
Bacterial vaginosis, 316
Bacteriuria, asymptomatic, 85
Barbiturate
abuse screen for, 322t, 323t
street names for, 331t
Benzathine penicillin G for syphilis,
305, 307
Benzodiazepine
abuse screen for, 322t, 323t
street names of, 331

Beta-adrenergic agonist, 142-143, 142t, 143t
Beta-mimetic, 138f, 139, 139t, 140, 140t-141t
Betamethasone for lung maturation, 282, 284t
Bicarbonate in diabetes, 41
Biliriubin, 106
Biophysical profile, fetal, 269, 270t, 271t, 272t
Biparietal diameter, 243f, 245f
Birth, definition of, 335
Birth rate, 335
Bishop score of inducibility of labor, 45t
Bleeding
    in peptic ulcer disease, 27
    in placenta previa, 182-184
    isoimmunization and, 112-113
    thrombocytopenia and, 77
Blood culture pyelonephritis, 86
Blood gas, fetal, 237f, 237t
Blood gases
    in asthma, 30
    neonatal, 238t, 239t
Blood group incompatibility, 101-113. See also Isoimmunization.
Blood pressure
    hypertension. See Hypertension.
    pregnancy-related changes in, 64t
Blood replacement products, 177t
Blood sampling
    in isoimmunization, 106, 112
    in thrombocytopenia, 78
Blood study
    in abruptio placentae, 172
    pregnancy-induced hypertension and, 157
Blood transfusion
    products for, 177t
    risks of, 178t
Bradycardia, fetal, 262t
Breast milk, antibodies in, 77
Bronchodilator, 33-34
Bronkosol, 33, 35

Bupivacaine, 221, 222t
Butorphanol, 215

C
Calcium carbonate, 26, 26t
Calcium-channel blocker, 150
Calcium gluconate, 147
Calcium in preeclampsia prevention, 163
Capillary glucose testing, 42
Carbamazepine for seizure, 80
Carbon dioxide, fetal, 237f
Cardiac auscultation in hypertension, 66t
Cardioactive agent, 322
Cardiovascular system
    fetal, 235f
    pancreatitis and, 24
    pregnancy-related changes in, 64t, 67f
Cartilage, cricoid, 221f
Catheterized urine specimen, 87
Caudal anesthesia, 222t
Caudal block, 216
Cefaclor in pyelonephritis, 87
Cephalosporin for group B streptococcus, 119
Cephapirin sodium for pyelonephritis, 86
Cerclage, cervical, 97, 98t, 99
Cervix
    culture of, 136
    incompetent, 95-100, 98t, 199
Cesarean delivery
    anesthesia for, 219
    fetal lung maturity and, 287
    in abruptio placentae, 176, 179
    in diabetic patient, 44-46, 45t
Chemotherapy, pregnancy loss caused by, 196
Chest x-ray
    in asthma, 33
    in hypertension, 66t
Chlamydia trachomatis, 314-316
Chloroprocaine, 221, 222t
Cholelithiasis, 20-22
Cholera vaccine, 295t
Cholescintigraphy, 21

Chorioamnionitis, 123-126, 124t, 125t
  group B streptococcus, 117
  premature rupture of membranes
    and, 127, 128
Chorionic gonadotropin, human, 91
Chorionic villus sampling, 112
Chromosomal abnormality, 196, 226t-
    227t
Chronic immunologic thrombocytopenia,
    73-77
Cimetidine, 27
Circulation
  fetal, 235f, 236f, 236t
  pregnancy-related changes in, 67f
Clindamycin
  for group B streptococcus, 119
  for vaginosis, 316
Coagulation
  abruptio placentae and, 173t
  disseminated intravascular, 169t
  thromboembolism and, 187
Cocaine, street names of, 331t
Codeine, street names of, 332t
Complete abortion, 198
Complete blood count, 172
Compression, umbilical cord, 128
Condyloma acuminata, 310-311, 312t
Congenital disorder
  anticonvulsant drug causing, 80
  diabetes-related, 38, 39t
  syphilis, 306-308
Consumptive coagulopathy, 178-179
Continuous infusion, insulin, 42, 45t
Contraction stress test, 269t, 270
Convulsion. See Seizure.
Corticosteroid
  for asthma, 26
  lung maturation and, 282-283,
    284t
  premature rupture of membranes
    and, 130
  thrombocytopenia and, 74-75, 77
Creatinine, 157
Cricoid cartilage pressure, 221f
Cromolyn sodium, 26
Cryotherapy, 311

Culture
  for group B streptococcus, 117
  in preterm labor, 136
  in pyelonephritis, 86
  premature rupture of membranes
    and, 129
Cystitis, 85
  group B streptococcus, 117

D

D-dimer, 192
D-isoimmunization, 101-113. See also
    Isoimmunization.
Death
  fetal, 200-203, 201t, 202t, 203t
    abruptio placentae and, 176,
      178-179
    antepartum, 3
    causes of, 202t
    evaluation of, 203
    intrapartum, 3
    reporting of, 201t
  neonatal
    causes of, 3
    prevention of, 4
  stillbirth, 200-203
  vital statistics on, 335-336
Deceleration
  early, 258f
  late, 260f
  prolonged, 263t
  variable, 259f, 263t
Deep venous thrombosis. See
    Thromboembolism.
Deformation syndrome, fetal, 128
Dehydration in diabetes, 42
Delivery
  analgesia/anesthesia for, 215-224.
    See also Analgesia/anesthesia.
  cesarean delivery. See also Cesarean
    delivery.
  chorioamnionitis and, 125
  isoimmunization and, 113
  premature rupture of membranes
    and, 130
  thrombocytopenia and, 76-77

Delta hepatitis, 56t, 60
Dexamethasone for lung maturation, 282, 284t
Diabetes, 37-48
    antepartum surveillance of, 43-44
    cesarean delivery and, 44-46
    congenital malformations with, 39t
    definition of, 37
    etiology of, 37
    evaluation of, 39-40
    glucola test for, 5
    incidence of, 37
    insulin administration in, 45t
    labor and delivery in, 44, 45t
    management of, 40-43
    morbidity/mortality in, 38-39
    White's classification of, 37, 38t
Diazepam, 81, 81t
Diffusing capacity, 33t
Dilantin, 80. See Phenytoin.
Diphenhydramine, 93
Direct maternal death, 336
Disaturated phosphatidylcholine test, 278t, 279t
Disseminated intravascular coagulation, 169t
Dissociative drug, 216
Documentation, admission note, 11-13
Doppler ultrasonography, 190
Doxylamine succinate, 92
Droperidol, 93
Drug abuse
    effects of, 325t-327t, 329t
    street names of drugs, 331t-333t
    urine screening for, 319, 320t-324t
Drug effects on fetal heart rate, 262t
Drug guidelines in pregnancy, 289
Dural puncture, 224

E

Early deceleration of fetal heart rate, 258f
Early syphilis, 304
Echocardiography, 66t
Eclampsia, 79, 156
Ectoparasitic infection, 316-317
Ectopic pregnancy, 112

Edema, pulmonary, tocolytic-related, 143, 144t
Effusion, pericardial, 106
Embolism, pulmonary. See also Thromboembolism.
    definition of, 187
    evaluation of, 189-190
    symptoms and signs of, 190t
Embolization in peptic ulcer disease, 27
Emergency
    cervical cerclage, 99
    hypertension, 68
Endometritis, 123
Endomyometritis
    definition of, 123
    group B streptococcus, 118
Endoscopy, 27
Epidural anesthesia, 222t
Epidural block, 216, 218
Epinephrine for asthma, 34
Erythroblastosis fetalis, 101
Erythromycin
    for chlamydial infection, 315
    for group B streptococcus, 119
    for syphilis, 307
Ester local anthestetic, 221, 222t
Estradiol, 91
Exophytic genital warts, 310-311, 312t
Expiratory reserve volume, 32t

F

Famotidine, 26
Fasting blood sugar, 41, 47
FDA drug guidelines, 289
Fentanyl, 215
Ferning, 128
Fertility rate, 335
Fetal death, 200-203
    abruptio placentae and, 176, 178-179
    antepartum, 3
    causes of, 202t
    evaluation of, 203
    intrapartum, 3
    reporting of, 201t
Fetal deformation syndrome, 128

Fetal distress
  Jarisch-Herxheimer reaction and, 306
  premature rupture of membranes and, 129
Fetal heart rate monitoring, 258f-260f, 261t-264t
Fetal lung maturity, 277-287. See also Lung maturity, fetal.
Fetal monitoring. See Fetal surveillance.
Fetal movement counts, 266
Fetal platelet count, 78
Fetal scalp blood sampling, 78
Fetal scalp pH, 264t
Fetal surveillance, 265-275
  amniotic fluid and, 274t
  biophysical profile in, 269, 270t, 271t, 272f
  contraction stress test in, 269, 270t
  fetal movement counts in, 266
  in diabetes, 43-44
  in hypertension, 66-67
  in seizure disorder, 81
  indications for, 265-266
  lung maturity, 277, 278t-280t, 281f, 282f
  nonstress test in, 266, 267f, 268f, 275f
  premature rupture of membranes and, 129
Fetus. See also Fetal entries.
  abruptio placentae and, 174-176
  acidemia in, 238t
  beta-adrenergic stimulation of, 142-143
  blood gases values in, 237f, 237t
  chromosomal abnormality in, 226t-227t
  circulation of, 235f, 236f
  growth of, 241f-245f
  isoimmunization and, 101, 102t-103t, 103-104, 107-108
  lung maturation effect and, 282
  placenta previa and, 182
  radiation exposure of, 229, 230t-232t, 233

Fever
  in chorioamnionitis, 124
  in Jarisch-Herxheimer reaction, 303
First-trimester pregnancy loss, 195-199
  definition of, 195
  etiology of, 196-197
  incidence of, 195
  management of, 197-199
Fluid, amniotic. See Amniotic fluid.
Foam stability test, 277, 283f, 284f
Follow-up prenatal care, 7-9
Food and Drug Administration
  drug guidelines in pregnancy, 289
  on tocolysis, 137
FTA-ABS test for syphilis, 307
Functional residual capacity, 32t

G

Gallbladder disease, 20-22, 22f
Gardnerella vaginalis, 316
  chorioamnionitis and, 124, 124t
General anesthesia, 219
Genetic disorder, 7
Genital herpes, 308-310
Genital warts, 310-311, 312t
Gestational age
  fetal growth and, 241f-245f
  lecithin/sphingomyelin ratio, 282f
  placenta previa and, 181
  premature rupture of membranes and, 129
Globulin, immune
  hepatitis B, 297t
  recommendations for, 297t-300t
Glucocorticoid
  for asthma, 35
  for fetal lung maturity, 282-283, 283t, 284f, 284t, 285, 285t
Glucola test
  for diabetes mellitus, 5
  hypertension and, 65
Glucose, 42, 43t
Glucose tolerance test
  normal, 37
  postpartum, 47

Gonadotropin, human chorionic, 91
Gonococcal infection, 312-314
    preterm labor and, 151
Grading
    of fetal heart rate deceleration, 263t, 264t
    placental, 253, 254f, 255t
Group B streptococcus infection, 115-119, 116t
    preterm labor and, 150-151
Growth, fetal, 241f-245f

H

Haemophilus vaginitis, 316
HBsAg, 54
Headache, postdural puncture, 224
Heart
    fetal, 235f
    isoimmunization and, 106
Heart rate monitoring, fetal, 258f-260f, 261t-264t
Hefner procedure for incompetent cervix, 98t
Helicobacter pylori, 25-26
HELLP syndrome
    in preeclampsia, 155
    management of, 163
Hematocrit, 168
Hematologic values in isoimmunization, 109t
Hemodynamic values, 161t
Hemoglobin, 168
Hemolysis, 101, 102t-103t
Hemorrhage, antepartum, 167-185
    assessment of, 167-168
    etiology of, 167
    in abruptio placentae, 168-179
    in placenta previa, 179-184
    in vasa previa, 184-185
    morbidity and mortality with, 167
Heparin therapy for thromboembolism, 192, 194
Hepatic circulation, fetal, 236f
Hepatitis, 49-62
    definition of, 49
    nomenclature of, 55t-56t

Hepatitis—cont'd
    prevention of, 49
    types of, 50t
Hepatitis A, 49-52
    diagnosis of, 50
    evaluation of, 49-50
    management of, 50, 52
    transmission of, 51t
Hepatitis A immune globulin, 299t
Hepatitis B
    evaluation of, 54, 54f, 57
    incidence of, 52
    management of, 57
    maternal morbidity/mortality in, 53
    perinatal morbidity/mortality in, 53
    prevention of, 57, 58t
    screening for, 53
    transmission of, 51t, 52-53
Hepatitis B immune globulin, 57, 58t, 297t
Hepatitis B vaccine, 57, 294t-295t
Hepatitis C, 59-60
    transmission of, 51t
Hepatitis D, 60
Hepatitis E, 61
Hepatitis G, 61-62
Hepatosplenomegaly, 106
Herpes simplex virus infection, 308-310
Histamine analog, 26
HIV/AIDS, 301-302
    syphilis in, 304
Hormone, thyrotropin-releasing, 283
Human chorionic gonadotropin, 91
Human immunodeficiency virus infection, 301-302
    isoimmunization and, 113
    syphilis in, 304
Human papillomavirus, 310-311, 312t
Hydralazine for hypertension, 68, 69t, 161
Hydration in asthma, 33
Hydrocortisone
    asthma and, 35
    fetal lung maturity and, 284t
Hydrops fetalis, 101

Hydroxyzine pamoate, 93
Hyperbilirubinemia, 101
Hyperemesis gravidarum, 91-94
Hyperglycemia in pancreatitis, 24
Hypertension
    chronic, 63-71
        definition of, 63
        etiology of, 63, 64t
        evaluation of, 63, 65-67
        morbidity and mortality with, 63
    pregnancy-induced, 155-163
        definition of, 155-156
        etiology of, 156
        evaluation of, 157
        incidence of, 156
        management of, 158, 159f, 160-
            163, 161t, 162t
        morbidity and mortality with,
            156-157
        prevention of, 163
        risk factors for, 156
Hypnotic, 321t
Hypocalcemia, 24
Hypotension, 223
Hypoxia, 6

I

Idiosyncratic asthma, 29
Immune globulin
    hepatitis B, 57, 58t
    hepatitis C, 59
    recommendations for, 297t-300t
Immunization
    hepatitis B, 57, 58t
    in pregnancy, 291, 292t-300t
Immunodeficiency disease, acquired,
        301-302
Immunoglobulin G
    for hepatitis A, 50, 52
    for thrombocytopenia, 75, 77
Immunologic thrombocytopenia, 73-77
Immunosuppressive therapy, 75-76
Incompetent cervix, 95-100
    definition of, 95
    etiology of, 95
    evaluation of, 95-96

Incompetent cervix—cont'd
    fetal loss and, 199
    management of, 97, 98t, 99-100
    morbidity/mortality with, 95
Incomplete abortion, 198
Incubation period
    for hepatitis A, 49
    for hepatitis B, 53
Index, amniotic fluid, 250f, 251f
Indirect maternal death, 336
Indomethacin
    cervical cerclage and, 99
    in preterm labor, 142t, 149-150
Induced labor
    in abruptio placentae, 179
    in diabetic patient, 44-46, 45t
Inevitable abortion, 197
Infection
    chorioamnionitis, 123-126
    group B streptococcus, 115-119, 116t
        tocolysis and, 150-151
    hepatitis, 49-62. See also Hepatitis.
    human immunodeficiency virus,
        301-302
        isoimmunization and, 113
        syphilis in, 304
    perinatal. See Perinatal infection.
    pregnancy loss caused by, 196, 199-
        200, 202t
    premature rupture of membranes
        and, 127-129
    preterm labor and, 136-137
    sexually transmitted, 301-317. See
        also Sexually transmitted
        disease.
    urinary tract, 85-87
Infiltration anesthesia, 222t
Influenza vaccine, 294t
Infusion
    insulin, 42
        administration of, 45t
        induced labor and, 44
    magnesium sulfate, 147
    terbutaline, 146
Inhalation anesthesia, 219
Inspiratory capacity, 32t

Insulin
   adjustment guidelines for, 42-43
   administration of, 40-41
   continuous infusion of, 42, 45t
   induced labor and, 44
Intraamniotic infection, 123-126
Intrapartum evaluation, 11-13
Intrapartum fetal death, 3
Intrapartum fetal monitoring, 258f-260f,
      261t-264t
Intravascular coagulation, disseminated,
      169t
Isoetharine, 34
Isoimmunization, 101-113
   antibodies causing, 102t-103t, 103
   definition of, 101
   differential diagnosis of, 104
   evaluation of, 105-107, 107f, 108f
   incidence of, 101, 103
   management of, 107-108, 110f-
      111f, 112
   morbidity and mortality from, 104
   pathophysiology of, 101
   prevention of, 112-113

J

Jarisch-Herxheimer reaction, 303, 306

K

Kell antibody, 103
Ketoacidosis, 41-42
Ketone, 41
Kleihauer-Betke test, 172

L

L/S ratio, 277, 278t, 279t, 280t
Labetalol, 68, 69t, 70
Labor
   analgesia/anesthesia in, 215-224.
         See also Analgesia/anesthesia.
   heparin therapy and, 194
   in diabetic patient, 44
   preterm. See Preterm labor.
   seizure disorder and, 82
Laboratory evaluation
   in appendicitis, 18t

Laboratory evaluation—cont'd
   in diabetes, 40
   in follow-up prenatal care, 8
   in hypertension, 65
   in isoimmunization, 109t
   in pregnancy-induced hypertension,
      162-163
   initial prenatal, 5t
Laboratory values in pregnancy, 209t-
      213t
Lash procedure for incompetent cervix,
      98t
Late deceleration of fetal heart rate,
      260f, 263t, 264t
Late syphilis, 304-305
Lecithin/sphingomyelin ratio, 277, 278t,
      279t, 280t
Leiomyoma, 199
Lice, 316-317
Lidocaine, 221, 222t
Lipase, 23
Lipids in amniotic fluid, 277, 278t,
      279t
Liquid nitrogen for genital warts, 311
Live birth, 335
Liver disease, 49-62. See also Hepatitis.
Liver enzyme in preeclampsia, 155
Local anesthetic, 220-221, 222t, 223-
      224
Low birth weight, 335
LSD, 332t
Lumadex-FSI, 278t, 279t
Lumbar epidural block, 216
Lumbar puncture in syphilis, 304
Luminal obstruction in peptic ulcer
      disease, 27
Lung maturity, fetal, 277-287
   assessment of, 277, 278t-280t,
      281f, 282f
   cesarean delivery and, 287
   glucocorticoid to accelerate, 282-283,
      283t, 284f, 284t, 285, 285t
   premature rupture of membranes
      and, 129
Lung profile, 278t, 279t
Lung volume, 32t

Lupus anticoagulant, 199, 200, 203
Lysergic acid diethylamide, 332t

M

Magnesium gluconate, 147
Magnesium hydroxide, 26, 26t
Magnesium sulfate
    for seizure prophylaxis, 160
    in preterm labor, 140t, 146-149, 148t
Malformation
    anticonvulsant drug causing, 80
    diabetes and, 38, 39t
Marijuana, 332t
Maternal morbidity/mortality
    abruptio placentae and, 171-172
    appendicitis and, 17
    asthma and, 30
    chorioamnionitis and, 123
    diabetes and, 38-39
    direct and indirect death, 336
    group B streptococcus causing, 116-
        117
    hepatitis A and, 49
    hepatitis B and, 53
    hyperemesis gravidarum and, 91
    in antepartum hemorrhage, 167
    isoimmunization and, 105
    peptic ulcer disease and, 25
    placenta previa and, 181-182
    pregnancy-induced hypertension
        and, 156-157
    premature rupture of membranes
        and, 127-128
    seizure disorder and, 79
    thrombocytopenia and, 73
    thromboembolism and, 188-189
McDonald procedure for incompetent
        cervix, 98t
Measles immune globulin, 300t
Measles vaccine, 292t
Membrane, amniotic
    infection of, 119, 123-126
    premature rupture of, 119, 127-131
Meperidine
    in labor, 215
    in pancreatitis, 24

Mepivacaine, 221, 222t, 223
Metabolic acidosis in asthma, 31t
Metabolic alkalosis in asthma, 31t
Metaproterenol, 33
Methamphetamine
    effects of, 329t
    street names of, 333t
Methyldopa, 67
Methylprednisolone, 35
Metoclopramide, 93
Metronidazole
    for vaginosis, 316
    premature rupture of membranes
        and, 129
Microviscosimetry, 277, 278t, 279t
Minute ventilation, 32t
Missed abortion, 198
Monitoring, fetal. *See* Fetal surveillance.
Monsomy X, 196
Muellerian fusion defect, 199
Mumps vaccine, 292t
Myometrial contractility, 138f

N

Nalbuphine, 215
Narcotic
    abuse screen for, 322t
    analgesia/anesthesia and, 215
Nasogastric suction in pancreatitis, 24
Neisseria gonorrhoeae, 312-314
Neonatal death, 335
    causes of, 3
    prevention of, 4
Neonatal infection
    chlamydial, 314-315
    group B streptococcus, 115-119, 116t
    HIV, 302
    pneumonia, 315-316
    syphilis, 306-308
Neonate
    accelerated lung maturation effects
        on, 282-283
    acidemia in, 238t
    hepatitis prevention for, 57, 58t
    seizure disorder and, 82-83
    thrombocytopenia in, 77

Nerve block
    classification of, 216-217
    complications of, 223-224
    dermatomes and, 218f
    effect of, on labor and delivery, 217-219
    spinal anatomy and, 219f
Neuroleptanalgesia, 216
Neurologic complications of anesthesia, 224
Neurosyphilis, 305
Nifedipine, 142t, 150
Nitrofurantoin, 87
Nitroglycerin, 69t, 71
Nitrous oxide, 219, 220
Nizatidine, 27
Nomenclature, hepatitis, 55t-56t
Nonmaternal death, 336
Nonpregnant patient
    appendicitis in, 18t
    hemodynamic values in, 161t
    incompetent cervix in, 97
Nonreactive nonstress test, 266, 268t
Nonstress test, 266, 267f, 268t, 275f
    premature rupture of membranes and, 129
Note, admission, 11-13

O
Obstruction
    peptic ulcer causing, 27
    ureteral, 87
Oligohydramnios
    findings in, 248t
    in premature rupture of membranes, 128
Ophthalmia neonatorum, 313
    chlamydial, 315
    gonococcal, 313
Optical density test, 278t, 279t
Oxygen, fetal, 237f
Oxytocin in abruptio placentae, 179

P
Pancreatitis, 23-25
Paracervical block, 216-217

Parenteral administration
    for analgesia/anesthesia, 215-216
    of sympathomimetics, 34
PCP, 333t
Pediculosis pubis, 316-317
Penicillin
    for gonococcal infection, 313
    for group B streptococcus, 118
    for syphilis, 303-304, 307
Peptic ulcer disease, 25-27, 26t
Percutaneous umbilical cord blood
        sampling, 106, 112
Percutaneous umbilical vein blood
        sampling, 78
Perforation, peptic ulcer, 27
Pericardial effusion, 106
Perinatal infection
    chlamydial, 314-315
    gonococcal, 313
    group B streptococcus, 115-119, 116t
    herpes, 309
    HIV, 302
    papillomavirus, 310
Perinatal morbidity/mortality
    abruptio placentae and, 170-171
    amniotic fluid levels and, 274t
    antepartum hemorrhage and, 167
    appendicitis and, 17
    asthma and, 29-30
    chorioamnionitis and, 123
    definition of, 335
    diabetes and, 38
    group B streptococcus causing, 116
    hepatitis A and, 49
    hepatitis B and, 53
    hyperemesis gravidarum and, 91
    isoimmunization and, 104
    peptic ulcer disease and, 25
    placenta previa and, 181
    pregnancy-induced hypertension
        and, 156
    premature rupture of membranes
        and, 127-128
    risk factors for, 6-7
    seizure disorder and, 79

Perinatal morbidity/mortality—cont'd
  thrombocytopenia and, 73
  thromboembolism and, 188
pH, neonatal, 238t, 239t
Phenaphthazine, 128
Phenobarbital for seizure, 82
Phenothiazine, 93, 323t
Phenytoin, 80, 160-161
Phosphatidylglycerol, 278t, 279t, 280t, 281f
Phospholipid in fetal lung maturity, 277, 281f
Placenta, isoimmunization and, 106
Placenta previa, 179-185
  definition of, 179-180, 180f
  etiology of, 180-181
  incidence of, 181
  morbidity and mortality with, 181-182
Placental grading, 253, 254f, 255t
Plague vaccine, 295t
Platelet count in preeclampsia, 155
Platelet disorder, 73-77
Pneumococcus vaccine, 295t-296t
Pneumonia, chlamydial, 315-316
Poliomyelitis vaccine, 292t-293t
Polyhydramnios
  incidence of, 249t
  isoimmunization and, 106
Polyploidy, 196
Postdural puncture headache, 224
Postpartum infection, 118
Postpartum management
  of diabetes, 46-47
  of thrombocytopenia, 78
  seizure disorder and, 82-83
Postterm infant, 336
Potassium in hypertension, 65
Preclinical pregnancy loss, 195
Prednisone
  asthma and, 35
  fetal lung maturity and, 284t
  thrombocytopenia and, 74-75
Preeclampsia, 155-156
Pregnancy-induced hypertension, 155-163. See also Hypertension, pregnancy-induced.

Pregnancy loss, 195-203
  first-trimester, 195-199
  preclinical, 195
  second-trimester, 199-200
  stillbirth, 200-203, 201t, 202t, 203t
Premature rupture of membranes, 127-131
  definition of, 127
  etiology of, 127
  evaluation of, 128-129
  group B streptococcus and, 119
  management of, 130-131
  morbidity with, 127-128
  preterm labor and, 130
Prematurity risk factors, 6-7
Prenatal evaluation, 3-9
  follow-up, 7-8
  patient history in, 4
  physical examination in, 5, 5t
  risk factor identification in, 6-7
Presentation, fetal, placenta previa and, 182
Pressure
  cricoid cartilage, 221f
  pulmonary artery wedge, 162t
Preterm infant
  definition of, 336
  pH and blood gas values for, 239t
Preterm labor, 135-151
  chorioamnionitis and, 124
  definition of, 135
  etiology of, 135
  evaluation of, 135-137
  group B streptococcus and, 117-118
  incidence of, 135
  Jarisch-Herxheimer reaction and, 306
  management of
    beta-adrenergic agonist and, 142-143
    beta-mimetics in, 138f, 139, 139t, 140, 140t-141t
    calcium-channel blocker in, 150
    group B streptococcus and, 150-151
    indomethacin in, 149-150

Preterm labor—cont'd
    management of—cont'd
        magnesium sulfate in, 146-149,
            148t
        pulmonary edema and, 143
        ritodrine in, 140t, 142, 145-146
        terbutaline in, 140t, 143, 145
        tocolysis in, 137-138
    morbidity and mortality with, 135
    prevention of, 151
    risk factors for, 135t, 136t
Probenecid, 305
Procaine, 221, 222t
Procaine penicillin for syphilis, 305
Profile, biophysical, 269, 270t, 271t,
    272f
PROM. See Premature rupture of
    membranes.
Promethazine, 92
Prophylaxis
    antibiotic
        for cervical cerclage, 99
        for group B streptococcus, 119-120
        for thromboembolism, 192, 194
        hepatitis B, 57, 58t
        seizure, 160
Protein C resistance, activated, 187
Prothrombin time in seizure disorder, 83
Pudendal block, 217
Pulmonary artery wedge pressure, 162t
Pulmonary edema, tocolytic-related,
    143, 144t
Pulmonary embolism
    angiographic categories of, 191t
    definition of, 187
    evaluation of, 189-190
    management of, 192, 193f, 194
    symptoms and signs of, 190t
Pulmonary function test, 30-31
Pyelonephritis, 85-86
    appendicitis vs, 19
Pyrethrin for lice, 316-317

R

Rabies immune globulin, 298t
Rabies vaccine, 294t

Rad, 233
Radiation exposure of fetus, 229, 230t-
    232t, 233
Radiographic evaluation, in cholecystitis,
    21
Ranitidine, 27
Ratio
    amylase/creatinine clearance, 22f
    lecithin/sphingomyelin, 277, 278t,
        279t, 280t
    surfactant/albumin, 277
Reactive nonstress test, 266, 267t
Recurrent abortion, 198-199
Red blood cell, isoimmunization and,
    101. See also Isoimmunization.
Regional anesthesia, 216-219, 217f, 218f
    complications of, 223-224
Rem, 233
Reporting of fetal death, 201t
Residual volume, 32t
Respiratory acidosis, 31t
Respiratory alkalosis, 31t
Respiratory disorder, 28-36. See also
    Asthma.
Respiratory distress, neonatal, 284f
Respiratory function in asthma, 33
Respiratory system, pancreatitis and, 24
Rh immunization, 101-113. See also
    Isoimmunization.
Risk factor
    for chorioamnionitis, 123
    for perinatal death, 6-7
Ritodrine, 140t, 142, 145-146
Roentgen, 233
Rubella vaccine, 293t
Rupture of membranes, premature,
    119, 127-131

S

Scabies, 317
Scalp blood sampling, fetal, 78
Scalp pH, fetal, 264t
Screening
    coagulopathy, 178-179
    diabetes, 37
    drug abuse, 319, 320t-324t

Screening—cont'd
  group B streptococcus, 118
  hepatitis B, 53
  syphilis, 305-306
Second-trimester pregnancy loss, 199-200
Sedative, 215, 321t, 323t
Seizure disorder, 79-83
  classification of, 79
  eclampsia, 156
  evaluation of, 79-80
  local anesthetic causing, 223-224
  management of, 80-83
  prophylaxis for, 160
  status epilepticus, 81t
Sepsis, group B streptococcus, 115
Serologic antigen, hepatitis B, 54
Serologic test for syphilis, 302-303
Sex chromosomal polysomy, 196
Sexually transmitted disease, 301-317
  bacterial vaginosis, 316
  chlamydial, 314-316
  ectoparasitic, 316-317
  genital herpes, 308-310
  genital warts, 310-311, 312t
  gonococcal, 312-314
  HIV/AIDS, 301-302
  syphilis, 302-308
Shake test of fetal lung maturity, 277, 280t, 283f, 284f
Shirodkar procedure for incompetent cervix, 98t
Shunt, fetal, 235f
Sodium bicarbonate, 26, 26t
Sodium nitroprusside, 70t, 71
Spinal anesthesia, 222t
  headache after, 224
  total, 223
Spinal block, 216
Splenectomy, 75
Spontaneous abortion, 195
Statistics, vital, 335-336
Status epilepticus, 81
Stillbirth, 200-203, 201t, 202t, 203t
  causes of, 265
  definition of, 335

Stillbirth rate, 335
Stimulation, acoustic, 266
Stone, cholelithiasis, 20-22
Streptococcus infection, group B, 115-119, 116t
  definition of, 115
  etiology of, 115-116
  evaluation of, 117
  incidence of, 115
  management of, 117-118
  morbidity and mortality with, 116-117
  prevention of, 118-119, 150-151
Stress test, contraction, 269t, 270
Subarachnoid block, 216
Surfactant/albumin ratio, 277
Surgery
  appendicitis, 19-20, 20t
  gallbladder, 22
  incompetent cervix, 97, 98t, 99
  peptic ulcer, 27
Surveillance
  fetal, 265-275. See also Fetal surveillance.
  in seizure disorder, 81
Symbols, 337
Sympathomimetic for asthma, 34-35
Syphilis, 302-308
  congenital, 306-308
  early, 304
  in pregnancy, 305-306
  late, 304-305
  neurosyphilis, 305
  penicillin for, 303-304
  serologic tests for, 302-303

T
Tachycardia, fetal, 261t
Tachypnea in thromboembolism, 189
Tap test of fetal lung maturity, 277
Temperature conversion chart, 207t
Terbutaline
  for asthma, 26, 35
  in preterm labor, 140t, 143, 145
Term infant, 335-336
Terminology
  abbreviations, 339-362

Terminology—cont'd
  hepatitis, 55t-56t
  symbols, 337
Tetanus-diphtheria toxoid, 297t
Tetanus immune globulin, 297t
Tetracaine, 222t
Theophylline, for asthma, 26, 35
Threatened abortion, 197
Thrombocytopenia, immunologic, 73-77
  differential diagnosis of, 73-74
  etiology of, 73
  evaluation of, 74
  management of, 74-77
  morbidity and mortality with, 73
Thromboembolism, 187-194
  definition of, 187
  differential diagnosis of, 189
  etiology of, 187
  evaluation of, 189-190, 190t, 191t,
    192
  incidence of, 187-188
  management of, 192, 193f, 194
  morbidity and mortality with, 188-
    189
Thrombolysis, 192
Thrombophilia syndrome, 188t
Thyrotropin-releasing hormone
  lung maturation and, 283
  premature rupture of membranes
    and, 131
Tidal volume, 32t
Titer, maternal antibody, 105
Tocolysis, 137-151
  beta-adrenergic agonist and, 142-
    143
  beta-mimetics in, 138f, 139, 139t,
    140, 140t-141t
  calcium-channel blocker in, 150
  group B streptococcus and, 150-151
  indomethacin in, 149-150
  magnesium sulfate in, 146-149, 148t
  premature rupture of membranes
    and, 130
  pulmonary edema and, 143
  ritodrine in, 140t, 142, 145-146
  terbutaline in, 140t, 143, 145

Tonic-clonic epilepsy, 81
Total spinal anesthesia, 223
Toxic, alum-precipitated, 172, 175t
Toxoid, tetanus-diphtheria, 297t
Tranquilizer, sedative, 215
Transfusion
  platelet, 75
  products for, 177t
Transmission
  of hepatitis A, 51t
  of hepatitis B, 51t, 52-53
  of hepatitis C, 59
  of hepatitis D, 60
  of hepatitis G, 61-62
Treponema pallidum infection, 302-308
Trichomoniasis, 129
Trimethadione for seizure, 80
Trisomy, 196
Typhoid vaccine, 296t

U
Ultrasonography
  abruptio placentae and, 172
  amniotic fluid volume and, 247t-
    249t, 250f, 251f
  cholecystitis and, 21
  fetal growth and, 241f-245f
  hypertension and, 66
  placenta previa and, 182-183
  placental grading via, 253, 254f,
    255t
  thromboembolism and, 190
Umbilical blood sampling
  blood gases and, 238t, 239t
  in isoimmunization, 106, 112
  in thrombocytopenia, 78
Umbilical circulation, 236f, 236t
Umbilical cord compression, 128
Ureteral obstruction, 87
Urinary tract infection, 85-87
Urine
  drugs detected in, 324t
  in antepartum hemorrhage, 168
  in pregnancy-induced hypertension,
    157
  in pyelonephritis, 87

Urine screening for drugs, 319, 320t-324t
Uterosacral-cardinal ligament cerclage, 98t
Uterus
    amniotic fluid index and, 250f, 251f
    nitrous oxide and, 219

V
Vaccination
    hepatitis B, 57, 58t
    in pregnancy, 291, 292t-300t
Vaginal bleeding. See Bleeding.
Vaginosis
    bacterial, 316
    chorioamnionitis and, 123-124
    premature rupture of membranes and, 129
Valacyclovir, 308
Valproic acid for seizure, 80
Variable deceleration of fetal heart rate, 259f
Varicella immune globulin, 297t
Vasa previa, 184-185, 185f
Venography, 192
Venous blood sampling, umbilical, 78
Venous thromboembolism, 187-194.
        See also Thromboembolism.

Ventilation, minute, 32t
Virus infection
    hepatitis, 49-62. See also Hepatitis.
    human immunodeficiency, 301-302
        isoimmunization and, 113
        syphilis with, 304
Vital capacity, 32t, 33t
Vital statistics, 335-336
Vitamin B$_6$, 92-93
Vitamin K, 81
Volume
    amniotic fluid, 247t-249t, 250f, 251f
    lung, 32t
Vomiting, 91-94

W
Warts, genital, 310-311, 312t
White blood cell, steroid effects on, 284t
White's classification of diabetes, 37, 38t

Y
Yellow fever vaccine, 293t

Z
Zidovudine, 302